THIRD EDITION

Principles and Techniques in Pediatric Nursing

GLORIA LEIFER, R.N., M.A.

Formerly, Department of Nursing Education,
Hunter College of the City University of New York;
Assistant Professor, Department of Nursing Education,
California State College,
Los Angeles, California

1977
W. B. SAUNDERS COMPANY
Philadelphia, London, Toronto

W. B. Saunders Company: West Washington Square
                          Philadelphia, PA   19105

                          1 St. Anne's Road
                          Eastbourne, East Sussex BN21 3UN, England

                          1 Goldthorne Avenue
                          Toronto, Ontario M8Z 5T9, Canada

Principles and Techniques in Pediatric Nursing   ISBN   0-7216-5713-3-Hard Cover
                                                    ISBN   0-7216-5719-2-Soft Cover

Last digit is the print number: 9   8   7   6   5   4   3   2   1

Dedicated to

SARAH MASEYAW LEIFER

A Nurse, Humanitarian and Mother

SPECIAL CONTRIBUTORS

WILLIAM S. ARNETT D.D.S.
Upland, California
(*Oral Hygiene*)

DOROTHY E. BAILEY
Director, Sensorimotor Program
First Baptist Preschool
Ontario, California
Vice President, W.E. Chapter
California Association for Neurologically Handicapped Children
Member, Advisory Board
Child Developmental Center
Casa Colina Hospital, California
(*The Handicapped Child*)

ALBERTO KADOSH D.D.S.
San Francisco, California
(*Oral Hygiene*)

INEZ L. KING TEEFY R.N., M.N.Ed.
Assistant Professor of Nursing
Texas Woman's University College of Nursing
Dallas, Texas
(*Calculating I.V. Flow; Mixing I.V. Solutions; CAM Tent; Mechanical Ventilators*)

PREFACE

The Need for This Book

The era of genetic medicine is with us today, and while awaiting the full benefits of this new age it is a nursing responsibility to do everything possible to maintain the lives and spirits of those entrusted to our care today. The continuing need for understanding and expert management will increasingly challenge nurses concerned with the growth and development of children and their care in health and illness.

This edition strives to maintain the goals expressed in the first and second editions. The increasing complexities of medical and nursing techniques have created a need for "specialty areas" in the field of nursing. The pediatric nurse must often cope with situations that differ from those in other services. Thus, pediatric nursing has gained recognition as one of the "specialty areas" of nursing. This fact, combined with the national trend in nursing education to decrease clinical experience in nursing courses, presents a problem to those concerned with the maintenance and improvement of nursing care in general hospitals. The practitioner of nursing does not cease to be a student upon graduation from nursing school.

The increased complexities of medical and nursing techniques are no longer limited to large medical centers. Nurses who practice in smaller institutions will soon come in contact with newer and more complex techniques of care; thus, increased knowledge and skills are required in order to maintain even the basic standards of child care.

This book has been designed as a comprehensive, self-explanatory reference book to bridge the gap between theoretical knowledge and practical skill in pediatric nursing.

Use of This Book

This book is designed for use by the practicing pediatric nurse as well as the new graduate nurse.

Teachers in in-service education programs, which often lack specialists in the field of pediatric nursing, can use this book as a valuable guide in teaching the nurse who has not been active on the pediatric unit, or the graduate nurse attracted to the pediatric staff.

This book may also be used as an adjunct to the standard textbook in student nurse education.

Format Design

A two-column format has been adopted so that the subject matter can be presented in a manner that permits rapid location of specific information. The two columns correlate principles with nursing responsibilities. An illustrated section concerning techniques of care follows in each chapter.

Content

This book deals with the practical aspects of nursing principles and the responsibilities and techniques that are essential to the practicing pediatric nurse. Basic nursing principles, common to *all* areas of nursing, are not included.

At the end of each chapter the reader will find an extensive bibliography of pediatric textbooks and current journal publications for independent study concerning further details of specific content or disease processes. The last chapter, providing a mini-review of common pediatric disorders, is designed to define the disorder and to assist the nurse in developing her own plan of individualized nursing care based upon nursing principles and responsibilities specific to that disease process.

In many hospitals the care of extramural newborns is delegated to the pediatric nurse. For this reason a special chapter dealing with the normal newborn is included.

New concepts of hospital care, equipment, and therapy are treated in terms of the principles and nursing responsibilities involved. Principles and techniques that apply to both older children and infants are grouped together to avoid duplication. This book is designed to familiarize the nurse with new items of equipment and to provide an understanding of how they influence the care of pediatric patients. It is not possible or desirable to discuss equipment manufactured by *all* companies or techniques in use at *all* institutions. The equipment selected for discussion in this book is a representative sample which incorporates principles applicable to similar equipment manufactured by other companies. The equipment discussed, therefore, was selected on the basis of principles of use rather than as an endorsement of a particular brand.

In this age of specialization, the many facets of nursing activities grow in scope and complexity. Therefore, it is necessary for texts either to expand their coverage or become more selective. Expanded texts, usually prohibitive in cost, generalize and skim over many specific details involved in the specialty area of pediatric nursing. This text is a *selective* text, designed to assist the nurse to *function* in a complex environment by helping her to understand the specific principles and nursing responsibilities involved in the *clinical setting*. Thus, any limitation or omission concerning topics such as disease processes does not imply that these aspects are less important, but rather that they are adequately covered in conventional *theoretical* textbooks. Current theoretical textbooks, however, do not provide the nurse with the understanding of principles and nursing responsibilities discussed in this *clinical* text. The nurse who works with children in the hospital is exposed to new and complex equipment and techniques. It is essential that she understand the principles and nursing responsibilities involved in the use of this equipment so that she can help the child adapt to its use.

Nursing techniques may vary from hospital to hospital, but the principles upon which these techniques are based generally remain stable. A nurse can function more effectively in the pediatric unit if she is not restricted by the ritualistic, procedure-centered techniques that are usually found in nursing procedure books. An essential feature of this book is the clear identification of selected principles designed to stimulate the nurse to use her judgment, within the bounds of acceptable standards, to best serve the patient's needs. I believe we must utilize the great wealth of creativity and ingenuity that exists in the nursing community if we are to develop and promulgate the best possible nursing care.

The author, the illustrator, and the publisher have coordinated their efforts to present this book in a manner which will stimulate nurses to achieve their maximum potential for professional performance in a complex clinical setting and to find a personal satisfaction in the maintenance of high standards in pediatric care.

This edition expands material related to nursing procedures in the intensive care unit, which has become an integral part of the pediatric hospital setting. A section concerning cardiopulmonary resuscitation of infants and children is a major addition and has been included because the technique differs considerably from that used with the adult owing to basic anatomical differences. The adult technique, if applied to infants or children, could prove fatal. An expanded section concerning inhalation therapy for infants and children has been added because this type of therapy is now commonly used in neonatal units as well as the pediatric ward, and more nurses will be involved with its use and will be responsible for a child receiving some type of inhalation therapy. Chest physiotherapy has been added at the request of our readers. It is currently practiced in conjunction with inhalation therapy rather than being limited to cystic fibrosis patients. Content concerning differences between the child and the adult has been expanded and is the focal point in the presentation of all material in this book, from complex intensive care to simple daily oral hygiene. Information on practices common to child and adult has been intentionally omitted in favor of presenting content that emphasizes the special nursing approach required because of basic differences between pediatric and adult patients.

Some examples of new and modern equipment used in pediatric care have been included in this edition; information concerning older models has been retained in the text only if my clinical research throughout this country has shown them to be still in popular use.

The section concerning administration of medications has been expanded to include an understanding of newer concepts upon which nursing approachs can be based. Drug-food interactions, drug-drug interactions, and the effect of drugs ingested by the mother on nursing infants are major additions to this text. Nursing responsibilities involved with the use of medicated or modified intravenous solutions are also discussed. Nursing responsibilities relating to the use of over-the-counter medications, the cultural aspects of pediatric pharmacology, and patient compliance have been integrated into this edition.

Nutrition of the pediatric patient has been expanded, not only in the chapter dealing directly with feeding infants and children, but also in the intensive care unit, where coffee is playing a major role in controlling apnea of prematures and in the outpatient section, where an understanding of food cults is essential in order to deal effectively with a growing number of pediatric patients.

Poisoning is still an outstanding pediatric problem in our complex environment. Toxicologists provide information concerning the physiologic changes induced by poisons; clinicians offer clues to effective diagnosis and management of poisonings; psychologists offer understanding of the drive to ingest in the various pediatric developmental levels, and the nurse must find a way to disseminate all this knowledge to children and to those who influence children. The clinic-office nurse is best suited to handle parent-child instruction concerning prophylaxis, as she often has contact with the child and the family in the nonstress health setting. The nurse may be the best qualified person to utilize information concerning the effective management of poisoning, as it occurs and she can also play an important role in preventing recurrent problems. The chapter on poisonings is designed to relate specifically to the pediatric patient from infancy through adolescence. The "sinister garden" emphasizes nature's poison, which is lurking in the "safe" back yard or picnic ground, as well as ingested household poisons and the approach to preventative and emergency care.

The section concerning oral hygiene for the pediatric patient has been expanded. To avoid duplication, some material concerning oral hygiene and emergency care of dental injuries has been placed in the clinic section, as it concerns the clinic nurse more often than the hospital nurse.

Material specific to the adolescent has been integrated throughout the book because the maturing adolescent is a pediatric patient often overlooked and he has needs specific to his developmental level.

Parents need occasional guidance along the path of life with the vital job of child rearing, and the clinic or office nurse is usually the first contact for promoting health and preventing disease. The clinic or office nurse can offer the reassurance necessary to build confidence in the new mother who has yet to identify positive responses in her infant. She can detect abnormalities early and offer prompt referral. She can observe firsthand interaction between parent and child and child and sibling, and can offer guidance based upon individual assessed needs. The clinic or office nurse is a most important link in the child health team. In my new chapter, the Pediatric Outpatient and the Clinic Nurse, I attempt to offer some illustrations of the role of the clinic nurse in pediatric care in health and disease. I attempt to show how a clinic or office nurse can transform wasted time into valuable time by effectively utilizing the waiting room for teaching or counseling. I illustrate how the clinic nurse can furnish the waiting room with valuable and interesting teaching aids, offering prophylactic or therapeutic health care values at no more cost than furnishing it with conventional third class magazines and comic books. The chapter is not meant to be all inclusive, but only to provide examples of the various responsibilities of the clinic nurse and is designed to motivate the reader to build upon this introduction to formulate individualized effective clinic nursing techniques. The chapter concerning the pediatric outpatient and the clinic nurse has been added as an integral section of this book because I believe the clinic nurse has long been subjected to textbook neglect. With proper initiative and utilization of time, the clinic nurse can help the pediatric outpatient reap the benefits of preventative health care that will improve the lives of the patient, the family, the community, and the next generation in our country.

GLORIA LEIFER HARTSTON

INTRODUCTION

The newest and most complex equipment to monitor, resuscitate, operate, and restore does not occupy as prominent a role in modern pediatric nursing as the skilled nurse who is alert, observant, and able to meet the individual needs of her pediatric patient.

The goal of pediatric nursing is to foster the growth and development of the child and promote an optimum state of health—physically, mentally and socially—so that he may function at the peak of his capacity.

This book presents current pediatric nursing techniques in terms of the principles involved and the nursing responsibilities inherent in them. The identification of principles and nursing responsibilities is purposely selective, so that the unique aspects of pediatric nursing may be brought into focus. Pediatric nursing and general adult nursing embrace many common principles. This book is designed to assist the nurse to identify and apply principles *specific* to the care of infants and children.

Definition of Terms Used in This Book

Principles are scientific facts upon which nursing activities are based. The principles presented in this book are selected to serve as guides for safe, effective clinical performance in the pediatric unit.

Nursing responsibilities may be classified as dependent or independent. Dependent responsibilities depend upon the physician's written requests. Independent responsibilities do not depend upon medical or administrative authority. It is the independent aspects of nursing responsibilities that contribute most significantly to professionalism in nursing. In this book, emphasis is placed upon the independent aspects of nursing responsibilities as the basis for nursing activities.

Psychological support, as used in this book, refers to nursing activities designed to meet the individual needs of the child and his family without violating their natural defenses or adaptive processes. The nurse does not attempt to judge or change responses, but attempts to assist the child and his family to obtain maximum gratification with minimum deprivation within the limitations imposed by the hospital environment and the child's disease process.

Follow-up care implies that continuity of care, beyond the hospital setting, is provided through referrals to available community agencies.

The *Mini-Review of Pediatric Disorders and their Nursing Responsibilities* is a nursing dictionary of technical terms and names of disease processes. The information in the mini-review is sufficiently extensive to provide a working knowledge of the terms or disease processes that will guide the nurse in planning related nursing activities.

I would like to thank the readers for the warm reception given the past editions of this book, and for the many letters comments and ideas that served to guide me in the preparation of this new edition.

As a parent I realize that a child is the most valuable possession one can have. With a little love and effort the child can outlast the best car, yacht, mansion, or any material thing many equate with happiness. The joys that a happy, healthy child can bring are quite unique. I would like to express a special gratitude to my children, Heidi, Barnet, Amos, and Eve-Danielle, who are passing through childhood relatively unscathed but who have taught me firsthand what it really means to be an anxious parent, thus in a sense, providing stimulation and motivation for the preparation of material in this edition that may prove to lessen the anxieties of other parents. My heartfelt appreciation is extended to my husband, Dr. Daniel Hartston, who made it possible for me to personally investigate the practices and problems of pediatric nursing care in the developed and underdeveloped areas of Africa, the Far East, the Middle East, and Europe, as well as in many parts of the United States. My appreciation is extended to the many members of the medical and nursing professions in these countries for their time and cooperation.

I wish to thank members of the nursing and medical staff of the New York City Department of Hospitals and other hospitals across the country for their generous time and helpful advice offered during my visits.

A special note of appreciation is extended to members of the medical and nursing staff of the Kaiser Permanente Medical Center in Fontana, California, who managed to find time in their busy schedules to work with me on studies that were basic to the revision of this text. Special acknowledgment goes to Bernadine Smith, R.N., of the Neonatal Intensive Care Unit and Mercedes Sgroi, R.N., Intensive Care Unit Supervisor for their assistance in research pertaining to the chapter on intensive care; and to Guy Hartman, M.D., for his encouragement and his editing of the section concerning plant poisoning. Fortunately, a most cooperative group of contributors, chosen because of their special interests and accomplishments, has made the task of revising this text more pleasant. My special thanks to Sarah Leifer, who, by her continued encouragement and detailed proofreading of the revised manuscript, made the revision of this book an enjoyable and painless experience.

I hope this book will fulfill the purpose for which it was planned. It is impossible to teach a nurse all the knowledge she must have to be an effective pediatric nurse in the short period of time delegated to pediatrics in most nursing schools. It appears to be sound practice, therefore, to place before the student and the graduate a book such as this, stating principles and nursing responsibilities that can form the basis for the independent study that should continue throughout professional life. It is hoped that the standards of care and the criteria for evaluating care developed and stated by the American Nurses Association coupled with continuing education, such as this text can provide, will help the nurse give high quality care to those entrusted to her.

CONTENTS

Chapter Four

OBSERVING, RECORDING, AND REPORTING 28

Chapter Five

ADMISSION OF INFANTS AND CHILDREN 32

Chapter Six

DAILY CARE OF NEWBORNS AND INFANTS 38

Chapter Ten

COLLECTION OF URINE AND STOOL SPECIMENS 71

Chapter Eleven

ADMINISTERING AN ENEMA TO INFANTS AND CHILDREN.. 75

Chapter Twelve

CARE OF A CHILD WITH A COMMUNICABLE DISEASE........... 78

Chapter Eighteen

ADMINISTRATION OF MEDICATIONS TO INFANTS AND CHILDREN

Chapter Nineteen

POISONING IN INFANTS AND CHILDREN

Chapter One

SOME UNIQUE ASPECTS
OF PEDIATRICS

Since the various responses of the child are influenced by the phases of growth and development, the age of the child is the most significant factor affecting nursing activities.

Illness can be a traumatic experience to the adult as well as to the child. However,
illness occurring at a specific phase of the developmental cycle may affect the developing personality. For example, a nursing procedure involving intrusion into a body orifice is more traumatic to a child five years of age, whose awareness of his body is keen,
than to an infant under one year of age, who is not yet aware of his own body. A fractured jaw may be more traumatic to a child under one year of age, who is in the oral
phase of development, than to a child five years of age, who has already passed this
phase. A school-age child who feels "different" from his peers because of a physical
handicap will suffer great psychological trauma that could affect his personality development. Separation from the family unit during hospitalization will cause anxiety in
any patient, but the integrity of the parent-child relationship may be severely impaired
by a sudden separation of a child from his parents.

The nurse can minimize the psychological trauma of a hospitalization experience
by helping the child to adjust to the situation rather than to repress his feelings. Play
therapy has a vital role in this area. Just as we adults "talk out" our problems, we must
let the child "play out" his problems. Therefore, in order to provide comprehensive care
to a pediatric patient, the nurse must clearly understand the effect of the illness and
hospitalization experience upon the growth and development process, and the effect of
the developmental status of the child upon his responses to therapy.

Since the child differs from the adult both anatomically and physiologically, differences in the response to therapy may be anticipated. An understanding of the normal
is essential in order to identify significant deviations. Some of the differences which
may affect nursing techniques and responsibilities are listed in the following section.

I. Some Physical Differences Between the Child and the Adult

Central nervous system

The central nervous system of the infant and young child is not fully mature. Certain reflexes present in the adult are absent in young children. The temperature regulating system of the newborn may be unstable.

Cardiovascular system

The cardiac output, blood pressure, and blood volume in a child differ from those in an adult. A blood loss of 30 cc. in an infant is more significant than a blood loss of 30 cc. in an adult.

Pulmonary system

The intercostal muscles that aid in respiration are not fully developed in the young child. Respiration in the newborn and the infant is often irregular. Due to the thinness of the chest wall, pressure or restraint on the chest may interfere with respiratory efforts. The lumen of the trachea is smaller in infants and children than in adults, and more easily occluded by mucous secretions. Irritation of the trachea by large catheters can cause laryngospasm and cardiac arrest in the young child.

Urinary system

Since the kidneys of the infant and young child are not fully mature, dehydration and overhydration occur more rapidly than in adults. Drug toxicity may also develop more frequently in the infant and young child who cannot excrete toxic substances as readily as an adult.

Gastrointestinal system

Infants tend to swallow air and are prone to develop gastric distention. Subsequent vomiting and aspiration of vomitus can be dangerous.

Nutritional needs

Nutritional needs are greater for infants and children because of the growth and development processes.

Susceptibility to disease

Infants and children are less resistant to disease than adults. Immunity passed via the placenta rarely lasts more than six months.

| Effect of trauma or disease | The effect of injury or disease upon growing tissue differs from the effect upon mature tissue. Therefore, the signs and symptoms of a specific disease manifested by a growing child differ from the signs and symptoms of the same disease manifested by an adult. |

The foregoing is only a partial listing of the physical differences between the child and the adult. These examples are cited particularly to alert the nurse to the physiological factors that influence the nursing care of infants and children.

II. Some Differences Between the Treatment of Child and Adult

Problems Presenting	Differences from Adult Therapy
Chest	
Abdominal distention and elevation of the diaphragm occur frequently with post-traumatic ileus and can interfere with breathing.	Respiratory failure can occur rapidly because elevation of the diaphragm poses a greater danger in relation to child's chest volume and ventilation.
Excessive bronchial secretions occur often in the ill or injured child.	A narrow tracheobronchial tree and weaker thoracic muscles make response to bronchial secretions more difficult, and requires prompt intervention and therapy such as endotracheal tubes, positive pressure therapy, and tracheostomy.
Tracheostomy	
An infant or child is often uncooperative and movement is unpredictable.	Accidental dislodgement must be prevented.
The infant or young child has a shorter neck than the adult.	The neck must be kept hyperextended to prevent obstruction of the airway.
Mucous plugs can obstruct the small lumen of the tracheostomy tube.	Humidity must be maintained and suctioning must be performed under sterile conditions.
Blood	
Blood loss often accompanies trauma or surgery.	Blood loss is a greater danger to the child because of the smaller blood volume, as compared to the adult. The loss of 50 cc. of blood in a newborn infant can precipitate shock.

Intravenous therapy

A rapid introduction of I.V. fluids can result in pulmonary edema, especially in children with congenital heart disease.

The rate of flow must be prescribed by the doctor and monitored with accuracy. The rate of flow is often 4 to 6 drops per minute, and special care and equipment is needed to maintain constant accuracy.

I.V. therapy can contribute to heat loss and can cause renal and cardiac problems.

Administration of cold blood or I.V. fluids can cause rapid heat loss and potentiate coagulation defects.

The smaller dosage for infants requires greater accuracy of administration to insure that the full dose is received.

When a total of 40 cc. of I.V. fluid is prescribed for an infant, the 10 cc. left in the tubing when the burette is empty is more significant than in an adult receiving I.V. therapy.

The I.V. set should be primed and air expelled from the tubing *before* the burette chamber is filled to the prescribed amount to be administered.

Fluids and electrolytes

Standard formulas are inadequate. Special mixtures of I.V. solutions are often required for infants and young children.

Accurate and constant monitoring of total serum solids, central venous pressure, urinary specific gravity, and intake and output is essential, as changes occur rapidly in infants and children.

An increased metabolic rate and renal immaturity play an important role in infants' and children's responses to illness and injury.

Fluid requirements can be calculated on the basis of weight, surface area, or caloric requirements. Signs of sodium retention must be observed and reported promptly.

Skin

Newborn infants have immature thermoregulatory systems, and a larger caloric expenditure is needed to compensate for heat loss.

Hypothermia is a greater threat to the child because the body surface area is larger compared to the weight. Measures to maintain environmental warmth must be taken during handling and therapy of infants and children.

Burns

Burns are a common injury in infants and children, owing to accidents or battered child problems.

A child's smaller airway, the difference in surface area distribution, and the labile metabolic responses of children mandate admission to a hospital for children with burns of more than 10 per cent of the surface area or critical areas such as the hands, face, or perineum.

Psychological

The developmental level of the child will affect his response to his illness and to his environment.

The evaluation of problems is more difficult in infants and children because of the difficulty in communicating. A greater insight is needed to enhance objective evaluation of the status of the child. It is more difficult to develop rapport and gain cooperation with pediatric patients. Separation from the family and familiar surroundings is more serious for the developing child than for the adult.

III.   Minimizing Psychological Trauma of a Hospitalization Experience

Psychological development is the interaction of the child's natural endowment with various environmental factors. The ability of a child to cope with a hospitalization is directly related to the type of illness he has, the therapeutic regimen, and his stage of development. Equally important is the adequacy of the care provided by the nurse. The nurse must have a clear understanding of the psychological development which takes place at each age level and should plan her nursing care and approach to meet the individual needs of the child. Table 1–1 presents a brief outline of some factors involved in developing an approach to pediatric nursing care.

TABLE 1–1.   A Guide to the Development of Nursing Approach

Level of Development	Effect of Hospital Environment	Nursing Approach
FIRST YEAR The infant is relaxed. He coos and smiles. Frustration initiates aggressive responses.	If the infant is improperly fed, restrained, or hurt, increasingly vigorous activity will be observed. If the nurse responds to the infant's aggressive action, no distress will result. However, if frustration and tension continue and increase, behavior will take on a destructive quality. If the child is at an age where he cannot direct his aggression to solve his needs, aggression will be expressed internally and may be manifested by later psychological disturbances.	Capacity for memory and anticipation begins in the first few months of life. Thus early experiences influence the reaction to later experiences and affect psychological growth and development. The nursing approach should strive to reduce tensions in the infant to tolerable limits. Do not allow him to cry for prolonged periods of time, without providing comfort and attempting to meet his needs. The use of a pacifier may be one method of meeting the needs of a young infant on parenteral feedings.
The need for emotional satisfaction is present in every infant from birth.	During family separation it is essential that a mother-infant relationship be established and maintained. A mother-substitute should be provided when the natural mother cannot participate in the care of the child (especially if the child is on mechanical monitors).	Cuddling, rocking, handling, bathing, and talking to the infant are important aspects of nursing care. Using visiting hours constructively and including mothers in the nursing care plan for the infant can meet these needs.
The sense of trust must the mastered during this stage of development.	The infant should not be made to feel "abandoned" in the hospital setting.	The nurse should spend time with the child and develop rapport with him in situations other than therapeutic activities so that the child will not develop a feeling of abandonment or loneliness.

TABLE 1–1.   (Continued)

Level of Development	Effect of Hospital Environment	Nursing Approach
PRESCHOOL The child increases his ability to understand and exercise self-control. Play and trial-acting are forerunners of thinking. Value judgments of right and wrong begin to develop.	The small child needs repeated explanations of limits in his new environment in order to prevent accidents. Increased demands and restraints can precipitate anger, rebellion, and aggression.	The child should be allowed to accept some responsibility for his own care in order to give him a sense of accomplishment. Judicious use of approval and disapproval is essential. Many therapeutic procedures can be presented in the form of play. The child should be encouraged to "play-out" and express his reaction to his experiences.
SCHOOL AGE Maturation of the central nervous system increases the child's ability to coordinate movements. Male-female identity emerges. A greater intellectual capacity emerges.	The hospital environment may precipitate feelings of inadequacy. The child should be adequately prepared for therapeutic experiences in an honest and clear manner.	The child should be encouraged to carry out everyday activities and participate in the procedures necessary in his treatment. Questions should be elicited and answered honestly. Children of the same sex should be grouped together.
ADOLESCENT A change in body configuration occurs with appearance of secondary sexual characteristics. Capacity for abstract thinking and reasoning develops to a keen level.	The adolescent is easily frustrated in a restrictive hospital setting. Emotional instability which may be evidenced should invite understanding rather than punishment in the hospital setting. An adolescent should be placed near children of his own age whenever possible.	Privacy is essential for the adolescent patient. The adolescent should be given greater responsibility for his care, but too much should not be expected of him. Rebellious or aggressive outbursts should be constructively diverted. It is desirable to provide some occupational therapy.

IV.   Assessing the Effects of Hospitalization Upon Growth and Development

When evaluating the growth and developmental problems of a child the nurse must also investigate the family history and history of prior hospitalization, as the stage of development in which the physical or psychological trauma occurred will determine the type of developmental problem presenting. For example, if the problem occurred during the critical phase of bladder control, bedwetting may be the primary manifestation seen, and it is often the first clue that there was ever a problem!

Selected Examples of Traumatizing Experiences

Separations.   Separation from family members due to death, divorce, hospitalization, or temporary travel:

a. If lasting more than 1 week can lead to nervous behavior.
b. Occurring before 5 years of age can lead to nervousness and aggressive behavior presenting as late as age 11 to 15 years.

Physical limitations occurring before 3 years of age.   Isolation for contagion, suturing, casts, or prolonged I.V. restraint can show adverse effects as late as adulthood.

Effects such as eating problems, toilet problems, sleep problems, and hyperactivity depend upon the developmental stage at which this event occurred. As an example, the Dennis-Braun splint used on the infant is often associated with speech problems by school age.

The *duration* of the restraint is of less importance than the *maturational level* at the time of the experience. Immobilization of long duration is usually associated with the development of problems relating to peer interrelationships. It should be remembered that physical limitation in the hospitalized ill child is often compounded by separation from the family, so both traumatic events will affect growth and development and later behavior of the child.

BIBLIOGRAPHY

Haller, J. A., Jr.: Newer Concepts of Emergency Care of Children. *Current Medical Dialogue, 41*:495, 1975.

Marlow, D.: *Textbook of Pediatric Nursing.* 4th Edition, W. B. Saunders Co., Philadelphia, 1973.

Miller, M. A., and Leavell, L. C.: *Kimber-Gray-Stackpole's Anatomy and Physiology.* 16th Edition, The Macmillan Co., New York, 1972.

Shaker, I. J., and Haller, A. J.: The Unique Problem of the Injured Child. *Modern Medicine, 43*:17:47, 1975.

Vaughn, V. C., III, and McKay, R. J.: *Nelson Textbook of Pediatrics.* 10th Edition, W. B. Saunders Co., Philadelphia, 1975.

Proceedings, XIII International Congress of Pediatrics, Vienna, Austria, 1971.

Chapter Two

EXTRAMURAL DELIVERY: ADMISSION AND IMMEDIATE CARE

Extramural delivery is defined as delivery of a live infant in any location other than the obstetrical unit. An infant that is not born under aseptic, controlled conditions must be admitted to a unit separate from the regular nursery. Since many hospitals delegate the care of "extramural" babies to the pediatric nurse, a section concerning the immediate care of the newborn is included in this book.

PRINCIPLES

I. Goals of Care

The goals of the immediate care of a newborn include: maintenance of a patent airway, provision for warmth, adequate identification, and prevention of infection.

II. Establishing Respiration

Anoxia in the newborn can cause serious brain damage. It is most important to clear the air passages, so that attempts at respiration will not result in aspiration of mucus.

NURSING RESPONSIBILITIES

Resuscitation, cord care, eye care, and identification are routinely initiated as soon as the infant enters the hospital admitting unit (unless his condition is critical and the doctor advises specific activities).

Immediate efforts to establish respiration are of utmost importance. The nurse must observe and record the time of the infant's first independent respiratory effort. The kind of cry, the skin color, and evidence of mucous secretions in the nose and mouth should be noted.

Suctioning

Mechanical aid to initiate respiration may be indicated to provide adequate ventilation.

Sterile DeLee suction and other infant resuscitation equipment should be available in the admitting and pediatric units. The pediatrician should be notified when an infant is in need of assistance in establishing respiration.

Excessive pull on the delicate mucous membranes of the newborn by suction may result in trauma of the tissues.

Suction should be gentle and intermittent. The suction catheter should not obliterate the airway.

III.   Cord Care

Prior to cutting the umbilical cord, a cord tie or clamp should be applied securely in order to prevent bleeding. The placement of a dressing on the cord stump is optional.

Sterile cord ties or clamps should be available in the ambulance, admitting, and pediatric units. Sterile scissors should also be available. The infant should be observed for signs of bleeding from the cord.

IV.   Eye Care

Special eye care is required by law in some states in order to prevent ophthalmia neonatorum.

Eye care should be provided as soon as possible. This procedure may easily be done in the admitting unit, and should be recorded on the chart.

Silver nitrate or Neosporin are the products most often used for this purpose, and should be instilled in the eyes as soon after birth as possible.

The equipment necessary for eye care should be kept available in the admitting and pediatric units and should include:
1. Medication
2. Sterile eye pack:
   a. Eye dropper or bulb syringe
   b. Sterile medicine glass and cotton
3. Solution used to irrigate the eye (if silver nitrate is used)

Discoloration of a liquid indicates that a chemical change has taken place which may alter the effectiveness of the substance.

The nurse should periodically check the silver nitrate ampule or stock bottle used, for discoloration, which may occur when the room temperature exceeds 70° F.

V.   Identification

An effective device for identifying the newborn infant must be affixed to each newborn and remain in place until his discharge from the hospital.

Equipment used for identifying infants should be kept on hand in the admitting and pediatric units.

The device used for identification must be waterproof, have smooth edges, and be made of a material that is not easily torn.

Identification bands should list the name, birth date, chart number, unit, and the full name of the mother. Each crib should be labeled with the name, birth date, and identification number of the infant assigned to it.

The footprints of the infant and the fingerprint of the mother should be imprinted on an approved form.

The footprinting should be performed by personnel specially trained in this technique, and the form should be affixed to the infant's chart.

Footprint plates should be stored at room temperature.

VI. Warmth

At birth the infant is not able to stabilize his body temperature and may require external measures to maintain body warmth.

The newborn infant should be warmly wrapped. The infant's body temperature should guide the nurse concerning the need for a heated crib until the infant's temperature is stabilized. All measures used to maintain the body warmth of the infant should be recorded in the nurse's note on the chart.

TECHNIQUES

I. Establishing Respiration

1. The infant's nose and mouth should be gently wiped with a clean or sterile material to remove obvious mucous secretions that may obstruct the air passage. Do *not* wipe the *inside* of the mouth with gauze.

2. The infant may be placed in the Trendelenburg position to facilitate drainage of mucus from the upper respiratory tract.

3. The trachea may be "milked" by stroking the neck in the direction of the mouth (Fig. 2–1).

4. Rubbing the infant's back or gently slapping the soles of his feet are techniques that may aid in initiating respiration, but should *not* be used *unless a patent airway has been established.*

Suctioning

Mucus in the nose and throat may be removed by suctioning, using a small catheter attached to a DeLee mucus trap. The catheter is placed in the infant's nose or mouth and the mouthpiece inserted between the nurse's lips. As the nurse sucks on the mouthpiece, a mild suction is created, drawing mucus through the catheter into the trap (Fig. 2–2).

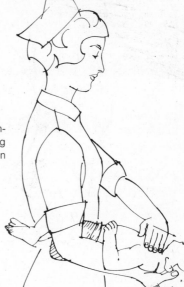

FIGURE 2–1. "Milking" the Trachea The infant is in Trendelenburg position. Arrows show movement of fingers when stroking the throat. The milking of the trachea should be followed by suction and resuscitation as necessary.

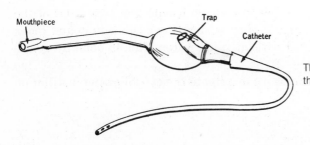

Mouthpiece   Trap   Catheter

FIGURE 2–2. The DeLee Suction Apparatus The mucus trap prevents the mucous secretions of the infant from reaching the mouthpiece.

A Kreiselman resuscitation machine may be utilized to clear the airway and administer oxygen (See Fig. 15–8, p. 141).

Deep or vigorous suctioning can cause vagal stimulation which will result in bradycardia and possible respiratory arrest.

II. Cord Care

A ligature (cord tie) is placed around the umbilical cord, approximately 1 inch from the abdominal wall, and tied securely in a square knot. A disposable clamp may be used in place of the cord tie. The cord may then be cut. The cord tie or clamp crushes the vessels within the cord and may be left in place until the cord dries and drops off.

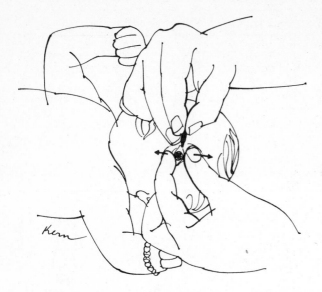

FIGURE 2–3. Technique of Instilling Eyedrops With the thumb and index finger in place as shown, use gentle pressure in opposite directions to open the eye of a newborn. The eyedrops should fall in the center of the lower conjunctival sac. The eye irrigation should be directed toward the outer canthus to prevent the spread of contamination to the lacrimal ducts. All equipment used for eyedrop instillation and eye irrigation should be sterile.

III. Eye Care

Wax ampules containing 1 per cent silver nitrate in a clear, colorless solution should be stored at room temperature. Normal saline should not be used in conjunction with silver nitrate solution, as precipitation may occur.

The infant's eyelids may be wiped with sterile cotton soaked with sterile water. The wax ampule of silver nitrate is punctured with a sterile needle and two drops of the solution dropped into each eye as the ampule is pressed between the thumb and index finger. The eyes should then be irrigated with distilled water. This is done by gentle pressure on a rubber bulb syringe (Fig. 2–3).

When Neosporin is used, it is not necessary to irrigate the eye following instillation of drops.

IV. Identification

The Clip-Seal Ident-A-Band® System

1. Fill out the required information on the Ident-A-Band card. With the clip up, so that the printing faces you, slide the card deep into the band (Fig. 2–4, A).

2. Holding the card firmly inside the band with the left hand, snap off the stub at the perforated red line (Fig. 2–4, B). Folding the card at the red line makes the stub snap off easily. Discard the empty stub.

3. Place the clip on top of the infant's wrist — so that the printing faces you — and wrap the band around the wrist (Fig. 2–4, C). (The band may be applied to the infant's ankle if you prefer.)

4. Feed the band squarely into the open clip and pull snugly to the baby's skin (Fig. 2–4, D). The band is applied snugly to the newborn, because they lose weight and the band will loosen. With infants and older children, a finger's width of space between the band and the wrist is necessary to avoid constriction of circulation.

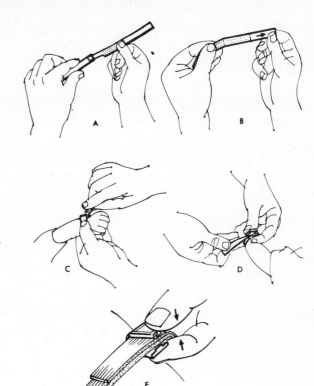

FIGURE 2–4. The Clip-Seal Ident-A-Band® identification bracelet.

5. Press the clip shut (Fig. 2–4, *E*). Trim the excess band with scissors. Slide the band so that the clip is at the outer edge of the infant's wrist or ankle to prevent skin trauma.

Footprinting of Infant

When properly done, skin prints are the only sure form of identification.

1. Remove vernix from the sole of the foot and wipe dry so that a clear footprint can be taken.

2. Lightly press the foot on the pre-inked plate, using a heel-to-toe motion.

3. Lightly press the foot on the approved ink-receptive form supplied for this purpose. Be sure the toe prints are included. Avoid dark, heavy footprints, as the skin lines on a newborn are very fine and may blur. Repeat the procedure for the other foot.

4. The footprint record should be attached to the infant's chart.

BIBLIOGRAPHY

A Caution on Aspiration of Infants. *Medical World News, 14*:5 April, 1971.

American Academy of Pediatrics: *Hospital Care of Newborn Infants.* Committee on Hospital Care, 1971.

Fuerst, E. V., Wolff, L., and Weitzel, M.: *Fundamentals of Nursing.* 5th Edition, J. B. Lippincott Co., Philadelphia, 1974.

Marlow, D.: *Textbook of Pediatric Nursing.* 4th Edition, W. B. Saunders Co., Philadelphia, 1973.

Vaughn, V. C., III, and McKay, R. J.: *Nelson Textbook of Pediatrics.* 10th Edition, W. B. Saunders Co., Philadelphia, 1975.

PRODUCT REFERENCES

C. R. Bard Inc., Murray-Hill, New Jersey: DeLee Mucus Trap.
Day-Baldwin Co., Hillside, New Jersey: "Directions for Use of Silver Nitrate Ophthalmic Solution."
Hollister Inc., Chicago, Illinois: "The Clip-Seal Ident-A-Band® System of Identification."

Chapter Three

OBSERVATION AND APPRAISAL OF THE NEWBORN

This brief review of the characteristics of the *normal* newborn infant is presented for the purpose of highlighting essential nursing observations. Accurate nursing observation within the first month of life is a vital factor in the survival and future development of the infant.

PRINCIPLES

The physiology of the newborn infant enables him to cope with the extrauterine environment, but the usual signs which accompany pathological processes may be concealed.

There are common, observable variations in the newborn which are nonpathological. An understanding of the variations will aid the nurse in relieving parental anxiety.

The nurse must have an understanding of the "range of normalcy" in order to identify the deviations from normal seen in her daily observations.

Knowing the gestational age of the newborn is important since premature and small-for-date newborns each have different and distinct needs that can be anticipated.

NURSING RESPONSIBILITIES

The nurse must understand the normal characteristics of the newborn infant in order to evaluate his status effectively. She should accurately record observations concerning an infant's behavior as well as his physiological status.

Most variations (illustrated in the following pages) will disappear within the first few months of life.

The variations observed should be charted and explained in simple terms to the parents.

Observations should be made and recorded after 24 hours of age when the infant is awake and between feedings.

TECHNIQUES

I.   Appraising the Newborn — Common Variations

Appraisal of the newborn infant in the mother's presence affords an excellent opportunity for teaching and guiding the parents concerning child development and care. Daily appraisal and recording should include:

Activity of Infant

The normal newborn exhibits uncoordinated movements of the arms and legs when awake. Tremors of the lips or extremities during periods of crying are commonly seen and are nonpathological. Constant tremors or tremors of the extremities during sleep may be of pathological significance and should be reported. The hands of the newborn infant are usually held in tightly clenched fists with the thumb under the other fingers.

Weight

See page 46.

Vital Signs

See page 41.

General Body Symmetry

General body symmetry and the movements of the extremities should be observed.

The Face

The face of the newborn is expressionless, and the lower mandible may quiver when stimulated. The cheeks should be full because of the presence of "sucking pads" of fat.

The Mouth

Salivation does not occur in the normal newborn infant. Excessive drooling may be indicative of a congenital anomaly and should be reported to the doctor. The palate should be examined for the presence of clefts or anomalies prior to the first feeding. Small white dots on the hard palate (Epstein's pearls) are caused by a normal accumulation of epithelial cells and disappear within a few weeks.

Eyes

The eye movements are not coordinated at birth because the neuromuscular system is immature. If the infant is held upright and tipped gently forward and backward, his eyes will open. Edema of the eyelids commonly occurs as a result of trauma during the normal birth process, or as a response to the medication instilled after birth. A small conjunctival hemorrhage or "blood spot" may be seen in the eye of a newborn, but it is not considered pathological unless symptoms of cerebral injury occur. The "blood spot" will disappear within the first six weeks of life. The size of the pupils of the eyes may not be equal during the first few weeks of life because of the immaturity of the neuromuscular system. Eye discharges should be considered abnormal and reported to the doctor without delay. Tears are normally absent in the crying newborn infant.

The Anterior Fontanel

This fontanel is diamond-shaped and should be flat. A sunken fontanel may indicate dehydration; a protruding fontanel may indicate increased intracranial pressure. It closes by 18 months of age.

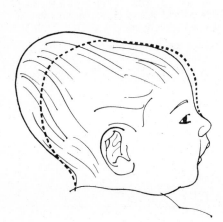

FIGURE 3-1. Molding Molding of the head occurs as a result of the overriding of the parietal bones as the head passes through the birth canal. The head appears longer than normal. This condition disappears without treatment within a few weeks. The dotted lines show the normal contour of the head as compared with the molded head of a newborn.

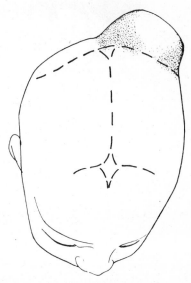

FIGURE 3-2. Cephalohematoma A subperiosteal hemorrhage resulting from trauma during delivery. Note that the swelling is limited to the boundaries of one cranial bone. The swelling feels "mushy" but does *not* pulsate or enlarge when the infant cries. Incision and drainage are contraindicated. This condition will disappear without treatment within six weeks.

Skin and Nails

The skin color should be pink. Fine hairs (lanugo) may appear on the skin, and some desquamation is common in the first four weeks of life. Excessive desquamation (peeling) of the skin should be reported to the doctor. A mottled or marbled appearance of the skin (cutis marmorata) and some cyanosis of the palms of the hands and soles of the feet are normal in the newborn and demonstrate sluggish peripheral circulation.

Pallor, jaundice, or cyanosis of the skin should be reported immediately. White, pin-head-sized papules appearing over the nose of the infant (milia) are common and are nonpathological. The nails usually protrude beyond the fingertips and may cause skin trauma in active infants.

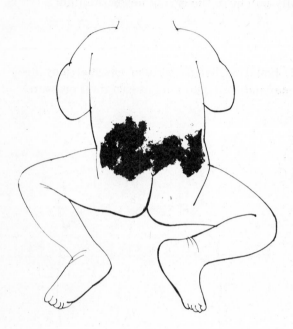

FIGURE 3–3. Mongolian Spots Well-demarcated areas of pigmentation, usually slate-blue in color, are known as mongolian spots. They usually appear on the buttocks or the back and occur most often in black infants. These markings are of no significance and usually disappear between the first and the fifth years of life.

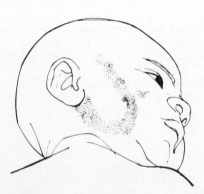

FIGURE 3–4. Forceps Marks An ecchymotic discoloration of the skin in the area of the face shown occurs as a result of a forceps delivery. The forceps marks may appear on one or both sides of the face and will disappear without treatment. Any breaks in the skin should be recorded and reported to the doctor.

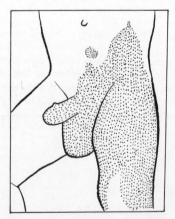

FIGURE 3–5. Port-Wine Stain (nevus flammeus) A red to purple discoloration usually observed at birth. It is not elevated, does not blanch on pressure, and.does not disappear spontaneously. Camouflage with cosmetics is usually the prescribed approach with small lesions. Port-wine stains distributed along the path of the trigeminal nerve may be associated with retinal or intracranial disease.

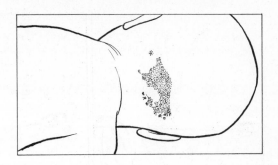

FIGURE 3–6.   Stork's Beak Mark   A pale pink spot seen frequently on the eyelids and occipital area of light-complexioned newborns infants. They are light in color, blanch on pressure and usually fade promptly, and disappear by one year of age.

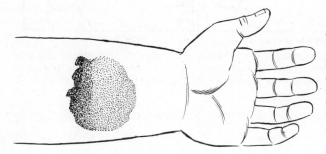

FIGURE 3–7.   Strawberry Mark (nevus vasculosus)   A raised, sharply demarcated, bright or dark red swelling present at birth or noticed during the first two months of age. After a period of variable growth, lesions become stationary in size (by eight months) and will disappear by seven years of age. Only those subject to repeated trauma are excised early.

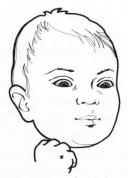

FIGURE 3–8.   Setting-sun Sign   In the setting-sun sign, the irises deviate downward and appear to sink beneath the lower eyelids. This transitory spontaneous phenomenon in the newborn can be elicited by quickly lowering the infant from a sitting to a supine position. Its *sustained* presence may be indicative of hydrocephalus or other brain disease.

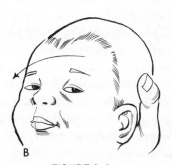

FIGURE 3–9.

Position of External Ear

Low set ears may be characteristic of specific congenital abnormalities, especially those related to the kidneys. Therefore, assessment of the position of the ear in relation to the eye is important.

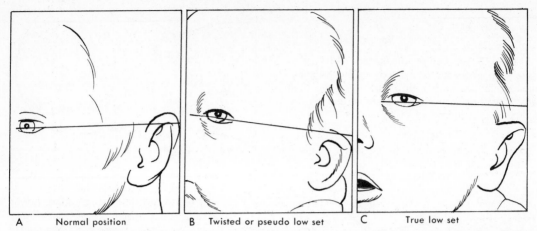

| A   Normal position | B   Twisted or pseudo low set | C   True low set |

FIGURE 3–10.   In the normal infant, the placement of the ear on the scalp falls on the extension of a line drawn across the inner and outer canthi of the eye. Incomplete helix development, commonly seen in prematures, and a normal variant in full-term infants can be mistaken for low set ears *(B)*. The helix of the ear assumes a normal shape as the baby matures.

Reflexes

Vital reflexes should be elicited and recorded. Certain reflexes are vital to the infant's life and many are protective. Absence of a reflex may indicate a pathological condition and should be reported to the doctor.

Rooting reflex.   The infant turns his head toward an object that touches his cheek. Because of this reflex, efforts at stablizing the infant's head by holding his cheeks between the thumb and forefinger will be met with great resistance.

Sucking reflex.   The infant initiates sucking movements when his lips are stimulated. This reflex is necessary for successful feeding and is usually accompanied by the swallowing and gag reflexes.

Moro reflex.   This symmetrical embracing movement of the arms is stimulated by sudden movements of the infant's head and demonstrates a sense of equilibrium. Absence of this reflex may indicate a neurological disorder, while a unilateral Moro reflex may indicate a local pathological condition such as a fractured clavicle.

Tongue retrusion reflex.   This normal reflex causes the infant to push out his tongue when an object is placed in his mouth. This reflex is often mistaken for a sign that the infant is refusing a bottle or solid food. (See Techniques of Feeding, Chapter 13, and Techniques of Oral Medication, Chapter 18.)

Reflexes may be easily elicited in a resting, quiet infant. A crying infant will not provide accurate responses.

Stool and Urine Output

The first stool of a normal newborn infant, passed within 24 hours after birth, appears greenish-black and tarry (meconium). The transitional stool, passed between the third to fifth days of life, appears greenish yellow and loose. Stools after the fifth day are normally yellow and pasty. When solid foods are offered to the child the stools turn

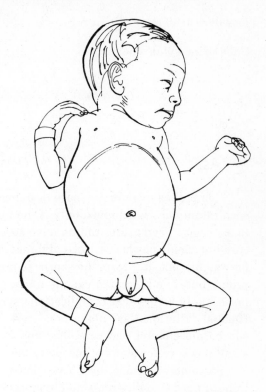

FIGURE 3–11. Abdominal Distention The thin muscles of the abdominal wall predispose the infant to distention, which may occur as a result of swallowing excess air. Sudden abdominal distention associated with vomiting, absence of stools, or cyanosis and choking are indicative of a pathological process and should be reported without delay. Note the fullness of the distended abdomen and the characteristic facial expression of the infant.

a brownish color. A small, hard, formed stool may indicate constipation; and a green, watery stool may indicate diarrhea. Both conditions should be reported to the doctor. The newborn infant normally passes two to four stools each day. (For average urine output of infants and children, see page 303.)

Retention of Feedings

The infant's ability to suck and to retain feedings should be noted and recorded.

Smelling the Newborn

Many metabolic disorders are associated with specific odors of the body or urine that should lead the nurse to suspect, report, and initiate investigation for early diagnosis and possible prevention of permanent damage to the infant.

Metabolic disorder	Characteristic odor
Ketoacidosis	Sweet, fruity odor to breath
Diabetes	
Starvation	
Vomiting	
Hyperpyrexia	
Phenylketonuria (PKU)	Musty, mousy odor to sweat and urine
Maple syrup urine disease	Maple syrup odor to urine
Methionine malabsorption syndrome	Yeastlike or dried celery-like odor to urine

Isovalericacidemia   Odor of sweaty feet to body and urine

Cat's urine syndrome   Urine smells like cat's urine

Trimethylaminuria   Fishlike odor to urine

Tyrosinemia   Rancid butter–like odor to body and
Fructosemia   urine

II. Assessing Maturity of the Newborn

Comprehensive nursing care designed to anticipate problems and meet the needs of each infant can be achieved only if the nurse can identify factors that influence the infant's needs. Premature infants have specific care requirements to assure survival. Mature but small newborns have different care requirements. For example, a small, underweight, but full-term newborn requires specialized care as does the premature, infant, but if he is treated exactly like a premature infant and is placed in an incubator he is likely to develop complications such as fever and rash. Neither weight nor estimated gestational age alone can determine maturity of the newborn. Specific problems can be anticipated and complications avoided if the nurse routinely examines every small newborn for signs of maturity level and reports her findings to the pediatrician.

Some observations the nurse should make that require little or no handling of the infant in order to differentiate the small but full-term infant from the premature infant are shown in the following illustrations.

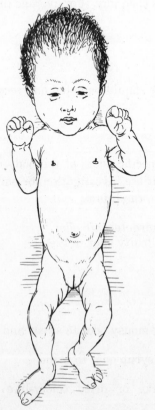

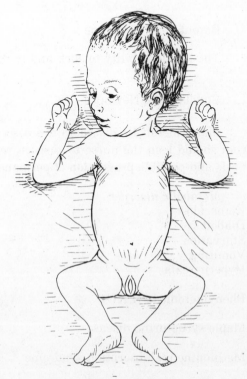

FIGURE 3–12. Full-term Underweight Newborn.   FIGURE 3–13. Premature Newborn.

Full-term Underweight Newborn

1. Infant appears long and skinny.

2. Head circumference is normal.

3. Each hair on head is distinct and separate.
4. Skin is dry, flaky, wrinkled.
5. Cartilage of external ear is rigid, less pliable.
6. Breast has palpable nodule, with erect nipple.
7. Lies with arms and legs drawn up to fetal position; elbows and knees elevated from mattress; head in line with trunk.
8. Testes descended; rugal folds and pigmentation of scrotal sac is present.
9. Labia major covers labia minora.

Premature Newborn

1. Infant has large trunk and short-appearing extremities.
2. Head circumference is less than normal.
3. Hair on head is fuzzy—tends to clump together.
4. Skin is transparent, less wrinkled.
5. Cartilage of external ear is soft, pliable.
6. No palpable nodule of breast tissue. Nipple is identifiable.
7. Lies flat in frog-like position with shoulders, elbows, and knees touching mattress and head turned to one side.
8. Testes undescended; rugal folds and pigmentation of scrotal sac are absent.
9. Labia major open and gaping.

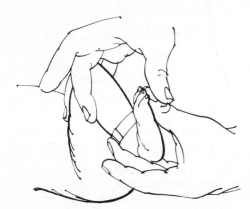

FIGURE 3–14.   In the full-term infant the foot can be pressed upward to lie flat against the anterior tibia.

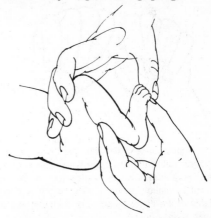

FIGURE 3–15.   In the premature infant the foot can be pressed upward only to form a 30-45 degree angle with the anterior tibia.

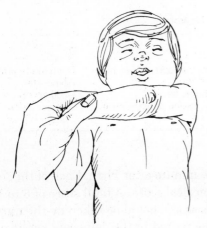

FIGURE 3–16.   In a full-term infant, when the arm is pulled across the chest, the elbow will go only as far as the chin in the midline. This is called the "scarf sign."

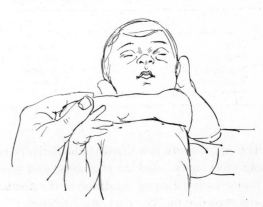

FIGURE 3–17.   In the premature infant, when the arm is pulled across the chest, it can be pulled into a straight line, the elbow passing the chin at the midline.

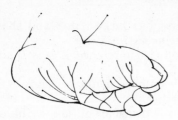

FIGURE 3-18. In the full-term infant, the sole of the foot has deep wrinkles and ridges.

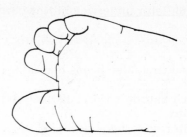

FIGURE 3-19. In the premature infant, the sole of the foot is smooth with few wrinkles.

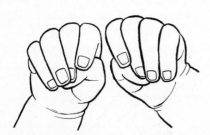

FIGURE 3-20. The Fisted Hand Newborn infants usually make a fist with the thumb pressed against the palm and enclosed within the fingers. If this phenomenon, known as "cortical thumb," persists as a sole position beyond three months of age, spasticity of the flexor muscles or corticospinal disease can be assumed.

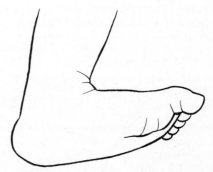

FIGURE 3-21. Flatfoot (pes valgus) Before the child begins to walk there may be no clear arch to the foot. Often, adipose tissue on the sole of the foot hides the arch or exaggerates weak muscles. If the condition persists beyond three years of age corrective shoes may be prescribed.

Apgar Scoring Chart for Newborn

Sign	0	1	2
Color	Blue or pale	Body pink, extremities blue	Completely pink
Heart rate	Absent	Below 100	Above 100
Respiratory effort	Absent	Irregular, weak	Good crying
Muscle tone	Limp	Some flexion of extremities	Active motion
Reflex irritability (catheter in nose)	None	Grimace	Cough, sneeze

The Apgar score is utilized in the delivery room, one minute after birth. Each of the five objective signs listed are evaluated and given a numerical score. A total score of 8 to 10 indicates satisfactory condition of the newborn. This score should be taken by the nurse and recorded on the chart. An Apgar chart should be posted in the delivery room to aid nurses in making an accurate Apgar evaluation of every newborn.

III.   Detecting Orthopedic Anomalies in the Newborn

Observation of musculoskeletal development at birth is essential to detect congenital orthopedic defects early and to minimize the degree of disability later. The purpose of this nursing observation is to recognize and report abnormal musculoskeletal findings rather than to diagnose specific pathological conditions. A quick and easy method of assessing the musculoskeletal status of the newborn is described in the following illustrations.

Examining the Neck and Chest

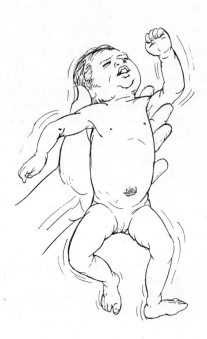

FIGURE 3–22.   Examining the Neck and Chest The neck of the newborn is generally not visible when he is lying on a flat surface. In order to observe the neck, lift the infant, with one hand supporting the back and shoulders, allowing the head to fall gently back into extension. This also makes the shoulders and thorax more prominent and stimulates the infant to move his upper extremities. Signs and symptoms of conditions which may be detected include sternocleidomastoid-muscle contracture, webbed neck, Sprengel's deformity, fractured clavicle, and asymmetry of the chest.

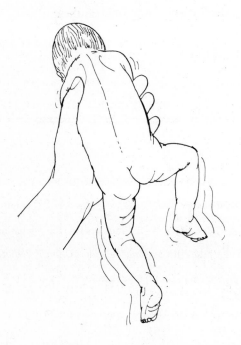

FIGURE 3–23.   Examining the Back When the infant is turned over and held in the palm of the hand he will slightly flex his back, facilitating observation of spinal anomalies such as meningocele, congenital scoliosis, and kyphosis. A tuft of hair, dimple, and palpable spinal bone defect of the spina bifida must be promptly reported. The infant will kick his legs when in this position unless pain or paralysis hinders activity. Asymmetry of the gluteal folds may indicate a congenital hip dislocation.

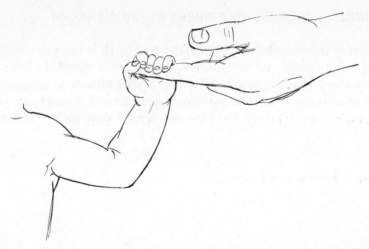

FIGURE 3–24.   Examining the Shoulder and Hand and Joints   In the first few weeks of life the infant's hip, knee, and elbow joints normally *cannot* be fully extended. Swelling and deformity of the shoulder may indicate fracture. A rough visual comparison of length and circumference of arms may help detect conditions such as agenesis or hypoplasia. Unilateral arm movements may indicate a brachial plexus injury. Permit the infant to grasp your finger and then gently rotate the shoulder externally and internally to assess muscle resistance. Erb or Klumpke's palsy may cause lack of resistance of muscles or muscle weakness. Examination of the hand can reveal extra digits, absence of digits, claw hand, or contractures.

IV.   Differentiating Seizures From Jitteriness

Seizures

1. Abnormal gaze is present. Extraocular movement.

2. Not responsive to stimulation.

3. Clonic jerking is present, local or general.

Jitteriness

1. Gaze unaffected. No extraocular movement.

2. Infant responds to stimulation.

3. Only a tremor is present, not clonic jerking.

BIBLIOGRAPHY

American Academy of Pediatrics: *Standards of Child Health Care.* Council on Pediatric Practice, Evanston, Illinois, 1971.

American Academy of Pediatrics: *Standards and Recommendations for Hospital Care of Newborns.* Committee on Fetus and Newborn, 1971.

Gellis, S., and Kagan, B. M. (Eds.): *Current Pediatric Therapy.* 7th Edition, W. B. Saunders Co., Philadelphia, 1976.

Mace, J., Goodman, S., Centerwall, W., and Chinnock, R.: The Child With an Unusual Odor. *Clinical Pediatrics, 15*:57–62, 1976.

Marlow, D.: *Textbook of Pediatric Nursing.* 4th Edition, W. B. Saunders Co., Philadelphia, 1973.

Proceedings, Annual Medical Symposium on Current Pediatric Therapy, Variety Children's Hospital, Miami, Florida, 1975–76.

Rao, P. S., and Strong, W. B.: Early Identification of Neonates With Heart Disease. *Journal of the Medical Association of Georgia, 63*:430–433, 1974.

Shirkey, H. C. (Ed.): *Pediatric Therapy;* 5th Edition, The C. V. Mosby Co., St. Louis, 1975.
Thompson, T., Swanson, R., and Weisner, P.: Gonococcal Ophthalmia Neonatorum. *Journal of the American Medical Association, 228* (2):186, 1974.
Vaughn, V. C., III, and McKay, R. J.: *Nelson Textbook of Pediatrics.* 10th Edition, W. B. Saunders Co., Philadelphia, 1975.

Chapter Four

OBSERVING, RECORDING, AND REPORTING

PRINCIPLES

The recordings in the nurse's note on the chart can help other members of the health team to build their plan of care.

In the field of pediatric nursing, keen observations are of the utmost importance because infants and young children cannot express their complaints or needs.

In most cases, the ability to observe bears a direct relationship to the knowledge of "what to look for." Failure to notice symptoms can cause errors that may be major impediments to the recovery of the pediatric patient.

NURSING RESPONSIBILITIES

One of the nurse's most important responsibilities is the analysis and recording of observations that are *significant to the individual patient.*

Through accurate observations and the analysis of those observations, the nurse can adapt nursing care plans to meet the individual patient's needs. The nurse should also work closely with auxiliary workers to motivate them to make observations that will aid and improve individualized care.

Nursing observations may be casually made or purposefully initiated during routine patient care. Observations should include general and specific factors. Positive as well as negative responses should be noted.

TECHNIQUES

Nursing observations must include factors concerning the pathophysiology of the disease, the effects of the prescribed therapy, and the developmental status of the child.

I. General Appearance

Throughout her association with the child, the nurse should be aware of his general appearance. General observations concerning height and weight in relation to age, symmetrical development of the body, general disabilities, color, fatigue or hyperactivity, posture, gait, apprehension, and facial expression should be recorded. The assessment of the general appearance of the infant or child can be the basis for deeper observations concerning specific problems. The following table may be used for recalling the average height and weight of children at various ages. This table provides *approximate* values and serves to aid the nurse in evaluating the growth and development status of the child. It is not suggested that the nurse should memorize these formulae, but rather should post the table in the clinic or ward for reference for the purpose of aiding the staff to better evaulate the status of the child.

TABLE 4–1.   Determining Average Height and Weight of Children*

WEIGHT:		
	Birth:	Weight (average) 7 ½ pounds
	3–12 months:	Weight = age in months + 11
	1–6 years:	Weight = (age in years × 5) + 17
	6–12 years:	Weight = (age in years × 7) + 5
HEIGHT:		
	2–14 years: Height in inches = (age in years × 2 ½) + 30	

*Adapted from Nelson, W.: *Textbook of Pediatrics.* 9th Edition, W. B. Saunders Co., Philadelphia, 1969.

II. Consciousness and Awareness of Surroundings

It is most important that the nurse assess the state of consciousness of the infant or young child. Infants and children respond more rapidly than adults to illness, and often more acutely. The nurse should check the infant's response to social smiles or toys or the response to pain stimuli. Manipulating the environment of the infant or young child can often stimulate responses if the level of consciousness is normal.

III. Muscle Tone

Many disease processes affect the muscle tone of the body. Inability to control eye movements, swallowing, or sucking should be reported to the doctor immediately. Any rigidity of a muscle should also be reported. For example, an infant or child should experience no discomfort when his neck is gently flexed so that his chin touches his chest. If acute pain (indicated by crying or resistance) is noted, the child has neck rigidity. In order to be accurate, however, the nurse should remember that observations of this nature must be made while the child is resting quietly. If the child is crying, any handling may increase his vocal outbursts and distort the observations.

IV. Vital Signs

The principles, nursing responsibilities, and techniques of observing vital signs in infants and children are discussed in detail on page 41. The nurse should be alert to

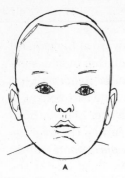 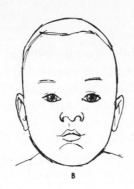

FIGURE 4–1. Flaring of the Nares   Normal respiration (A) does not alter the size of the nares. Wide flaring of the nares (B) during inspiration indicates deviation from normal and should be reported.

overt symptoms of deviations in the vital signs of infants and children. Early dyspnea, for example, may be detected by observing flaring of the nares or substernal retraction during the respiratory cycle. The nurse must keep in mind that the rhythm of respiration in the young infant is often irregular. However, irregularities of respiration in older children should be considered as a deviation from normal.

V.   Skin

The skin should be observed for color, eruptions, cyanosis, erythema, icterus, petechiae, cysts, trauma, and scars. An accurate description of the condition that is observed is much more valuable than an interpretation of the observation. For example, pallor is not necessarily indicative of an anemic state. The nurse may observe a fairly good skin color of the face, but notice circumoral pallor or circumoral cyanosis. Circumoral cyanosis may be noted during activities such as feeding and should be promptly reported to the doctor. A cyanotic child is not necessarily bluish from head to toe!

The nurse must accurately describe what she sees. A vague statement such as "a rash is noted over the trunk of the body" is not very helpful to other members of the health team, as an evaluation of this undescribed rash is impossible. The statement should have said, "a maculopapular rash with an erythematous base over the trunk of the body." Then the nurses and doctors on the following tours of duty can evaluate the progress of the rash. The development of pustules would then be quite significant.

Icterus is most easily detected by observing the skin under natural light or observing the sclera of the eye.

VI.   Developmental Status

Although the nurse should assess the child's developmental status, she should avoid labeling a child as "retarded" without substantial evidence. The stages of growth and development follow a definite sequence, but it must be understood that the time of accomplishment falls within a "range of normalcy." Many factors influence the developmental status of the child. A deprived child may not have mastered some developmental tasks because of a lack in his environment or supervision.

After the nurse assesses the developmental status of the child, nursing care activities may be planned in a fashion that will foster his growth and development. Nothing is more frustrating to a child than an adult who treats him as if he were at a level lower than his real status. Did you ever say a four-and-one-half-year-old child was four years old? What was the child's reply? However, it is natural for some children to regress to a certain extent when they are separated from their parents and hospitalized. It is unwise to stop a child from crying by saying "don't act like a baby." Crying in the pediatric unit should be accepted with understanding, and techniques such as diversion should be used rather than reprimand.

VII. The Disease Process

The nurse should have an understanding of the symptoms of the disease process of each child in her charge. Positive as well as negative responses should be noted on the chart. For example, if an epileptic child has a convulsion, the nurse would make a notation on the chart describing the seizure. This would constitute a *negative* response of the child. However, if a day passes without a convulsion, the nurse should note that "no convulsions or tremors were noted." This constitutes a *positive* response of the child. Thus the absence as well as the presence of pathological symptoms is an important observation.

If observations specific to the disease process are not recorded on the chart, then legally speaking the observation was not made, and nursing neglect can be assumed. Too often in the case of the convalescent child or the child who "poses no problem," the nurse's notes are recorded on a weekly basis. Surely some daily observations were made but not recorded. The unrecorded observation is of no value and constitutes a definite neglect of nursing responsibility.

VIII. Therapy

The nurse should observe and record the child's responses to the therapy prescribed. The positive as well as the negative responses to positioning, ambulation, bed rest, etc., should be noted and recorded. Responses to the medications received should also be recorded on a daily basis.

BIBLIOGRAPHY

Chambers, W.: Nursing Diagnosis. *American Journal of Nursing, 62*:102, 1962.

Gellis, S., and Kagan, B. (Eds.): *Current Pediatric Therapy.* 7th Edition. Philadelphia, W. B. Saunders Co., 1976.

Vaughn, V. C., III, and McKay, R. J.: *Nelson Textbook of Pediatrics.* 10th Edition, Philadelphia, W. B. Saunders Co., 1975.

Stedman, D. J.: The Application of Learning Principles in Pediatric Practice. *Pediatric Clinics of North America, 17*:427, 1970.

Chapter Five

ADMISSION OF INFANTS AND CHILDREN

PRINCIPLES

I. Arrival at the Unit

Facilities for receiving a new admission should be available at all times.

The admitting unit usually notifies the ward of the new admission via phone.

Parental anxiety concerning the health and treatment of the child require special consideration.

II. Identification

An effective means of identifying the child should be affixed upon admission and remain in place until the child is discharged.

III. Obtaining Information

A friendly, reassuring manner enables the nurse to elicit pertinent information and relieve some of the parent's anxiety.

NURSING RESPONSIBILITIES

Units in the admitting room should be clean and ready for use.

The nurse answering the phone should obtain the following information:
1. Age of child
2. Diagnosis of child's illness
3. Special needs (such as oxygen)

The nurse should greet the parents and child by name and spend time with them to develop a positive nurse-parent-child relationship.

The nurse should check the identification of the child, record his name and age and the diagnosis, and place a bed card in the child's unit.

The nurse should record the habits of the child (see Habit Record, Fig. 5–1):
1. Eating   5. Motor ability
2. Sleeping   6. Allergy
3. Elimination 7. Drugs
4. Verbal ability

Assessing the child's physical status and identifying his immediate needs will facilitate the initiation of an individualized nursing-care plan.

The nurse should examine the child's body and record lesions, scars, etc. Property such as eyeglasses should be listed. All pertinent observations should be recorded on the chart.

IV. Recording Information

An accurate nurse's record will be helpful in evaluating the progress of the child.

Information recorded on admission should include:
1. Temperature, pulse, respiration
2. Weight
3. Time of admission and method of transportation
4. Observations: color, activity, state of consciousness, distress

V. Maintaining Safety

The nurse is responsible for the environmental safety of children on the unit. The behavior of children is often unpredictable.

A crib net or jacket restraint should be applied to any child *who is capable* of climbing over the side rails. Restraints are not necessary for children in youth beds unless specifically indicated.

The level of the child's growth and development is the key factor in determining specific activities necessary to maintain safety.

The nurse must be constantly alert to maintain a safe environment for the child in the hospital.

Play is an essential part of a child's day, and appropriate toys should be provided for children of all ages.

Toys should be inspected for safety before being left with a child. Toys should:
1. Have no sharp edges
2. Be allergy-free
3. Have no small, removable parts
4. Be unbreakable
5. Be washable
6. Be lead-free

VI. Assisting the Doctor

The nurse is responsible for assisting the doctor with diagnostic procedures and transcribing his written orders.

The nurse should promptly carry out the written orders of the doctor and initial each order she carries out.

TECHNIQUES

I. Arrival at the Unit

The nurse should assign the appropriate unit for the reception of the child. The selection of a unit should be based upon the child's age and the diagnosis. Children with open wounds, such as burns, should be admitted to a private unit whenever possible. Children under five years of age should be placed in a crib and children over five years of age may be placed in a youth bed. Side rails should be used on the beds of all infants and children. The regulations of the hospital concerning visiting hours should be discussed with the parents.

Parents should be encouraged to stay with their child for a while for the purpose of: (1) developing a positive nurse-parent-child relationship, and (2) providing necessary history and information.

Clothing may be taken home by the parents or listed and sent to the hospital clothing room.

The nurse should interview the parents to determine if the child has any unusual problems, habits, or anxieties which may require specific arrangements in order that the child's individual needs be met.

II.   Identification

See Identification technique, page 12.

III.   Obtaining Information

1. Take the child's temperature, pulse, and respiration.
2. Weigh the child.
3. Obtain oxygen and suction if necessary.
4. If a Catholic child is placed on the critical list, notify the priest.
5. Record all the above information on the chart. (See page 35.)

IV.   Toys

Toys or books for diversional therapy may be obtained from the playroom. (See Diversional Therapy, Chapter 24.) To prevent the spread of infection, all toys should be washed or cleaned if found on the floor and before being given to another child.

V.   Carrying Out Orders

All doctor's orders should be clearly written on an approved hospital form. An order must be carried out without deviation. If a doctor prescribes a drug using a brand name, the nurse may not substitute another brand of the same chemical preparation without the doctor's consent.

Medications

"Stat" medications should be administered immediately and recorded. Routine medications are transferred to a medicine ticket (see page 182), which is placed in the area provided.

CHILD'S NAME_____ BIRTH DATE_____

We want to make your child as comfortable and happy as possible. If we know about his or her nickname, favorite friends, pets, food preferences and, above all, normal pattern of living, we can help your child feel more at home. Won't you please help by telling us about your child.

Nickname _____ _____ Parent's name_____

Address and phone number_____Child's religion_____ Baptized _____.

Names and ages of your other children _____ Does your child need help with dressing_____

Washing face _____Combing hair _____ Brushing teeth _____ Has your child been in a hospital before_____

Does the child know why he or she is being admitted to the hospital _____

Does your child seem to make friends with unfamiliar grownups easily_____

EATING HABITS

Is your child breast fed _____ _____ Uses bottle _____ Spoon_____ Cup _____ Feeds self alone _____.

Feeds self with help ____ _____ ____ If on a schedule, at what hours_____What is his present formula_____

_____ _____ What fruit juices does your child drink_____

_____ _____ From bottle _____ From cup_____ Is your child allergic to any foods_____

What foods does your child especially like _____

or dislike_____ Are there any other feeding routines or

aids that we should know about ___ _____

ELIMINATION

Is your child toilet trained for bowel movement_____ For urination_____ For how long _____ Does your child wear diapers_____ Does your child use a toilet

chair or toilet_____ What is word used for urination_____ Bowel movement_____ Is child taken to toilet at night_____ If so, at what time_____

SLEEPING HABITS

Is your child a heavy sleeper _____ When is bedtime _____ Are naps taken _____ If so, at what time _____

Does your child sleep alone _____ Crib _____ Bed with sides _____ Adult bed_____ Does your child climb out of bed_____

Describe any special bedtime routine, e.g., having prayers heard, taking teddy bear or doll to bed, etc. _____

_____

PLAY

Has your child a favorite toy_____ Did you bring it along_____ Any favorite games _____

Is the child used to playing alone _____ With other children _____ With grownups_____

Does your child have a pet at home _____ What is it _____ What is its name_____

SCHOOL

Does your child attend nursery school_____ Grade school_____ Name of school _____

Grade _____ Name of best friend(s) _____

Name of favorite teacher_____List any special interests (hobbies,

favorite books, favorite TV, radio programs, etc.) _____

Is there anything else about your child that you feel we should know to make his or her hospital stay as pleasant as possible?_____

_____

FIGURE 5–1. A Sample Habit Record (Courtesy of Ross Laboratories) Information recorded on the habit record should be transferred to the chart. A complete habit record will facilitate the planning of individualized nursing care.

Treatments

All daily treatments prescribed should be transferred to a treatment sheet or Kardex file and checked by the nursing personnel on each tour of duty.

Laboratory Tests

X-ray or laboratory request slips should be filled out and forwarded to the proper department according to hospital policy. Emergency laboratory tests will require immediate phoning of the service involved.

Diet

The diet prescribed is transferred to a daily diet slip and sent to the dietary department. The diet prescribed should be explained to the parents and the child.

VI. Consents

In some hospitals, one consent upon admission is sufficient for any and all procedures performed upon the child during his hospitalization. Other hospitals require an individual consent for each therapeutic or surgical procedure. The nurse should be guided by the policy of her hospital concerning the consents necessary prior to treatment.

A consent from the parent or guardian is usually required for the following procedures:
1. Suturing of a facial laceration
2. Dental extraction
3. Blood transfusion
4. Bronchoscopy, gastroscopy, sigmoidoscopy, and similar procedures
5. Vaginal examination
6. Ventriculography
7. Spinal tap
8. Paracentesis
9. All operative procedures performed in the operating room

A separate consent should be obtained for each surgical procedure, even when multiple-stage operations are involved. Consents over 30 days old should not be honored. All consents should be written in the place allocated on the child's chart, and witnessed by the doctor.

Consents are not usually required for the following procedures:
1. Angiogram
2. Cast application
3. Hypothermia
4. Phlebotomy
5. Sternal bone-marrow puncture

It may be helpful if the nurse interprets the doctor's explanations to the parents so that the parents are fully aware of the nature of the treatment to be given.

VII. Accident Prevention

In the pediatric unit, accident risks increase because the young patient lacks coordination, understanding, and obedience, has a short attention span, and is hyperactive. A few areas requiring special consideration for accident prevention will be discussed.

1. Electricity is used in every part of a hospital to power a number of fixed and mobile machines. Extension cords sometimes seem to be inadvertently designed to trip nurses and patients! The nurse carrying an infant in the intensive care unit where many machines are in operation within a small area runs a high risk of accident. Special precautions are essential when carrying infants within a unit. The use of extension cords should be kept at a minimum.

2. Static electricity and explosive gases are a deadly combination present in many hospital units. Use of cotton blankets for infants and cotton underslips for nurses is advisable.

3. Falls from cribs, youthbeds, wheelchairs, stretchers, highchairs, and even from the arms of aides and nurses can be prevented if safety belts are used and if patients are carefully supervised.

4. Sharp objects, such as scissors, knives, and needles, and breakable objects within the reach of a curious child can cause serious accidents. Children should not be near the medicine cabinet, and medicines and equipment should not be left on a bedside stand.

5. Potent poisons left within reach of children who may wander into a utility room can cause serious problems. Utility room doors should be kept closed and children should not be allowed to wander unless adequately supervised.

6. Administering medication to a child who does not have proper and adequate identification increases the risk of administering a medicine to the wrong child, especially if the child cannot confirm his name verbally. Just because a child is in a bed with a name tag on the bed does not mean he is the child who belongs there. Children enjoy "swapping beds." Every child should wear a name tag and it should be checked daily.

Patient safety is a nursing responsibility. Awareness of the causes of accidents is necessary in order to institute preventative measures.

BIBLIOGRAPHY

American Academy of Pediatrics: *Care of Children in Hospitals.* Committee on Hospital Care, 1971.
Blake, F., Wright, H., and Waechter, E.: *Nursing Care of Children.* 8th Edition, Lippincott, Philadelphia, 1970.
Hershey, N.: Formularies, Formulary Systems and the Law. *American Journal of Nursing, 64*:118, 1964.
Marlow, D.: *Textbook of Pediatric Nursing.* 4th Edition, W. B. Saunders Co., Philadelphia, 1973.
Mellish, P.: Preparation of the Child for Hospitalization and Surgery. *Pediatric Clinics of North America, 16*:543, 1969.
Pickett, L. K.: Hospital Environment for the Pediatric Surgical Patient. *Pediatric Clinics of North America, 16*:531, 1969.

Chapter Six

DAILY CARE
OF NEWBORNS
AND INFANTS

PRINCIPLES

I. Environmental Temperature

The newborn infant has an unstable heat regulating system, and his body temperature may be influenced by the environmental temperature.

II. Spiritual Needs

The spiritual needs of the infant and his family should be respected when death is imminent.

III. Observation of Vital Signs

The vital signs of the newborn and the infant will reflect his status and adjustment to extrauterine life.

An individual thermometer reserved for the exclusive use of each infant reduces the possibility of cross-infection.

NURSING RESPONSIBILITIES

A temperature of 72° F. (22.2° C.) and a relative humidity of 35 to 40 per cent is recommended for pediatric units. The temperature should not fall below 68° F. (20° C.). The nurse should check the temperature of the room during each tour of duty.

If an infant is critically ill, a clergyman should be notified, as baptism may be necessary. Baptism may be performed by the nurse in an emergency.

The temperature, pulse, and respiration of the infant should be taken twice a day. If a deviation from normal is noted, more frequent recordings are required. Pulses are routinely taken on infants older than one year of age and on younger infants who are receiving drugs affecting the circulation. An axillary or rectal temperature may be taken.

The temperature of an infant may be altered by the bath, due to evaporation of water from the skin.

An infant's temperature should be taken before the bath is given.

IV. Weighing the Infant

The weight of the infant reflects his status and is the basis for determining his nutritional needs and medication dosages. Accurate weights should be recorded at regular intervals during hospitalization. An infant or child with a kidney disease or a nutritional disorder requires a daily weight record.

Policies establishing the regular intervals for weighing infants and children should be posted in a conspicuous place by the head nurse. The weights should be recorded on each infant's chart.

The weighing scale should be draped separately for each infant to prevent the spread of infection.

Sterile impervious paper must be draped over the scale basket before each infant is placed on the scale.

Linen should not be used to drape the scale, as fluids such as urine may seep through the material and contaminate the scale.

The use of paper barriers will prevent the indirect spread of infection.

Paper barriers should be kept available near the scale.

V. Bath and Skin Care

The newborn infant has few defense mechanisms against unfavorable circumstances in his environment. He must therefore be protected from sources of infection. Strict aseptic technique should be maintained in all phases of infant care.

A crib should be assigned for the exclusive use of an infant in order to prevent cross-contamination. Individual supplies should be stored in the space provided in each bassinet. Equipment should include:
1. Disposable cups for bath water
2. Chix or soft cloths
3. Thermometer
4. Diapers and linen

The less the skin is handled, the better its condition will be. Some hospitals do not require the removal of vernix from the skin at birth; others advocate use of pHisoHex or another cleanser. The nurse should be guided by the philosophy of her hospital.

Routine baths must be given in each infant's individual crib.

Using powder with oil will tend to form a paste that retains body secretions and may precipitate skin irritation.

Powder should not be used for infants in a hospital unit. An approved baby oil may be applied to areas of the skin which may be dry, cracked, or peeling.

Particles of powder may be inhaled by the infant and have an irritating effect upon respiratory tract.

The daily care should be planned so that the growth and development of the child are fostered.

Independence should be encouraged in older children who may assume partial responsibility for their baths. Tub baths may be given with the approval of the doctor, with consideration given as to facilities available, the diagnosis, and the level of activity allowed.

VI. Clothing

The amount of clothing an infant or child needs depends upon the temperature of the room, the infant's temperature, the therapeutic measures in use (such as oxygen), the disease process involved, and the levels of activity allowed.

The circulation of the newborn is not completely established at birth, and the hands and feet may be expected to be cooler than the rest of the body.

Nursing activities should be designed to foster the growth and development of the child.

When an infant is awake or crying, there is movement of the entire body, and restraint will arouse resistance.

Open pins are a potential source of danger when left within the reach of the child.

Cleanliness is a major factor in the prevention of diaper rash and skin infections. Diaper rash may be precipitated by stagnant urine.

Shirts, diapers, and gowns should be available in the pediatric unit. During the winter months infant socks may be advisable. Socks should be 1/2 inch longer than the infant's foot to prevent cramping of the toes.

Determination of body warmth should be based upon the body temperature or the skin temperature of the trunk of the body rather than by feeling the hands and feet.

Diapers may be omitted when the child is capable of controlling urination and defecation. Pajamas only would then be used.

While tight clothing will restrain the activity of the infant, excessively loose clothing may cause him to smother.

Safety pins should be closed when removed from the diaper and placed out of the sight and reach of infants and children.

Articles of clothing should not be washed by personnel in the pediatric unit. Plastic pants, which tend to retain heat and aid in urine stagnation, should *not* be used in pediatric units. Appropriate receptacles should be available for soiled clothing. Soiled linen should not be placed on the floor or in the rungs of the crib sides.

VII. Cord Care

In the newborn, the umbilical area provides a portal of entry through which infection can be carried throughout the child's system.

The umbilical cord should be observed for bleeding or signs of infection which include:
1. Redness
2. Odor
3. Discharge

Care should be taken to avoid contaminating the umbilical stump with urine or feces.

A tub bath should not be given before the cord falls off.

The umbilical cord will dry and fall off during the first week of life.

It is not necessary to place a dressing over the cord stump. The nurse should record the condition of the cord stump in the nurse's notes on the chart.

TECHNIQUES

I. Observation of Vital Signs

Rectal Thermometer Technique

1. Remove the infant's diaper.
2. Grasp the infant's ankles firmly, placing your index finger between the ankle bones to prevent skin trauma (Fig. 6–1).
3. Lubrication of the thermometer is optional.
4. Place the bulb of the thermometer in the anus and hold it securely in place for three minutes.
5. Read and record the temperature.
6. The hands should be washed following this procedure.

Note: Gently pressing the infant's buttocks together may inhibit the reflex response of the rectum to the thermometer and prevent defecation during the procedure.

Axillary Thermometer Technique

Hold the thermometer firmly against the unwashed axilla, with the infant's arm pressed against his side, for ten minutes. When recording the temperature, the nurse should note the method used.

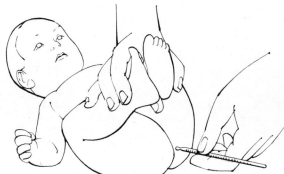

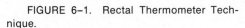
FIGURE 6–1. Rectal Thermometer Technique.

II. Types of Thermometers

1. Glass thermometers that are resterilizable.
2. Thermometers that are disposable.
3. Thermometers that are reusable for one patient and then disposable.
4. Thermometers that have electric probes covered with a disposable sheath.

The type of thermometer to use is determined by its advantages, such as rapid, clear reading, disposability, and breakage difficulty, or disadvantages such as expense and inability to use rectally.

Conventional glass thermometer (Fig. 6–2 *A*).   Reusable; washable; easily available; may be used at home.

Uni-temp (Fig. 6–2 *B*).   Uses a sensitive chemical dot that turns blue when heated. Dots are arranged in increments of .2° F. from 96° to 104° F. Can be used repeatedly by one patient and then discarded. The axillary unit with adhesive backing can be affixed to axilla for constant readings.

IPCO Temp-Stix (Fig. 6–2 *C*).   This has a reusable plastic dial and a throwaway probe containing the temperature-sensitive coil. Oral and axillary readings are made in one minute and rectal readings in 30 seconds.

AMI thermometer (Fig. 6–2 *D*).   Electronic thermometer connected by a wire to a read-out meter that performs on a battery. It has a disposable plastic sheath. The unit should be calibrated before each reading.

Using an electronic thermometer.   If the oral probe is too large to fit into the child's mouth, an accurate reading can still be obtained even if the mouth is not closed, *as long as the probe is in the area of the sublingual artery.* The probe is relatively bite-proof. An oral or rectal temperature can be taken with an electronic thermometer.

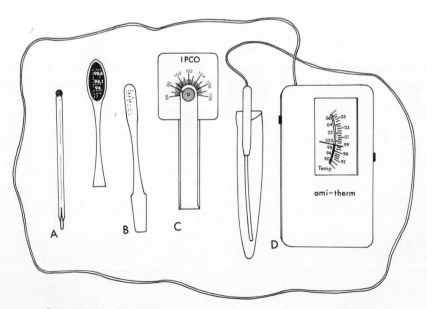

FIGURE 6–2. Thermometers   (See text for uses of each instrument.)

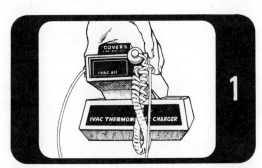

Remove the thermometer from the charger and place the carrying strap around your neck.

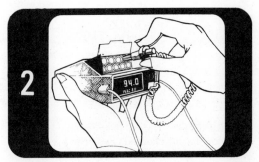

Grasp probe by the large ring at the top. Attach a disposable probe cover by inserting probe firmly into the probe cover. Do not push top — it is the ejection button.

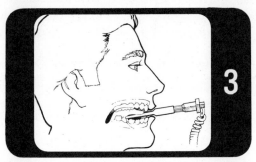

For oral temperatures*, *slowly* slide probe under the front of the patient's tongue and along the gum line, to the sublingual pocket at the base of the tongue. Patient's lips should come to rest at the step on the probe cover.

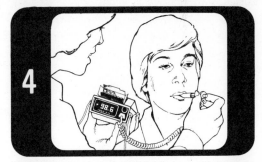

Hold the probe! Do not watch the digital display panel but watch the position of the probe in the patient until audible signal notifies you that the patient's temperature has been reached and is displayed.

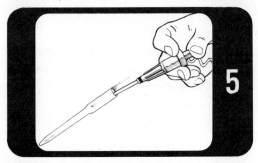

Remove probe from patient's mouth. Discard probe cover by pushing ejection button with thumb.

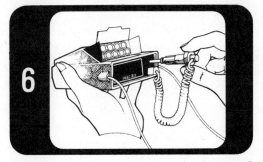

After reading and recording temperature, return probe to its storage well. This will automatically turn the thermometer off. After completing temperature rounds, return thermometer to charging base.

*For rectal temperatures, follow similar technique, except use red colored probe. Use current techniques for penetration.

FIGURE 6–3.   Using an Electronic Thermometer   (Courtesy of IVAC Corporation)

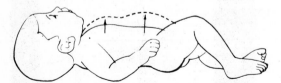

FIGURE 6–4. Normal Respiration The dotted lines show that the chest and abdomen rise together, with no retractions. The chin does not lag, and there are no audible sounds during inspiration or expiration. An active child indicates that all his energy is not reserved for respiratory efforts.

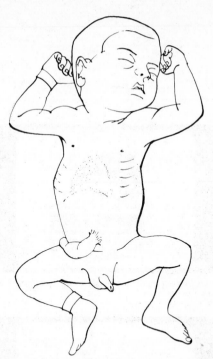

FIGURE 6–5. Sternal Retraction Note the triangular indentation over the sternal area of the chest indicating marked retraction during inspiration. The chin may lag, and the minimal activity of the infant indicates that all energy is being used for respiratory efforts.

Observing Respiration

Respiration may be observed by watching the movements of the abdomen, as the diaphragm and abdominal muscles play a large role in respiratory activity. In the newborn, respiration may be irregular in rate, depth, and rhythm. Irregularities in the respiration of an older infant or child should be reported immediately.

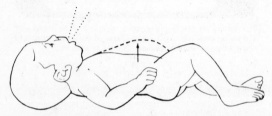

FIGURE 6–6. See-saw Respiration The dotted lines show that the chest does not rise in unison with the abdomen. Sternal retraction may be present. The chin will lag, and an audible grunt may be heard during the respiratory cycle. The child's activity is minimal.

TABLE 6–1. Approximate Respiratory Rates At Various Ages

Age	Rate per minute
Newborn	30–50
2 years	24–32
6 years	22–28
10 years	20–26
12 years	18–24
Adult	16–22

Taking the Pulse

A pulse may be obtained at any of the peripheral pulse points, the temporal area being the most popular for infants and young children. The pulse should be taken routinely on infants and children over one year of age, or on any baby who is receiving a drug or who has a disease affecting the circulatory system.

TABLE 6-2.   Average Pulse Rates At Various Ages*

Age	Rate per minute	Age	Rate per minute
Newborn	120	6 years	100
1–11 months	120	8 years	90
2 years	110	10 years	90
4 years	100	14 years	80
		Adult	70

*Adapted from Nelson, W.: *Textbook of Pediatrics*, 9th Edition, W. B. Saunders Co., Philadelphia, 1969.

Taking the Blood Pressure

Blood pressure readings are taken only when specifically ordered by the doctor. In order to obtain accurate blood pressure readings, it is important that the correct size of cuff be used. A narrow cuff will produce a reading higher than it really is, and a wide cuff will produce a reading lower than it actually is. The blood pressure cuff should be 20 per cent wider than the diameter of the arm:

Birth to 1 year—use 1 to 1 1/2 inch cuff

2 to 8 years—use 3 inch cuff

8 to 12 years—use 4 inch cuff

Methods of Taking the Blood Pressure

The child should be quiet and in a supine position. The best method for obtaining the blood pressure of infants and children is the method that provides *both* a systolic and diastolic reading—then the pulse pressure is known. Knowledge of the purpose for which blood pressure readings are taken may make techniques that provide systolic readings only adequate for achieving the intended goal.

Auscultation. The stethoscope head must be small enough and the arm cuff should cover two thirds of the upper arm. The cuff technique used on the legs provides readings that are usually 20 mm. Hg higher than in the arms. The conventional blood pressure technique may be used with cuff and stethoscope of the proper size.

Doppler method. This method uses a transducer in the cuff to transmit and receive ultrasound waves. It detects movement in the arterial wall to provide an accurate measure of blood pressure (see Fig. 6–7).

Palpatory method. Using the proper size blood pressure cuff (see p. 45), the point at which the pulse distal to the cuff reappears upon deflation of the cuff provides a systolic reading of blood pressure.

Flush method. A blood pressure cuff is placed on the wrist or ankle. The part of the extremity distal to the cuff is compressed by firm wrapping. The cuff is inflated to

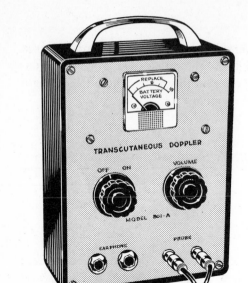

Transducer

FIGURE 6–7.   The Doppler Blood Pressure Technique The Doppler replaces the stethoscope for accurate blood pressure readings of infants and prematures. Place the flat transducer (filled with aqueous coupling gel) over the brachial artery or the radial artery at the point at which it comes closest to the surface and tape it in place. Take up any loose skin to prevent the transducer from shifting off the artery. Apply a blood pressure cuff of proper size. The transducer cable runs up the arm near the infant's head where it is plugged into the instrument. Pump up blood pressure cuff in the usual manner. Release cuff pressure, and using earphones or the speaker option, read the blood pressure manometer for systolic pressure when first sound is heard. Systolic pressure readings as low as 10 mm. Hg can be made on infants by using this machine with the standard sphygmomanometer and cuff.

200 mm Hg and the wrapping removed. The cuff is deflated slowly until the blanched part of the extremity flushes. The systolic pressure is read at the point at which flushing occurs.

TABLE 6–3.   Some Average Blood Pressure Readings*

Weight of child	Normal reading	Weight of child	Normal reading
8 lb.	75/50	36 lb.	110/70
10 lb.	90/60	85 lb.	115/75
12 lb.	95/60	Adult	120/80
15 lb.	100/70		

*Adapted from Dripps, R. D., Eckenhoff, J. E., and Vandam, L.: *Introduction to Anesthesia: The Principles of Safe Practice*, 4th Edition, W. B. Saunders Co., Philadelphia, 1972.

II. Weighing the Infant

1. Drape and balance the scale.
2. Remove the infant's clothing.*
3. Gently lift the infant from his crib and place him in the scale basket.

---

*If a situation contraindicates the removal of clothing during the weighing procedure, the infant may be weighed with his clothes on and the weight of the clothing (weighed after it is removed) deducted from the total weight reading to determine the infant's naked weight.

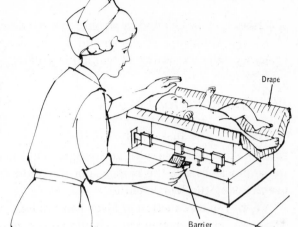

FIGURE 6-8. Weighing the Infant. Note that the drape covers the entire scale basket. The nurse is using a paper barrier to adjust the weights. One hand is held over the infant's body as a safety measure.

4. For reasons of safety hold one hand over the body of the infant (not touching him).

5. Using a paper barrier, adjust the weight to balance the scale.

6. Return the infant to his crib.

7. Take an accurate reading of the weight and record it on the chart.

8. Remove and discard the draping.

A marked change in weight should be reported to the doctor and recorded on the chart.

III. Bath and Skin Care

Avoid chilling by exposing only part of the infant's body during the bathing procedure. The temperature of the water should be 100° to 105° F. (37.7° to 40.5° C.) and a soft cloth should be used to wash and dry the infant. Daily care involves washing the skin in the creases of the body with tap water only. pHisoHex or another approved solution may be used to wash selected areas of the body where dried blood, meconium or secretions may have accumulated. Soap may be used for older children.

Care of the Genitalia

Special care should be given to the genitalia: In females the labia should be cleansed with a front to back motion, avoiding contamination of the vaginal and urethral areas. In uncircumcised males the prepuce of the penis should be gently retracted, cleansed, and replaced. (Failure to replace the retracted foreskin may cause paraphimosis.)

Mouth Care

The tissues of the mouth are delicate and prone to infection. An infant's mouth may be cleansed by offering sterile water feedings. Children should be encouraged to brush their teeth daily except when brushing is contraindicated (scurvy). (See Chapter 7 for techniques of oral hygiene.)

Eye Care

Eyes may be cleaned by stroking with a damp cloth, from the inner canthus outward.

Note: Applicator sticks should not be used to clean the nose, ears, or other body orifices, as the possibility of trauma is great.

IV. Sponging for Fever

Sponging reduces body temperature by promoting evaporation. A tepid water sponge bath combined with antipyretic drugs is the safest method of reducing fever. The nurse must observe the response of the child during and after the sponge bath. Avoid overdressing the febrile child.

Very rapid reduction of fever can produce vascular collapse in a seriously ill child. The water of the sponge bath should be warm enough to avoid producing shivering. Ice water sponges should not be used routinely as acute toxic reactions can occur in children.

V. Clothing

Shirts

To place an infant's arm through a sleeve, the nurse should put her fingers through the bottom of the sleeve and grasp the infant's hand through the armhole. While holding his hand, she can then gently pull the sleeve up toward the infant's shoulder.

Gowns

The lower portion of an infant's gown should be folded and secured around him so that he does not smother or lie upon the gown and wet it when he voids. With infants and children who are experiencing respiratory difficulty, avoid tight wrapping of the gown around the chest and abdomen.

Diapers

One half of the folded diaper is placed under the buttocks of the infant and the remainder drawn over the lower abdomen and pinned securely on both sides. Females

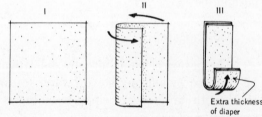

FIGURE 6–9. Folding the Diaper to Provide **Extra Thickness** I. Place the diaper on a flat surface. II. Fold it in thirds. III. Fold the bottom third to the midway point of the diaper.

Extra thickness of diaper

may require an extra thickness at the posterior area, while male infants require extra thickness over the anterior area, because of patterns of urine flow (Fig. 6–9).

Pinning the diaper securely around the leg area prevents contamination of linen and fingers with fecal matter. Long socks may be pinned to the lateral edge of the diaper. When placing a pin in the diaper, the point should be directed toward the back or the mattress. This provides a safety factor in case the pin opens. When not in use, pins should be closed and placed out of the sight and reach of the infant.

VI. Cord Care

A weeping cord stump may require daily topical applications of a solution which is antiseptic and drying. The infant's diaper should be placed below the cord site, as urine will spread on the cloth of the diaper and could reach the borders. An infant who has an infection of the cord stump should be isolated from other infants.

BIBLIOGRAPHY

Alexander, H., Cohen, M. L., and Steinfeld, L.: The Measurement of Blood Pressure in Neonates—The Criteria for Choice of an Occluding Cuff. Paper presented at the 25th Annual Conference of Engineering in Medical Biology. October, 1972.

American Academy of Pediatrics: *Care of Children in Hospitals.* Committee on Hospital Care, 1971.

Dripps, R. D., Eckenhoff, J. E., and Vandom, L.: *Introduction to Anesthesia: The Principles of Safe Practice.* 4th Edition, W. B. Saunders Co., Philadelphia, 1972.

Harmer, B., and Henderson, V.: *Textbook of the Principles and Practice of Nursing.* 5th Edition, The Macmillan Co., New York, 1970.

Marlow, D.: *Textbook of Pediatric, Nursing.* 4th Edition, W. B. Saunders Co., Philadelphia, 1973.

Moss, A., and Dixon, H.: The Optimum Size Blood-Pressure Cuff. *American Journal of the Diseases of Children, 100*:617, 1960.

Vaughn, V. C., III, and McKay, R. J.: *Nelson Textbook of Pediatrics.* 10th Edition. W. B. Saunders Co., Philadelphia, 1975.

PRODUCT REFERENCES

AMI Medical Electronics, New York, New York: AMI Thermometer.
BioKinetics Corp., New York, New York: IPCO Temp-Stix.
IVAC Corp., San Diego, California: IVAC Thermometer.
Liquid Crystal Inc., New York, New York: Unitemp Thermometer.
Parks Electronics Laboratories, Beaverton, Oregon: Doppler blood pressure apparatus.

Chapter Seven

ORAL HYGIENE FOR INFANTS AND CHILDREN

PRINCIPLES

A child must be sufficiently motivated if he is to accept and carry out daily oral hygiene.

Healthy tissues and the presence of antibacterial enzymes in the saliva provide natural defense mechanisms against oral infection.

The oral cavity contains a balanced biological system of microorganisms. Oral antibiotics can upset this balance and increase susceptibility to oral infection. Food and tissue debris on the surface of the teeth provide a reservoir for microorganisms.

Oral hygiene is primarily a mechanical cleaning process. The muscular action of the tongue, lips, and cheek; saliva; mastication; and a detergent diet aid in the natural cleansing of the mouth. Chronic illness, malocclusion of the teeth, and a nondetergent diet may necessitate more frequent oral care.

Brushing the teeth and rinsing the mouth stimulates gingival health by increasing local circulation.

The toothbrush should be small enough to be effective in the small mouth of a

NURSING RESPONSIBILITIES

Teaching the patient and his parents concerning dental care and oral hygiene is an integral part of meeting the comprehensive needs of pediatric patients.

General health and a well balanced diet including detergent foods aid in maintaining good oral hygiene.

Oral care should be designed to remove retained food debris rather than to remove all organisms from the mouth.

Examples of detergent foods are zwieback, raw apples, and other fruit. A diet rich in soft or sticky foods will necessitate frequent attention to oral hygiene to maintain healthy oral tissues.

Gingival massage should be included when brushing the teeth.

The preferred toothbrush for a child should have a short head and handle,

child. Long, soft bristles enable the brush to clean better between teeth.

Nylon bristles are smoother than natural bristles but provide somewhat less gingival stimulation. Hard bristles are thought to contribute to gum recession and tooth abrasion when used with some abrasive dentrifices and a horizontal brushing technique. Worn bristles irritate the gums and are less effective in achieving the goal of oral care.

The newborn retains poorly keratinized gingival tissue until hard foods are eaten. The oral mucosa is thin and easily injured in an infant and young child.

The mechanical stimulation that results from brushing may aggravate certain inflammatory diseases of the mouth, blood dyscrasias, and other disease processes.

Safeguarding the health of the primary teeth will greatly contribute to the proper eruption and occlusion of the permanent teeth.

Tooth decay occurs as a result of bacterial action on food debris. Particles of food lodged between the teeth can result in decay and periodontal disease.

Fluorides change the chemical composition of tooth enamel and make it more resistant to decay.

and soft bristles. The brush should have two or three rows of six tufts of bristles and should be a half inch in depth.

When selecting a toothbrush, flexibility and softness are most important. Nylon bristles are recommended. A toothbrush should be replaced when the bristles are worn or missing.

Regular brushing of the teeth should be started by three years of age. Routine dental checkups are advised from age three through adulthood. In infants, an adequate intake of water before or after feedings provides satisfactory oral hygiene.

The nurse must be aware of the diagnosis of the patient's disease in order to determine when brushing is contraindicated. However, meticulous oral hygiene is essential for the child with blood dyscrasia in order to avoid the need for therapeutic and surgical dentistry.

Parents should be instructed that although the child's teeth are primary, they are just as important as his permanent teeth and deserve equal attention.

Children can be encouraged to brush properly by playing the red tablet test game. Parents can obtain "disclosing" tablets at a drug store. When dissolved in the mouth, these tablets will temporarily leave red spots where the child is not brushing well.

Mechanical, pulsating, oral irrigating devices, when used with proper supervision, effectively remove lodged particles between the teeth and aid in massaging the gum tissues.

Drinking fluoridated water, brushing the teeth with a toothpaste containing fluoride, or regular, topical application of fluoride to the teeth by a dentist or dental hygienist should be recommended to parents.

TECHNIQUES

There are many recommended techniques for brushing the teeth. Parents and children need guidance in learning the most effective brushing technique. Some modern electrical toothbrushes provide adequate gingival stimulation.

I. The Preferred Toothbrush

The preferred toothbrush for a child (Fig. 7–1) has soft, flexible bristles, a straight head, and a short handle.

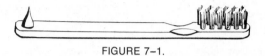

FIGURE 7–1.

II. Toothbrushing Technique

The sequence of areas to be brushed is considered here (see Fig. 7–2) because the young child's attention span is characteristically short. Since a child is more alert at the beginning of the procedure, the area to receive initial attention should be the area least obvious and most often neglected.

Both the exposed portion of the teeth and the inner apsect (facing the tongue) should receive attention during the toothbrushing process. Sorrin recommends the following toothbrushing technique (see Figures 7–3 to 7–6*):

Step 1.   Wet the bristles of the toothbrush. Place the brush flat against the teeth with the bristles parallel to the long axis of the teeth and pointing toward the gum line. The bristles should cover the teeth and extend slightly over the gum line.

---

*Figures 7–3 to 7–6 are adapted from Sorrin, S.: *The Practice of Periodontia,* McGraw-Hill Book Co., Inc., New York, 1960.

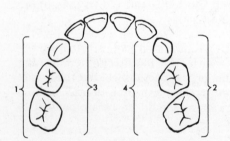

FIGURE 7–2.   In brushing the teeth, one should brush the areas enclosed in the brackets first.

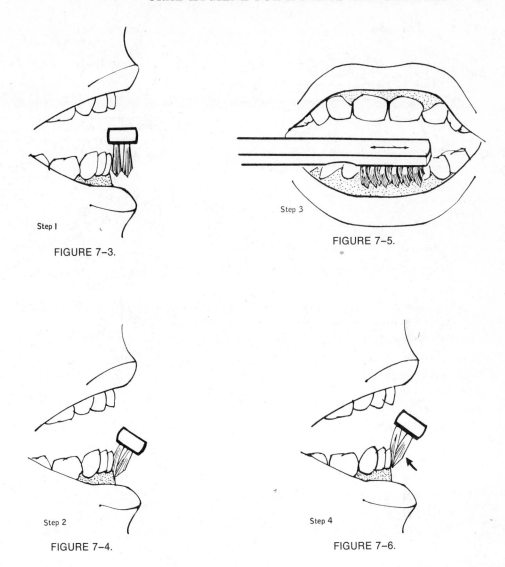

Step 1

FIGURE 7–3.

Step 3

FIGURE 7–5.

Step 2

FIGURE 7–4.

Step 4

FIGURE 7–6.

Step 2. Turn the brush to an angle of 45 degrees, applying pressure on the teeth and gums. (This pressure may cause gingival tissue to become temporarily ischemic.)

Step 3. *Maintaining the position of the bristles,* gently sway the brush to each side to provide a "pumping" action. Enough pressure should be maintained to keep the bristles bent.

Step 4. Maintaining the same pressure and angulation of the brush, gradually move the bristles towards the top or biting surface of the teeth.

The four steps described should be repeated several times before moving to the next area to be brushed.

Figure 7–7 illustrates the proper application of the toothbrush in preparation for step 1 when brushing the inner surface (facing the tongue) of the upper posterior teeth.

The chewing surface of the teeth should not be brushed with a sliding motion. The bristles should be placed directly upon the chewing surface of the teeth and given a slight rotary motion as shown in Figure 7–8.

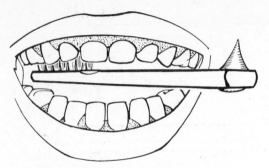

FIGURE 7–7. Position for brushing inner surface of the teeth.

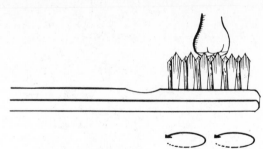

FIGURE 7–8. Technique for brushing chewing surface of the teeth.

The "tell, show, and do" method of teaching children is most effective but requires close supervision to reinforce learning.

The nurse may use a Kelly clamp or forceps to guide and assist the child in learning the proper toothbrushing techniques (Fig. 7–9).

Stimulation of the areas between the teeth that are inaccessible to the toothbrush may be accomplished by the use of rubber tips, plastic wedges, dental floss, or dental tape. Insert the rubber tip horizontally between the teeth. Hold it with the tip pointing downward toward the biting surface of the teeth and at a 45 degree angle to avoid tissue trauma. Gently rotate the tip four of five times to produce a massaging action.

Most commercial toothpaste preparations adhere to rigid standards and are not harmful. Salt or sodium bicarbonate in water may be used as a dentifrice when other preparations are not available.

Although the use of a fluoride-containing toothpaste is recommended, it is the *brushing technique* and not the toothpaste that is the most essential part of the oral hygiene program.

The use of fluoride dentifrices is not the most effective fluoride therapy for preventive dental care. Vitamins containing fluoride can be administered to children, even in

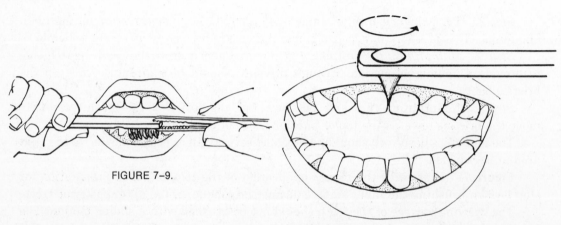

FIGURE 7–9.

FIGURE 7–10. Proper insertion of a rubber tip for between-the-teeth massage.

areas where the local water contains fluoride, as long as the total fluoride content administered does not exceed 1 ppm. The local health source, the dentist, or the pediatrician should be consulted. Systemic fluoride (water or vitamins) plus 6 months topical application at the dentist's office until 8 to 10 years of age is considered the best method of preventative care.

Between meal snacks should generally be discouraged, but when given, should consist of sucrose-free edibles such as potato chips, corn chips, celery sticks, carrot sticks, cheese, peanuts, sunflower seeds, or sugarless gum.

Teaching the Child About Flossing the Teeth

Children can be taught to floss their teeth by making believe the fingers of their open hands are the teeth. The nurse can demonstrate that the brush will not remove the "junk" between the fingers, hence the floss on each side of the tooth is needed. Figure 7–11 shows how dental floss is drawn down one side and up the other using the hand to demonstrate the technique of dental flossing.

III. Care of the Toothbrush

Following the general rules for the care of a toothbrush will aid in achieving the goals of oral hygiene.
1. Avoid rinsing the bristles in hot water.
2. Hang the brush to dry after use.
3. Avoid the use of closed containers for storage.
4. Discard the brush when the bristles soften and lose their resiliency.
5. Children should not exchange toothbrushes. Brushes should be discarded after the child has been discharged from the hospital, as resterilization is not effective or desirable.

IV. Mouthwashes

Rinsing the mouth with a lukewarm solution, using pressure, aids in dislodging food debris. This is most essential for children who wear dental braces. The child should force liquid between the teeth by the alternate ballooning and contraction of the cheeks.

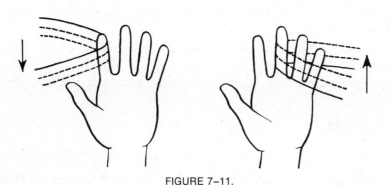

FIGURE 7–11.

Many commercial mouthwash preparations are available on the market. Some antiseptic mouthwashes must be diluted with water to prevent irritation of soft tissues. A pleasant refreshing taste in the mouth contributes significantly to the comfort of a sick child.

V. Oral Hygiene for the Seriously Ill Child

The nurse provides oral hygiene for the seriously ill child. She may cleanse the oral muscosa and teeth for a disabled child by placing gauze over a tongue depressor (Fig. 7–12). The gauze may be soaked in saline solution, a mild antiseptic, or sodium bicarbonate.

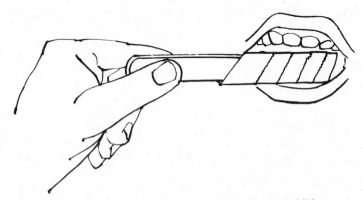

FIGURE 7–12.   Cleansing the teeth for a disabled child.

VI.   Oral Hygiene for the Child Receiving Radiotherapy

Rapid tooth decay in children receiving radiotherapy is usually the result of a drastic reduction in saliva secretion because of radiation fibrosis and necrosis in the parotid gland. Special oral care includes:

1. Brush with fluoride toothpaste.
2. Floss between the teeth.
3. Intensive short-term topical therapy. (Application of a topical fluoride gel once or twice a day for two weeks or application of a 0.4 per cent stannous fluoride gel with a toothbrush at bedtime.)
4. Wash mouth with a calcium phosphate solution three times a day to supply minerals normally secreted in saliva.
5. Chew sugarless gum to stimulate salivary secretion.

BIBLIOGRAPHY

Aasenden, R., and Peebles, T. C.: Effects of Fluoride Supplementation from Birth on Deciduous and Permanent Teeth. *Archives of Oral Biology, 19*:321–26, 1974.
Caldwell, R. C., and Stallard, R. E.: *Textbook of Preventive Dentistry.* W. B. Saunders Co., Philadelphia, 1976.

Council on Dental Therapeutics, American Dental Association. Accepted Dental Therapeutics. Edition 35, Chicago, American Dental Association, 1973.

Finn, S. B.: *Clinical Periodontics.* 4th Edition, W. B. Saunders Co., Philadelphia, 1973.

Glickman, I.: *Clinical Periodontology.* W. B. Saunders Co., Philadelphia, 1965.

Goldman, H., Forrest, S., Byrd, D. L., and McDonald, R.: *Current Therapy in Dentistry,* C. V. Mosby Co., St. Louis, 1968, Volume 3.

Guggenheimer, J.: Radiation Therapy Can Harm the Teeth. *Modern Medicine, 44*:123, 1976.

Nizel, A. E.: *Preventive Dentistry.* W. B. Saunders Co., Philadelphia, 1972.

Webster, W., Roberts, H., and Penick, G.: Dental Care of Patients with Hereditary Disorders of Blood Coagulation. *Modern Treatment,* Jan., 1968, pp. 93–109.

No Caries for Radiology Patients. *Medical World News, 16*:42, 1975.

Revised Statement on Fluoridation. *Journal of the American Medical Association, 231*:1167, 1975.

Value of Fluoride Supplements in Prevention of Dental Caries. *Journal of the American Medical Association, 234*:312, 1975.

Chapter Eight

TRANSPORTATION OF INFANTS AND CHILDREN

PRINCIPLES

Identification is necessary to assure the return of a patient to his proper location within the hospital and to establish his or her identity unequivocally.

When infants are moved, each infant should be transported separately to prevent cross-contamination.

Provisions for the safety of the child during transit are essential.

A doctor's approval is required to transport an infant from the unit when to do so requires the interruption of therapeutic measures (such as oxygen).

The temperature of the corridors will be lower than the temperature in the pediatric unit.

NURSING RESPONSIBILITIES

The nurse must be sure that appropriate identification is affixed to an infant before he leaves his crib. The infant's identification should be rechecked before he is replaced in his crib.

A special stretcher or bassinet should be reserved for the transportation of infants to areas outside the pediatric unit. Each time it is used the crib or stretcher should be draped with clean linen to prevent cross-contamination.

A responsible staff member should accompany the infant at all times.

Adequate restraint (a stretcher strap or crib net) should be used.

A record should be entered on the chart indicating where the child was taken, why, and for how long he left the unit.

The infant's therapeutic needs should be considered before removing him from his crib.

The child should be adequately clothed and covered to prevent chilling during transportation.

58

The technique of carrying an infant is based upon his anatomic structure and motor ability. The principles of safety must be observed.

Head and back support is necessary in young infants. Since an infant's movements are unpredictable, the nurse must hold the child securely to protect him from injury.

TECHNIQUES

I. Carrying the Infant

The Cradle Position

When an infant is carried in the cradle position (Fig. 8–1), his head and back are supported adequately by the nurse's arm *(A)*. Note that she grasps his thigh with her hand *(A)* to insure a secure hold. Her other arm *(B)* is free for activity.

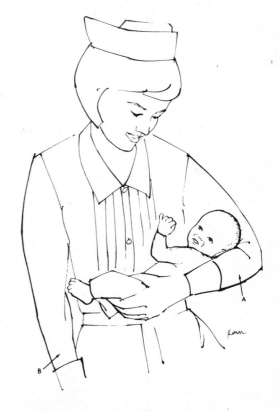

FIGURE 8–1.   The Cradle Position.

The Upright Position

The infant's head must be supported until he is able to do so by himself. The upright position (illustrated in Fig. 8–2) is not recommended when the nurse desires to have her other arm *(B)* free for activity. If only one hand is used, this hold will not allow for the infant's unexpected movement, and there is danger of resultant back strain. The infant's head should not come in contact with the nurse's face.

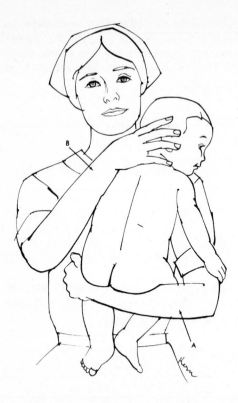

FIGURE 8–2.   The Upright Position.

In the football hold (see Fig. 8–3) the head is supported with the hand, the back is supported by the forearm, and security is maintained by gently pressing the infant's buttocks between the nurse's elbow and her hip. This position is useful when the nurse wishes to have one hand free for other activity.

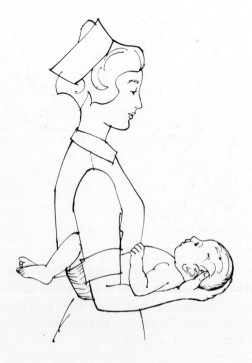

FIGURE 8–3.   The Football Position.

TRANSPORTATION OF INFANTS AND CHILDREN

When an infant or child must be transferred from one unit to another within the same hospital or from one hospital to another hospital, the nurse has specific responsibilities she must carry out before releasing the child for transfer. It is a nursing responsibility to assess the needs of the child and determine that the equipment and environment during transportation is safe and adequate to meet the child's individual needs.

GENERAL NURSING RESPONSIBILITIES

1. Positioning and restraining the child to prevent falls is essential. A restraining strap should be used when transporting children on stretchers or in wheelchairs.

2. The body temperature should be maintained by means of blankets or equipment such as portable incubators.

3. Adequate means of identification should be attached to the patient. (See p. 12.)

4. A copy of the patient's records or chart should accompany him to maintain communication between the sending and receiving units.

5. During ambulance transfer, a light should be available to facilitate observation. Equipment to maintain warmth and prevent hypothermia, and a clean area should be provided to minimize exposure to contaminants.

I. Transporting Patients in Shock

Equipment necessary to measure and record blood pressure must be available. If intravenous replacement fluids are running, equipment for administering the fluid under pressure may be required because elevation of I.V. bottles to a desirable level in an ambulance may be limited.

II. Transporting Patients in Respiratory Distress

An unobstructed airway must be maintained. The child's stomach should be empty or a nasogastric tube should be inserted prior to transportation. Do not feed a child immediately prior to a planned ambulance transfer. Suction equipment should be on hand in case vomiting occurs. The child should be positioned and restrained so that he can be turned if vomiting occurs. Airways, an Ambu bag or portable resuscitator (see Chapter 15), and full oxygen tanks should accompany the child who is in respiratory distress.

III. Transporting Children with Head Injuries

A nasogastric tube to prevent vomiting and aspiration should be in place when transporting children with head injuries. The head should be slightly elevated to minimize increased intracranial venous pressure. Body alignment should be maintained when positioning and moving the child.

BIBLIOGRAPHY

American Academy of Pediatrics: *Care of Children in Hospitals.* Committee on Hospital Care, 1971.
Bean, W.: The Transportation of Sick Infants. *Current Medical Dialogue, 10*:731, 1973.
Marlow, D.: *Textbook of Pediatric Nursing.* 4th Edition, W. B. Saunders Co., Philadelphia, 1973.
Morse, T.: Transportation of Critically Ill or Injured Children. *Pediatric Clinics of North America, 16*:565, 1969.

Chapter Nine

RESTRAINING AND POSITIONING INFANTS AND CHILDREN

PRINCIPLES

Various restraints, to facilitate examination or maintain safety, are essential in the care and treatment of pediatric patients.

Restraints are used only when necessary and never as a substitute for careful observation.

Improperly applied restraints can cause skin irritation and impair circulation.

NURSING RESPONSIBILITIES

Whenever possible, explain the reason for the restraint to the parents and the child.

The use of restraints is essential when the infant or child is in a high chair or wheel chair.

Any kind of restraint must be checked every 15 minutes and removed periodically.

Adequate padding under wrist and ankle restraints is essential to prevent skin irritation.

TECHNIQUES

I. The Mummy Restraint

The mummy restraint may be used during many procedures such as gastric washing; eye, ear, or throat examinations; etc. To apply this restraint:

1. Place a blanket or drawsheet flat on the bed.

2. Place the infant on his back on the sheet with the top of the sheet at the infant's shoulderline and the bottom of the sheet extending approximately 10 to 12 inches beyond his feet.

3. Place the infant's arm at his side in anatomical position.

4. Fold the sheet over the body and under the arm at the opposite side, tucking the excess securely under the infant (see Fig. 9–1, *A*).

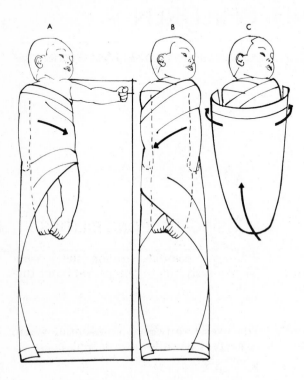

FIGURE 9–1. The Mummy Restraint.

5. Place the other arm in anatomical position.

6. Fold the sheet over the body and tuck the excess under the infant (see Fig. 9–1, *B*).

7. Separate the corners of the bottom portion of the sheet to give it width and fold it up toward the shoulder. Tuck both sides of the sheet under the infant's body (see Fig. 9–1, *C*) and secure by crossing one side over the other in the back and tucking in the excess.

II. The Crib-net Restraint

A crib net should be applied to the crib of any infant *capable of climbing over the crib sides.* The crib net is applied snugly over the top and sides of the crib. It should be secured to the mattress *spring* so that the crib sides may be lowered without removing the crib net. When the child stands in the crib, the net will stretch to accommodate his size, but he will not be able to climb over the side rail. Note that all knots are tied in a manner that permits quick release.

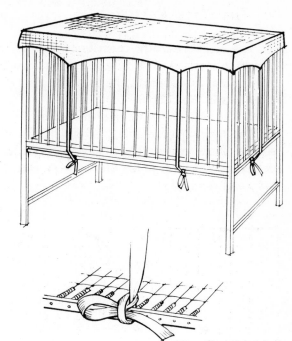

FIGURE 9–2.   The Crib-net Restraint.

III.   The Jacket Restraint

The jacket restraint may be applied in place of a crib-net restraint. The jacket is put on with the ties in the back so that the child cannot remove it himself. The long tapes at each side of the jacket are loosely secured to the spring *underneath* the mattress. The nurse must be alert to prevent the infant from entangling himself in the long tapes, especially if he is restless. This restraint may also be used for children in high chairs or wheel chairs.

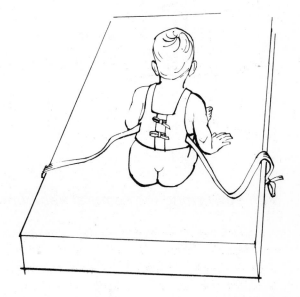

FIGURE 9–3.   The Jacket Restraint.

IV.   The Elbow Restraint

The elbow restraint consists of a piece of material into which tongue depressors have been inserted at various intervals. (See Fig. 9–4, A.)

1. Place the elbow in the center of the restraint and wrap the restraint around the infant's arm. (See Fig. 9–4, B.)

2. The restraint may be anchored by means of string or safety pins.

The tongue depressors prevent flexion of the elbow but otherwise do not limit freedom of movement. The elbow restraint may be used for infants who are receiving scalp-vein infusions, those who have eczema of the face or body, and infants who have had a cleft-lip repair.

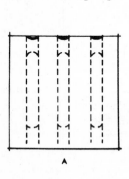 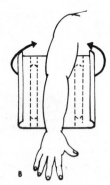

FIGURE 9–4.   The Elbow Restraint.

V.   Positioning for Jugular Venipuncture

The external jugular vein is frequently used to obtain blood samples from infants and young children. Place the child in a mummy restraint and lower his head over the side of the bed, stabilizing his head with your hands. (See Fig. 9–5).

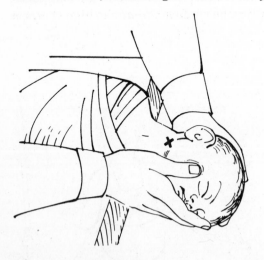

FIGURE 9–5.   A Child Positioned for Jugular Venipuncture.

VI.   Positioning for Femoral Venipuncture

For femoral venipuncture the infant is placed on his back and his legs spread apart in a froglike fashion. Restrain and stabilize his legs by placing your hands at the knee area as shown in Figure 9–6. Note that the nurse's face is in an advantageous position to soothe the infant by talking and smiling. This technique favors maintenance of the nurse-infant relationship. The genitals should be covered with a diaper to prevent contamination of the puncture site by urine. The infant should be observed for signs and symptoms of arteriospasm.

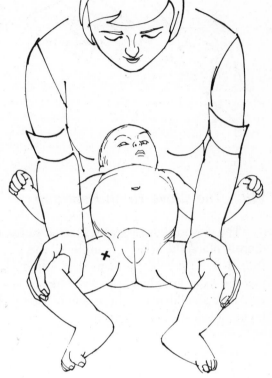

FIGURE 9–6.   Position for Femoral Venipuncture.

VII.   Positioning for Lumbar Puncture

When positioning an infant for lumbar puncture, restrain his lower limbs with a sheet and hold him as shown in Figure 9–7. The infant's knees and neck are in a flexed position. The sitting position for spinal lumbar puncture is often used in premature infants who have a lower cerebrospinal fluid pressure.

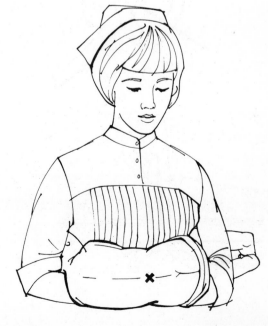

FIGURE 9–7.   Child in Position for Lumbar Puncture.

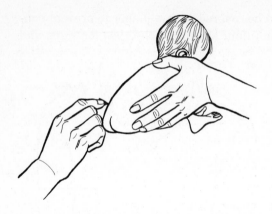

FIGURE 9–8. The sitting position for spinal lumbar puncture is often used in premature infants who have a low cerebrospinal fluid pressure.

VIII.   The Clove-Hitch Restraint

The clove-hitch restraint is used to restrain one limb or all four. Using gauze or a diaper, place the wrist or ankle in the loops as shown in the illustration. The arrow (Fig. 9–9, *A*) shows the loops that are placed together before the wrist is inserted. Adjust the loops snugly to the wrist or ankle and tie the ends to the *mattress spring*. The restraint should not tighten when both ends are pulled taut if it is properly applied. Padding the skin is essential.

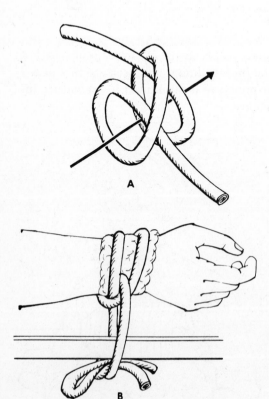

FIGURE 9–9.   The Clove-Hitch Restraint.

IX. The Diaper Sling

1. Place the crib mattress in Fowler's position so that the weight of the infant's body will rest on the buttocks.

2. Place the rolled diaper (see Fig. 9–10, *A* and *B*) in a "U" shape on the crib mattress and secure the ends to the sheet.

3. Set the baby in the folded diaper as if it were a swing (see Fig. 9–11). This position prevents strain of the abdominal muscles and is most often used with infants who have had Ramstedt surgery.

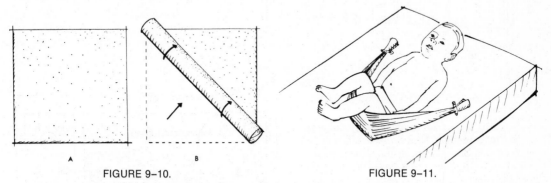

FIGURE 9–10.   FIGURE 9–11.

FIGURES 9–10 and 9–11.   The Diaper Sling   (*A*) Place the diaper on a flat surface. (*B*) Roll it to obtain the greatest length.

X.   Placing the Infant in Fowler's or the Trendelenburg Position

In standard-size adult beds, a gatch lever facilitates adjustment of the mattress to Fowler's or the Trendelenburg position. Infant bassinets, cribs, and incubators are not equipped with gatch adjustments, but the mattress may be placed in Fowler's or the Trendelenburg position as shown in Figures 9–12 and 9–13.

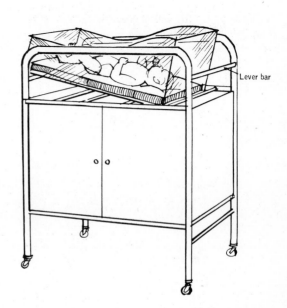

Lever bar

FIGURE 9–12.   The Bassinet in the Trendelenburg Position   To place an infant in the Trendelenburg position, elevate the foot of the bassinet basket and let it rest on and extend over the lever bar of the bassinet table. To obtain Fowler's position, elevate the opposite end of the bassinet basket.

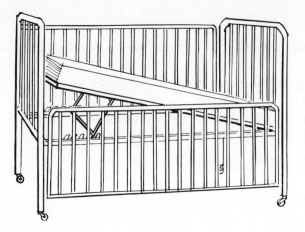

FIGURE 9-13.   The Crib in Fowler's Position   Elevate the head portion of the mattress and bedspring of the crib and place the supporting bar grooves to obtain the desired level. Elevate the foot portion of the mattress and bedspring to obtain the Trendelenburg position. A bar under the bedspring fits into grooves to support the mattress at the desired level.

FIGURE 9-14.   An Infant in an Incubator in the Trendelenburg Position   The infant in an incubator may be placed in the Trendelenburg position by raising the board under the foot portion of the mattress and supporting it with a rolled towel or wooden block wedge. The 15° prone Trendelenburg position is used for postural drainage.

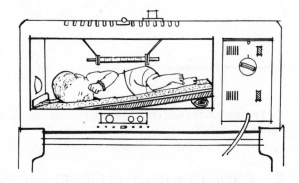

BIBLIOGRAPHY

Marlow, D.: *Textbook of Pediatric Nursing.* 4th Edition, W. B. Saunders Co., Philadelphia, 1973.
Shirkey, H. C. (ed.): *Pediatric Therapy.* 5th Edition, The C. V. Mosby Co., St. Louis, 1975.
Vaughn, V. C., III, and McKay, R. J.: *Nelson Textbook of Pediatrics.* 10th Edition, W. B. Saunders Co., Philadelphia, 1975.

Chapter Ten

COLLECTION OF URINE AND STOOL SPECIMENS

PRINCIPLES

The excretory products are often a vital clue to the child's physiologic state.

Organisms present in collecting containers can contaminate urine or stool specimens and distort the results of laboratory analysis.

The infant must be protected from injury during collection of specimens.

NURSING RESPONSIBILITIES

Careful collection, labeling and handling of urine and stool specimens are essential to facilitate accurate laboratory analysis.

The infant's perianal area should be cleansed prior to the collection of urine or stool specimens. The specimen bottle should be aseptically clean or sterile.

When a glass tube is used to collect urine specimens, the infant must be restrained to prevent breakage of the glass.

TECHNIQUES

The labels for urine and stool specimens should contain the following information:
The child's name
The ward unit
The nature of the specimen
The date and hour of collection
The type of analysis requested by the doctor
Routine urine and stool specimens should be collected in the morning. Since a freshly passed specimen facilitates more accurate analysis, specimens should be taken to the laboratory as soon as possible.

I.   The Cellophane Diaper

In some hospitals, a disposable cellophane diaper is used to collect urine specimens from infants and children. The cellophane diaper is applied instead of the regular diaper, with the point of the diaper between the infant's legs. The head of the crib mattress should be elevated in Fowler's position to facilitate drainage of urine to the collection portion of the diaper. When the urine specimen has been passed, the diaper is removed, the point cut with scissors and the urine transferred to a specimen bottle.

II.   Use of the Plastic Disposable Urine Collector

The type of plastic disposable urine collector illustrated in Figure 10–1 may be affixed to the perineal region to facilitate the collection of a urine specimen. Peel off the gummed backing (A) and place the adhesive portion firmly against the perineum of the infant. The adhesive will adhere to the skin. Place the infant in Fowler's position to aid the flow of urine by gravity. Check the bag frequently until the desired amount of urine is obtained. Remove the bag by peeling the adhesive gently from the skin. Transfer the specimen to a urine bottle, label, and send it to the laboratory.

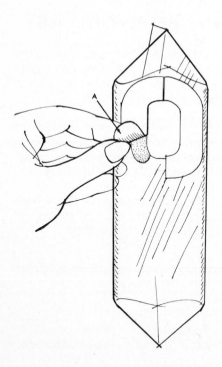

FIGURE 10–1.   Plastic Disposable Urine Collector.

III.   Test Tube Method of Collecting Urine

To use a test tube to collect urine, line the edges of the test tube with adhesive tape. Insert the penis in the tube and secure the adhesive tape to the pubis as shown in Figure 10–2. The infant's legs should be restrained for safety. Place the infant in Fowler's position to aid the flow of urine by gravity. Remove the test tube by peeling the adhesive from the skin. Transfer the urine to a specimen bottle, label it and send it to the laboratory. This method should be used only when plastic disposable urine collectors are not available.

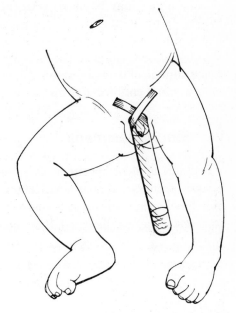

FIGURE 10-2.   Test Tube Method of Collecting Urine.

IV.   Suprapubic Aspiration of Urine

Needle aspiration of urine is used when an adequate clean urine specimen is desired and other methods have failed. Some pediatricians prefer a suprapubic needle aspiration to a catheterization procedure. The bladder tap provides unequivocal information concerning the bacteriology of the urine.

Nursing Responsibilities

1. The procedure should be performed at least one hour after the patient has voided. A sterile technique is used.
2. The child lies supine with the legs held in a froglike position.
3. The doctor palpates the bladder and the nurse may be requested to compress the infant's urethra. (In the male infant this is accomplished by pressure on the penis; in the female, by pressure upward through the rectum.) Compression of the urethra serves to prevent urination during the procedure.
4. The suprapubic area is cleansed with iodine and alcohol.
5. A 20 cc. syringe, with a 20 gauge 1 1/2-inch needle attached, is used by the doctor to pierce the abdominal wall approximately 1 to 2 inches above the symphysis pubis.
6. The aspirated urine is placed in a sterile tube, labeled, and sent to the laboratory.
7. No dressing is required following the procedure.
The nurse should observe the child for signs of hematuria following the procedure and report positive findings to the doctor.

V. Measuring Hourly Urine Output

When the doctor requests an accurate hourly recording of urine output, and a catheter is not inserted, the nurse must devise a method to collect all urine passed. A plastic diaper may be used, with the collecting point of the diaper affixed to drainage tubing. In male infants, a finger cot may be placed over the penis (with a hole cut in the end of the finger cot) and the end portion affixed to drainage tubing. The drainage tubing should be secured to the side of the bed so that looping of the distal end is avoided and drainage of urine by gravity is promoted. The distal end of the drainage tubing may empty into a calibrated drainage bag which is secured to the bedframe.

VI. Stool Specimens

When a stool specimen is requested, the infant's freshly passed stool may be scraped from the diaper with tongue blades and placed in a covered waxed specimen cup. Stool specimens must not be contaminated by urine or the results of specific laboratory tests may be distorted. Stool specimens should be labeled as described on page 71.

BIBLIOGRAPHY

Harmer, B., and Henderson, V.: *Textbook of the Principles and Practice of Nursing.* 5th Edition. The Macmillan Co., New York, 1970.
Klein, J., and Gellis, S.: Diagnostic Needle Aspiration in Pediatric Practice. *Pediatric Clinics of North America, 18*:219, 1971.
Vaughn, V. C., III, and Mckay, R. J.: *Nelson Textbook of Pediatrics.* 10th Edition. W. B. Saunders Co., Philadelphia, 1975.
Saccharow, L., and Pyrles, C.: Further Experience with the Use of Percutaneous Suprapubic Aspiration of Urinary Bladder: Bacteriological Studies in 654 Infants and Children. *Pediatrics, 43*:1018, 1969.

PRODUCT REFERENCE

Aloe Medical, St. Louis, Missouri: Plastic Disposable Urine Collector.

Chapter Eleven

ADMINISTERING AN ENEMA
TO INFANTS AND CHILDREN

PRINCIPLES

Enemas may be given to promote the expulsion of feces or flatus, soothe mucous membranes, soften stools, or provide therapeutic systemic effects. The purpose of the enema is the determining factor in selecting the fluid to be used and the type of enema to be given.

The infant's body must be supported in alignment while he is on a bedpan.

When a child with megacolon (congenital Hirschsprung's disease) receives an enema, the enlarged tissue surface of the bowel increases the absorption of the fluid. *Tap water must never be used with infants suspected of having megacolon.*

Heat or cold affects the tissues and nerves in the rectal mucosa, producing specific responses.

An accurate record of all treatments and responses to therapy should be kept.

NURSING RESPONSIBILITIES

An enema requires a doctor's written order. The order should state the amount and type of solution to be used. The nurse must understand:
1. The purpose of the enema
2. The amount, type, and temperature of the solution to be used

Rubber or plastic-covered pillows should be used to position the infant. The bed may be protected with an extra rubber sheet.

The nurse must *never assume* that an enema involves the use of tap water. The doctor's orders must be specific. No more than 300 cc. of solution should be given to an infant or child unless it is specifically ordered.

Unless an ice-water enema is ordered to reduce fever, the enema solution should be prepared at a temperature of 105° F. and should enter the rectum at body temperature.

The nurse should record in the nurse's notes:
1. Date and time of the enema
2. Amount and type of solution used
3. Response of the infant
4. Accurate description of the returns

A retention enema usually involves the use of an oil solution. It differs from other enemas in that stimulation of peristalsis is avoided.

The nurse must understand the purpose of the treatment and the developmental abilities of the infant. (Infants and young children are unable to retain the solution voluntarily.)

TECHNIQUES

I. The Cleansing Enema

When ordered, a pediatric, prepared, disposable enema may be used and administered directly from the disposable container. When an enema can and tubing are used, they should be aseptically clean. An isotonic saline solution can be made from 1 tsp. salt to 1 quart of water. Suggested amounts of solution to prepare are: Infant, 150 ml. to 250 ml.; 18 months to 10 years, 250 ml. to 500 ml.; 10 years to 14 years, 250 ml. to 750 ml.

II. Positioning an Infant for an Enema

1. Place a pillow under the infant's head and back to maintain body alignment.
2. Pad an infant-size bedpan and place it under the buttocks.
3. A diaper or folded sheet may be placed under the bedpan, brought over the thighs, and pinned to secure the positioning.

III. Administering the Enema

1. Expel air by running the solution through the tubing.
2. Lubricate and slowly insert a small catheter 1 1/2 to 3 inches into the rectum (depending on the size of the infant).
3. Elevate the enema can to a point where the solution begins to flow into the rectum by gravity (not above 18 inches). A 50 ml. syringe barrel attached to a catheter may be used for very small children.
4. After the returns are completed, the infant should be cleaned and allowed to rest. Only small quantities of the total solution should be instilled, and time should be allowed for some return. As little solution as possible should be used to obtain a satisfactory result.
5. After use, all equipment should be cleaned and sterilized.

IV. The Retention Enema

1. Position the infant as described above, lubricate a small French catheter, and insert it into the rectum.
2. Using a funnel, allow the prescribed amount of oil at about 100° F. (37.7° C.) to flow slowly through the catheter into the rectum.

3. Pressure over the anus is necessary during and following the administration of oil so that the solution will not be immediately expelled. (Press the buttocks together.)

4. A cleansing enema may be given 30 to 45 minutes after an oil retention enema, if ordered by the doctor.

5. All equipment used should be cleaned and sterilized.

BIBLIOGRAPHY

Harmer, B., and Henderson, V.: *The Textbook of the Principles and Practice of Nursing.* 5th Edition, The Macmillan Co., New York, 1970.

Kestenberg, J. H.: Psychosexual Impact of Childhood Enemas. *Human Sexuality,* Jan. 1976, p. 173.

Marlow, D.: *Textbook of Pediatric Nursing.* 4th Edition, W. B. Saunders Co., Philadelphia, 1973.

Vaughn, V. C., III, and McKay, R. J.: *Nelson Textbook of Pediatrics.* 10th Edition, W. B. Saunders Co., Philadelphia, 1975.

Chapter Twelve

CARE OF A CHILD WITH
A COMMUNICABLE DISEASE

PRINCIPLES

I. Placement in the Unit

The admission of a child with a communicable disease to a general hospital is safe if proper facilities are available.

II. Preparing for Isolation

Adequate isolation technique is an integral part of the care of a patient with a communicable disease and is essential in preventing cross-contamination. Cleanliness is basic to the prevention of communicable diseases.

Medical aseptic technique can be successful only when *all* persons who come in contact with the child adhere to the technique.

III. Preventing the Spread of Infection

Communicable diseases are transmitted in the following ways:
1. Via the respiratory tract (such as staphylococcic infections, measles, meningitis, diphtheria)
2. Via the gastrointestinal tract (such as polio, dysentery, typhoid)

NURSING RESPONSIBILITIES

When assigning a unit for a child with a communicable disease, the nurse must consider the welfare of the child and each of his contacts.

The nurse must establish interdepartmental cooperation. Instruction of the staff and supervision of the technique used in caring for the isolated child are the responsibilities of the nurse in charge of the pediatric unit.

The nurse must know the causative organism, the mode of transmission of the disease, and the portals of entry and exit of the organism in order to plan effective standards for the techniques involved in the nursing care. It is essential to obtain a history of the patient's exposure to in-

3. Via dermal contact (such as impetigo, venereal diseases)
4. Via parenteral contact (such as hepatitis, syphilis)

fectious diseases and his immunization record. Family contacts may be referred to a public health agency. (See page 268.)

IV. Facilities

The existing facilities should be reviewed in order to establish effective techniques.

Each member of the staff should be instructed as to the areas considered "clean" or "contaminated."

V. Specific Precautions

Transmission via the respiratory tract. Infectious diseases transmitted by droplets of moisture (as in coughing or sneezing) are highly communicable.

A private room is desirable to prevent the droplet spread of infection.

Diseases transmitted via the gastrointestinal tract. House flies act as vectors in the spread of G.I. tract diseases.

Adequate screening of doors and windows is essential. Insect control can be obtained by calling the hospital exterminator.

Transmission by dermal contact. Gloves are not necessary when caring for a patient with a communicable disease.

Adequate handwashing technique is essential when caring for patients with dermal lesions.

Parenterally transmitted diseases. All items which come in contact with the blood of the patient should be cleaned and sterilized before routine reprocessing.

Disposable equipment should be used when it is available.

Isolation gowns. The isolation gown is not an effective barrier to the spread of disease when it is used by several people during a prolonged period of time.

When hospital policy requires the use of an isolation gown, the gown should be discarded after being used once.

Isolation masks. The use of masks is not generally recommended, except when dealing with droplet-borne infections.

The decision to use masks should be based upon the individual diagnosis and the age of the child. Clean masks should be kept in a covered container, and the container for soiled masks should be clearly labeled.

Care of dishes and utensils. When dishwashing machines are used, the high temperature makes it unnecessary to keep contaminated dishes and utensils separate.

The nurse should notify the dietary department when paper dishes are desired. Contaminated nipples and bottles should be cleaned before they are returned to the formula kitchen.

Care of linen. Patients and hospital workers must be protected from sources of infection.

Laundry bags used for contaminated soiled linen should be properly labeled.

Floors and environment. Dry sweeping of floors should be avoided as dust will not adhere to a dry broom.

The nurse should foster interdepartmental cooperation concerning all activities involved in the maintenance of isolation units.

Visitors. Parents should be encouraged to participate in the care of their children whenever it is practicable.

Individual gowns should be provided for parents when indicated.

Use of clean equipment in contaminated areas. Clean equipment, unless it comes in contact with contaminated areas, will remain clean.

The nurse must be alert to the contamination that may occur and take action to clean articles adequately before re-use.

Terminal disinfection. All equipment should be cleaned and sterilized after use. An approved solution may be used to disinfect items that cannot be sterilized.

The room contents should be cleaned and the room aired for 24 hours before re-use. Screens and curtains should be sent to the laundry. Toys may be washed with soap and water and returned for general use.

TECHNIQUES

I. Placement in the Unit

Children with the following conditions may be isolated in a cubicle in the general ward area: anthrax, cholera, dysentery, epidemic diarrhea, gas gangrene, impetigo, infectious hepatitis, meningitis, polio, typhoid, paratyphoid, and venereal diseases. Children with communicable diseases such as chickenpox, diphtheria, measles, mumps, pertussis, and tuberculosis should be placed in a separate unit.

II. Preparation for Isolation

The linen coordinator may be called upon to supply needed isolation gowns, extra linen, and masks. The housekeeping department should be notified so that proper cleaning of the isolation unit may be performed with minimal hazard to the porter. The nursing supervisor should be consulted concerning the use of personnel, to prevent the spread of infection. Personnel with upper respiratory infections or skin lesions should not be assigned to give direct bedside care to children with communicable diseases.

III. Facilities

"Clean" areas may include the hallway, the nurses' station, the medicine area, the kitchen, and the utility area of the ward. "Contaminated" areas may include the floors everywhere, the child's room and its contents, the inside of sinks and hoppers, and the inside of refuse containers.

Room facilities should include:
1. Facilities for handwashing, preferably a sink
2. Separate utility space for cleaning and soaking used equipment
3. Separate covered containers for soiled linen and diapers
4. Individual equipment for the child
5. Barriers (paper towels)

The beds should be at least three feet apart.

IV. Specific Precautions

Isolation techniques are based upon the mode of transmission of the disease (see Specific Precautions, page 79).

A report of certain communicable diseases must be filed with the city health department upon the admission of the child.

Personnel giving direct care to the child with a communicable disease should seek protection when immunization measures are available. Frequent handwashing is essential.

Isolation Gowns

When isolation gowns are used, a fresh gown should be used for each patient contact. Organization of activities is essential for the economical use of supplies.

Isolation Masks

If a mask is used, it should cover both the nose and the mouth, be worn no longer than 30 minutes, and be discarded immediately after use.

Disposal of Wastes

Paper bags for the disposal of tissues should be available within the unit. All contaminated waste should be wrapped securely and discarded in a special receptacle marked "isolation."

Bedpans may be emptied into the community sewage system, using the bedpan flusher. The flusher should be handled with paper barriers.

Waste cans should be lined with paper and kept covered.

All reusable equipment should be cleaned, wrapped, labeled "isolation," and sterilized before routine reprocessing. Infusion bottles should be discarded after use.

Care of Dishes

Disposable dishes may be requested through the dietary department. If regular dishes are used, they should be returned to the kitchen for processing in the dishwashing machine. Formula bottles should be washed and returned to the reception area of the formula kitchen.

Care of Linen

All used linen should be placed in a special laundry bag and labeled. Diapers should be placed in a covered receptacle. Laundry bags should be closed, tied, and labeled "isolation."

Laundry bags which have been contaminated on the outside should be placed in a separate, clean bag. The technique for doing this is:

1. Have a "clean" nurse hold the clean bag with the top cuffed over her hands.
2. The "contaminated" nurse places the full bag into the clean bag.
3. The "clean" nurse then ties and labels the bag for pickup by laundry personnel.

Use of Clean Equipment in a Contaminated Area

A stretcher may be protected from contamination by covering the stretcher pad with a sheet and folding the sheet over the child. Stretchers used to transport deceased patients who had a communicable disease should be washed and aired before reuse.

When taking the blood pressure of a child with virulent skin lesions, the cuff should be applied over the sleeve of the child's gown.

A barrier should be placed on the bedside stand and clean equipment placed on the barrier. After her hands are contaminated, the nurse should use paper barriers to touch the equipment or its parts. After the nurse washes her hands, she may discard the paper barrier and return the equipment for general use.

Otoscopes and stethoscopes may be washed with an alcohol sponge, using friction, and returned for general use.

V. Providing a "Sterile Environment"

New methods are being developed to protect the infection-prone patient from organisms which commonly plague hospital environments.

One new device, now in experimental use, eliminates the need for gowns and masks, reduces the spread of air-borne infection, and aids in defining "clean" and "contaminated" areas in the unit. Known as the "RES-System" this apparatus consists of equipment which resembles an oxygen tent. The plastic canopy fits over the entire bed, however, and contains a large opening for introducing and removing equipment and supplies for nursing care. Conventional zipper openings in the canopy are replaced by long plastic sleeves and detachable gloves. The slight positive pressure within the tent gives the canopy a "ballooned-out" appearance. The apparatus filters the air at the intake and the outlet, clearing the room of the usual air-borne organisms.

The principles involved in the care of a patient in this unit are similar to those involved in the care of a patient in an incubator or oxygen tent, except that movement around the bed is not quite so limited. All equipment placed in this tent should be sterile, including dishes and utensils.

The standard-sized beds used for experimental research with this unit were specially designed to include the "bedside stand" within the tent setup. This unit may soon prove to be a boon in the care of patients in isolation and aid in reducing the psychological trauma resulting from conventional isolation techniques.

BIBLIOGRAPHY

American Academy of Pediatrics: *Care of Children in Hospitals,* Committee on Hospital Care, Evanston, Illinois, 1971.

American Academy of Pediatrics: *Control of Infectious Diseases,* Committee Report, 14th Edition, Evanston, Illinois, 1970.

California State Department of Public Health: *Manual for Control of Communicable Diseases in California,* 1971.

Department of Health, Education and Welfare: *Isolation Techniques for Use in Hospitals.* Publication 75-8043, United States Government Printing Office, Washington, D.C., 1975.

Marlow, D.: *Textbook of Pediatric Nursing.* 4th Edition, W. B. Saunders Co., Philadelphia, 1973.

Harmer, B., and Henderson, V.: *Textbook of the Principles and Practice of Nursing.* 5th Edition, The Macmillan Co., New York, 1970.

Vaughn, V. C., III, and McKay, R. J.: *Nelson Textbook of Pediatrics.* 10th Edition, W. B. Saunders Co., Philadelphia, 1975.

Chapter Thirteen

FEEDING INFANTS AND CHILDREN

Breast feeding is not discussed in this chapter because the newborn referred to was born extramurally or is a newborn excluded from the regular nursery because of his health status.

PRINCIPLES

NURSING RESPONSIBILITIES

I. The Newborn

During the first twelve hours of life, the fluid balance and nutritional state are such that food and fluids are not necessary.

Feedings are usually initiated within six to twelve hours following birth.

The newborn presents clues that indicate his ability and readiness to nurse (rooting reflex, sucking reflex, etc.).

Glucose is usually offered as the first feeding for a newborn infant. The nurse must appraise the infant's response to feedings, as occult congenital anomalies may exist.

Respiratory difficulty or brain damage in the newborn infant may affect his ability to suck and swallow.

II. Carrying Out the Doctor's Order

The doctor orders the formula or diet which is based upon:
1. Age of the child
2. His habit history
3. Disease process

The nurse may consult with the dietician in planning individual diets to meet the needs of infants and children.

84

There are variations in the needs of infants in respect to the amount of food and the frequency of feedings.

The number of feedings decreases as the infant grows older.

The early establishment of good eating habits will contribute to the personality development of the infant. Feedings should not be forced.

III. Formula Feedings

Formula prepared in the hospital must be stored in an environment of 50° F. (10° C.) or lower to prevent the growth of pathogens. Formula prepared and sealed by the manufacturer does not require refrigeration.

The nurse should check the temperature of the formula refrigerator daily and report deviations to the supervisor.

Since various age groups and disease processes are present in the pediatric unit, there may be different diet prescriptions for each infant.

The name of the infant should be checked with the name on the bottle cap to insure that the proper baby receives the proper formula.

IV. Positioning

The effectiveness of feedings is influenced by:
1. Position of the baby
2. Position of the nipple in the mouth
3. Position of the bottle
4. Environment and attitude
A calm, unhurried atmosphere is conducive to successful feeding. Infants need to satisfy their sucking urge.

All infants should be picked up and held during feedings. The infant's head and back should be supported.

The nurse should plan at least one half hour for each infant feeding. However, prolonged feeding times are undesirable, as they will not foster favorable eating habits.

V. Burping

The swallowing of air during feeding leads to abdominal distention and discomfort which inhibits sucking. Frequent burping enables the infant to consume the maximum amount of formula offered.

The baby should be bubbled or burped after every ounce and at the end of the feeding.

When an infant is held in an upright position, the air bubbles rise to the top of the stomach, reaching a free passage for the exit of the air swallowed.

A sitting position is preferred for burping an infant because it facilitates continuous observation of his responses.

VI. Charting

An accurate record of the consumption and retention of feedings will aid in evaluating the progress of the infant.

The nurse should chart:
1. Type of formula offered to the infant
2. Amount taken by the infant

3. Amount retained by the infant

A note concerning the color, activity, sucking and swallowing abilities, and fatigue of the infant should be recorded in the nurse's note on the chart.

VII. Solid Foods

Solid foods may be started as early as the second or third week of life, depending upon the doctor's order.

Feeding techniques should foster growth and development.

The tongue retrusion reflex must not be mistaken for the infant's refusal of food. Patience is essential when infants are developing the skills involved in eating solid foods.

Unless medically contraindicated, independence should be fostered during mealtime.

It is important to provide the proper texture and consistency of foods for young children.

Young children prefer foods at moderate temperatures.

New foods should be introduced one at a time to facilitate detection of allergic responses.

Jars of baby foods should be stored in a dry, moderately cool location.

The nurse should foster growth and development during feeding time by using her judgment to:
1. Feed solid foods via spoon, not mixed with formula
2. Initiate cup feedings
3. Offer hard toast, zweiback, or crackers when teeth appear (if not medically contraindicated)
4. Allow the infant to assist with feedings (the use of "finger foods" for preschool-age children)

The nurse should use the "habit record" as a guide to determine the amount of assistance necessary during mealtime (see p. 35).

"Finger foods" such as carrot sticks should be encouraged for the preschool child.

Cold foods should be served with the chill removed.

New foods should be introduced in small amounts (1 to 1 1/2 tsp.) early in the day to allow ample opportunity to observe the child's responses.

Before opening a jar of baby food, the top of the jar should be wiped clean to avoid contamination of the food. Partially used cans or jars may be covered and stored in the refrigerator for no longer than 3 days.

VIII.   Feeding Problems

A hospitalized toddler, often negativistic, may present a feeding problem when a therapeutic diet is of prime importance in the recovery phase of his illness. Anxiety may develop in the nurse, the parent, and the child unless a planned approach is initiated.

The mealtime environment plays a vital part in stimulating the appetite of children. Since children enjoy sharing experiences and mimicking adults, a group table headed by a staff member will provide a "natural" atmosphere conducive to eating.

The motto, "mealtime is happy time," should be basic to the plan of care for a hospitalized child.

The nurse should consult with the doctor so that therapy may be planned with consideration for nutritional needs. The child should not be "snatched away" from the table for a short but painful treatment. Visiting hours that coincide with mealtime are desirable.

IX. Teaching the Parents and the Child

Instruction concerning the nutritional needs of childhood will be more meaningful if visual aids are used.

Many food manufacturing companies will provide sample jars or bottles of food upon request. The nurse should plan to use sample jars of baby food or wax food models as teaching aids to stimulate interest in learning about nutrition.

The solute or osmolar load of formulas derives from the electrolyte and sodium content. The highest solute load is found in undiluted cow's milk and the lowest in human milk. If the solute load fed to the infant exceeds available body water for renal excretion, hypertonic or hypernatremic dehydration will result. It is known that low fat milk, when boiled for 5 to 15 minutes will at least double in sodium content.

Mothers who use boiled skim milk for infants with diarrhea should be cautioned to dilute this milk and not offer it full strength to a sick infant. Reinterpreting and clarifying doctors orders for use of skim milk is a nursing responsibility.

Mothers who use regular skim milk routinely in place of whole milk should be urged to include foods rich in vitamin A and D in the infant's diet.

TECHNIQUES

I. Carrying Out the Doctor's Order

A file card containing the formula prescription for each child should be kept in the formula kitchen and used as a guide for the daily preparation of formulas.

II. Formula Feedings

The formula bottle is obtained from the refrigerator and may be warmed prior to feeding if this is hospital policy. It is *not* harmful to feed premature or full-term infants cold milk. The nipple, with holes of sufficient size to suit the individual child, should be checked for patency. Holes that are too large may cause choking; holes that are too small may cause fatigue. After feeding, the unused portion of formula should be imme-

```
┌─────────────────────────────────────────────────────────────────────┐
│                                                                       │
│   Ward: 12A                                         Date: 9/4/71      │
│                                                                       │
│      Name: John Jones                                                 │
│                                                                       │
│      Formula: Evaporated milk 7 oz.                                   │
│                                                                       │
│             Water 14 oz.                      3 1/2 oz. × 6 feedings  │
│                                                                       │
│             Dextra-maltose 3 tbsp.                                    │
│                                                                       │
│      Hours:   10-2-6-10-2-6                                           │
│                                                                       │
│      No. of feedings: 6                                               │
│                                                                       │
│   Doctor: Brown                                    Nurse: J. Doe      │
│                                                                       │
└─────────────────────────────────────────────────────────────────────┘
```

FIGURE 13-1. Sample Formula Prescription for a Newborn   This file card should be filled out by the nurse and kept in the formula kitchen. All information on this card was prescribed by the doctor.

diately discarded. A rewarmed formula or a formula that has been left standing for a long time provides media for the growth of pathogenic organisms and should not be used.

III. Positioning and Feeding the Infant

The nurse washes her hands and dons a gown before feeding an infant to prevent cross-contamination. Note that the nurse's hand grasps the thigh area to insure safe positioning (see Fig. 13–2). The nurse observes the infant's tolerance and response to feedings.

1. Wrap the infant warmly and hold him in a slight Flower's position to aid in swallowing.

2. Place the entire nipple in the infant's mouth.

3. Formula must always fill the entire nipple area, or discomfort will occur due to the swallowing of air.

4. Place a quilted pad on your lap (under the infant's buttocks) to avoid soiling your uniform as a result of the gastrocolic reflex that is stimulated by feeding.

IV. Burping

Holding the infant in a sitting position to burp him will allow for observation of his responses.

1. Seat the infant upright on your lap with his head and body tilted slightly forward.

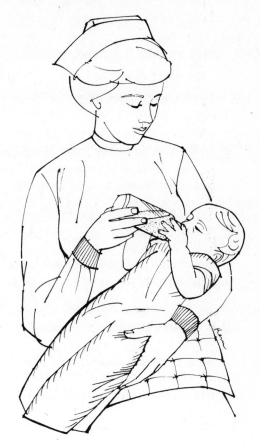

FIGURE 13–2.   Positioning and Feeding of an Infant.

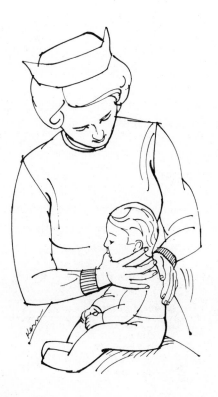

FIGURE 13–3.   Burping an Infant.

2. Support his head and chest by placing your fingers over the *mandible bone* of his face.

3. With your free hand, gently pat or massage his back until the infant burps.

V. Adjuvant Feedings

Adjuvant feedings may be prescribed by the doctor to supplement formula feedings.
1. Pablum and baby foods should be offered *before* the formula.
2. The cereal may be mixed with formula to obtain the desired consistency.
3. Cereal should always be fed with a *spoon,* not in a bottle.

VI. Junior Foods

Junior and chopped foods are usually offered at regular meal hours and are sent to the ward already prepared by the dietary department.

VII. Solid Foods

Solid foods are usually introduced into the diet at 2 1/2 to 3 1/2 months. Earlier feeding of solid foods is of little nutritional or psychological value.

Unless medically contraindicated, the usual pattern of introducing new foods to the infants is:

Cereal — 2 to 3 months of age
Fruits and vegetables — 2 to 3 months of age
Egg yolk — 4 months of age
Meat — 6 months of age
Potato — 9 months of age

VIII. Typical Dietary Pattern for a Six-Month-Old Infant

A six-month-old infant usually follows a dietary pattern such as:
Morning: Baby cereal, baby fruit, and formula.
Noon: Baby meat, baby vegetable, pudding, and formula.
Evening: Egg yolk, baby vegetable, baby fruit, and formula.
Bedtime: Formula.

Offering the young child adult-sized portions of food is not conducive to the development of good eating habits.

TABLE 13–1.   Amounts Eaten at One Meal at Various Ages

Food	Age 2 years	Age 4 years
Milk	1 cup	1 cup
Egg	3 tbsp	1/2 cup
Meat	3 tbsp	1/2 cup
Vegetable	1/4 cup	1/2 cup
Fruit	1/3 cup	2/3 cup

IX. Supplementary Fluids

In many hospitals, between-meal nourishment is a routine part of nursing care. The nurse may use Table 13–2 as a guide in selecting oral fluids that will best meet the needs of the individual child. For example, the child who loses body fluids or electrolytes from a draining meningocele or through diaphoresis in fibrocystic disease may require sodium-containing fluids, while a child who loses fluids and electrolytes in diarrhea or alkalosis may require a fluid rich in potassium. Oral fluids should be selected on the basis of therapeutic value, based upon a knowledge of the pathophysiology of the disease process. Clear water by mouth is not always the best fluid to offer a child and in some cases may be harmful. Offering clear water to a thirsty child contributes to a state known as "water intoxication" and may defeat the goal of hypertonic parenteral therapy.

The nurse should remember that the hospitalized child is ill, and many illnesses directly affect the fluid and electrolyte balance. Selection of supplementary fluids allowed in the diet should therefore be based upon dietary needs, water and electrolyte needs, taste appeal, and variety. Although the nurse cannot diagnose and prescribe for electrolyte needs, she can seek the doctor's guidance so that her selection of fluids for oral administration can be based upon sound principles rather than haphazard choice.

TABLE 13–2.   Electrolyte Values of Common Fluids*

Fluid	Calories per liter	Na.	(mEq./l.) K.	HCO_3.
Milk (whole)	670	22	36	30
Ginger ale	360	3.5	0.1	3.6
Coca-Cola	435	0.4	13	13.4
Pepsi-Cola	480	6.5	0.8	7.3
Orange juice (sweetened)	540	0.2	49	50
Grape juice	670	0.4	31	32
Tomato juice (canned, salted)	210	100	59	10
Lytren	280	50	20	34

*Adapted from Nelson, W.: *Textbook of Pediatrics*. 9th Edition, W. B. Saunders Co., Philadelphia, 1969, page 231.

X. Forced Feedings

Although professional dietitians are responsible for planning and preparing meals for pediatric hospital units, the nurse is often called upon to provide supplementary feedings or "forced feedings." "Forced feedings" should be considered a challenge to the nurse to use ingenuity and creativity in encouraging consumption of food. Too often the term "force feeding" or "force fluids" is interpreted as a physical contest between the nurse's efforts and the child's resistance.

The recipes listed in the following section contain ingredients commonly found in the kitchens of pediatric units, combined in a unique or different manner to provide an attractive, nourishing supplementary feeding for the toddler or older child.

XI. *Recipes for Supplementary Nourishing Feedings**

1. *Four-in-one milk shake*
   1 cup whole milk
   1 container strained fruit
   1 egg
   2–3 tbsp. cereal
   Combine ingredients, blend, and serve.
2. *Tomato-meat soup*
   3 1/2 tbsp. strained meat
   1 cup tomato juice
   1 tbsp. lemon juice
   Salt to taste
   Blend ingredients, beat, and serve.
3. *Cereal milk shake*
   1/4 cup cereal
   1 1/3 cups milk
   2 scoops ice cream
   Blend or beat, and serve.
4. *Ice-cream puff*
   1 container strained fruit
   1 egg
   1 scoop ice cream
   1/2 cup ginger ale
   Combine fruit, egg, and ice cream in a jar; cover and shake. Add ginger ale and serve.

These four examples of supplementary feedings may also be used to provide a child with cereal, meat, or broth that, in simple form, may be refused. Occasionally, an older child may require a baby-food diet because of injuries such as a fractured jaw, ruptured intestine, etc. Baby-food diets for older children may prove tiresome and repetitious, and the stimulation of appetite is a real nursing challenge. Often, with the doctor's consent, the nurse may modify the preparation of the baby-food diet and make mealtime more "grown-up" and pleasing. Daily personal touches and "surprises" can dress up a dull meal and make mealtime an occasion for happy anticipation for a convalescent child.

XII. *Special Diets*

Providing special diets for chronically ill children is a challenge. It is difficult to provide adequate nutrition and caloric intake to meet the growth needs of children who may be on a restricted diet, who may not have a good appetite, and who may have likes and dislikes to cope with. Consultations among doctors, nurses, nutritionists, and parents can often help in planning special diets to meet individual needs. As an example, a child with renal insufficiency must restrict intake of phosphorus. This may require restricting intake of milk and other proteins which are necessary for adequate

---

*Recipes are supplied by courtesy of Gerber Products Company.

nutrition. When a drug such as aluminum hydroxide gel is given *during* meals, it combines with phosphorus in the intestine, permitting a greater intake of a variety of foods. A palatable form of aluminum hydroxide gel may be obtained in the following recipe:

*Amphojel cookies:**

One cookie is equivalent to 2 tablets Amphojel.

1 cup salt-free butter

1 1/2 cups white sugar

1 1/2 cups cake flour

3/4 cup cornstarch

1 egg

3 tsp. vanilla

100 tablets (ground) Amphojel

Mix ingredients, drop batter well apart on ungreased cookie sheet, and press flat with floured fork. Bake at 350°F. until done. Yields 50 cookies.

Sample Recipe for a Bland Diet

Mock poached egg:

　　1 potato

　　Butter, milk, or cream

　　Salt

　　Strained carrots

Mash potatoes with butter, milk, or cream. Beat until fluffy and season with salt. Heat strained carrots seasoned with butter and serve in the center of a mound of mashed potato.

Sample Recipe for a Low Residue Diet

Aspic salad:

　　1 pkg. lemon gelatin

　　1 cup hot tomato juice

　　1 cup cold tomato juice

　　1 container strained mixed vegetables

　　1 tsp. salt

Dissolve gelatin and salt in hot tomato juice. Add cold tomato juice. Chill until thick. Fold in strained vegetables, pour into mold, and chill.

XIII.　The Elimination Diet

In an elimination diet, foods to which the child may be allergic are completely eliminated from the diet. Handling food or being exposed to the odor of food containing the suspected allergen is undesirable. When allergic symptoms subside, the doctor may order the addition of new foods, one at a time. If signs and symptoms of allergy occur, the specific food should be eliminated from the diet.

---

*Recipe from Vaughn, V. C., III, and McKay, R. J.: Nelson Textbook of Pediatrics. 10th Edition, W. B. Saunders Co., Philadelphia, 1975.

XIV. The P. K. U. Diet

The dietary restrictions for the child with phenylketonuria are designed to prevent an excessive accumulation of phenylalanine in the blood. The child on this diet requires close and frequent medical supervision over a long period of time. The diet is usually terminated by the time the child is 5 years of age and is replaced by a normal diet with close follow-up. Behavior problems have been associated with abrupt violation of the dietary regime, and permanent brain damage can result if the phenylalanine content of the diet is not restricted. Nearly every food in the average diet contains phenylalanine.

The challenge involved in the "P.K.U." diet revolves around the fact that, although an excess of phenylalanine will be harmful, a deficiency will also be harmful. Lofenalac, a Mead Johnson product used in "P.K.U." diets, is a synthetic commercial milk that may be served as a formula or a pudding. Lofenalac, although essential, is not the sole source of nutrition for the child. The diet may include:

1. Lofenalac (which may give a green color to the stool)
2. A small amount of natural foods of estimated phenylalanine content
3. Vitamins
4. Iron
5. Water
6. Sugar and fat (energy sources)

Phenylalanine-free foods include: water, refined sugar, pure starch, and pure oils.

During periods of illness and rapid growth, dietary adjustments are necessary. The phenylalanine blood level should not exceed 3 to 7 mg. per 100 cc. of serum.

XV. Diet in Renal Failure

Acute Renal Failure

Reduction of urine output requires fluid restriction to prevent overhydration and pulmonary edema. Therefore, adequate caloric intake is often a problem. Hyperalimentation (see p. 209) may be indicated to provide required nutritional needs. The usual restriction during acute renal failure is:

Protein 0.5 gm/kg./day
Sodium 12 mEq./M²/day
Potassium 25 mEq./M²/day or less
Fluid 600 ml./M²/day

Low protein electrolyte foods minimize catabolism and its resultant intercellular potassium, phosphate, and hydrogen ion buildup. Low solute formulas for oral feeding include Similac PM 60/40 (Ross) and SMA S-26 (Wyeth). Hycal (Beecham) and salt-free butter balls (General Mills) add calories when oral feeding is permitted.

Chronic Renal Failure

Protein may be restricted to 0.5 to 1.5 gm./kg./day only if renal insufficiency is evident. Eggs, meat, fish, cheese, and milk are considered quality protein sources. Intake should be designed to match the loss from the kidneys. Procedures such as dialysis result in protein losses that should be replaced. Carbohydrates taken within four hours of protein ingestion may prevent catabolism of protein and amino acids. Controlyte, Cal-power, and Hycal prepared in beverages, cookies, jelly, and popsicles provide high carbohydrate, low electrolyte calories.

Salt restriction is usually not prescribed unless severe hypertension and edema are clinically present. Routine restriction of salt in all renal patients can result in contraction of the extracellular fluid volume and can cause further reduction of renal function.

Fluid restriction is not routinely advised and is based upon results of intake and output, control of hypertension, and monitoring of electrolytes.

Vitamin supplements including folic acid are often advised. Diseased kidneys fail to convert vitamin D to the metabolite that aids in calcium absorption from the gastrointestinal tract. Therefore, parenteral vitamin D and oral calcium lactate or carbonate are also prescribed.

Aluminum hydroxide is often prescribed to bind dietary phosphate and decrease phosphate absorption, thus minimizing the need to eliminate milk from the diet.

XVI. Nutritional Content of Prepared Milks

The goal of all prepared milks is to simulate the nutritional properties of human milk and meet the individual needs of infants. A number of these products with their nutritional content are listed in Table 13–3.

TABLE 13–3. Nutritional Content of Prepared Milks*

Milk	*Dilution*	*Cal. per oz.*	*Protein* *gram*	*CHO.* *per*	*Fat* *100 ml.*	*Na.*	*K.* *mEq./L.*	*Ca.*
Alacta (Mead Johnson)	1:9	14	3.6	5.1	1.2	21.7	43.5	69.8
Bremil (Borden)	1:1	20	1.5	7.0	3.5	13	22	35
Carnalac (Carnation)	1:1	20	2.2	8.2	2.6	17.3	24.3	42.1
Cow's	—	20	3.3	4.8	3.5	25	35	62
Enfamil (Mead Johnson)	1:1	20	1.5	7.0	3.7	10.9	17.9	32.4
Evaporated	1:1	22	3.6	5.3	4.2	27	37	65
Human	—	20	1.1	6.8	4.5	6.5	14	16.5
Lactum (Mead)	1:1	20	2.7	7.8	2.8	17.4	28.1	50
Lofenalac (Mead Johnson)	1:7	20	2.2	8.5	2.7	26.1	34.1	48
Meat Base Formula (Gerber)	13:19	17.4	2.8	4.1	3.2	17	12	52
Modilac (Gerber)	1:1	20	2.1	7.6	2.6	17	21	42
Mull-Soy powder (Borden)	1:8	20	3.1	4.5	4.0	26	35	65
Nutramigen (Mead Johnson)	1:6	20	2.2	8.5	2.7	17.4	25.6	50
Olac (Mead Johnson)	1:1	20	3.4	7.5	2.7	21.7	40.9	59.8
Similac (Ross)	1:6	20	1.7	6.6	3.4	11.2	18.2	33.6
Similac PM 60/40 (Ross)	1:8	20	1.5	7.2	3.4	6.5	14.1	16.5
Skim milk	1:10	10	3.4	4.8	0.05	22	38	62
SMA S–26 (Wyeth)	1:1	20	1.5	7.2	3.6	6.5	14.1	21.5

*Adapted from Nelson, W.: *Textbook of Pediatrics*. 9th Edition, W.B. Saunders Co., Philadelphia, 1969, p. 154.

Note: Alacta and skim milk are examples of high protein, low fat formulas. Neo-Mull-Soy, MBF (Meat Base Formula), and Nutramigen are examples of hypoallergenic formulas. Lofenalac is an example of a low phenylalanine formula.

Feeding a high protein formula to prematures or newborns can cause tyrosinemia, which may have permanent deleterious effects on intellectual function, in particular, the area of visual perception, producing a minimally brain damaged (MBD) child with school learning problems. Therefore, high protein feedings should be used with extreme caution.

XVII.   Teaching Parents About Feeding Newborns and Infants

With the early discharge of the newborn from the hospital and the popular use of concentrated infant formulas there is an increased need to instruct the mother carefully prior to discharge from the hospital. Numerous types of formulas can be found on the supermarket shelves: some are in concentrated form, some are to be fed without dilution, and others are to be diluted with varied amounts of water. Since many of the containers look alike it is necessary to read carefully and understand the directions on the label in order to prevent fatalities that can result if the formula is improperly diluted or prepared. Such problems are especially prevalent in non-English speaking or poorly educated groups of mothers who fail to read and follow directions carefully. The nurse must watch for these problems and carefully interview the mother at each clinic visit to elicit detailed information regarding feeding practices.

Food selection should be based upon nutritional value. Limiting excessive caloric intake in the young will prevent obesity in later years. Commercially prepared soups and meat and vegetable combination baby foods are high in carbohydrates and are not the best protein sources. Home prepared soups do not have the best food value and many vitamins are lost by overcooking. Foods with artificial flavors and colors should be avoided as they are most often associated with allergies and behavior changes. Diets high in fats cause a delay in gastric emptying, resulting in distention and abdominal discomfort as well as excessive weight gain. Diets high in carbohydrate cause increased fermentation in the intestine causing distention, flatulence, and excessive weight gain. Good eating habits, including a balanced selection of food from the essential food groups, should be initiated early, as food habits are formed before 2 years of age.

Principles of Fostering Good Nutrition

1. Children will learn to eat and enjoy nutritious foods offered to them.
2. Children can learn to enjoy even an unpalatable taste if it is presented in a positive setting.
3. A sweet taste will cause a child to select that food over others presented.
4. Parents and television often teach a child what "tastes good" and they have a definite impact on developing eating habits.

XVIII.   Recommended Daily Dietary Allowances for Infants and Children

Eating habits are developed early in life. They are influenced by posture at the table, the emotional atmosphere during mealtime, the time allowed for meal consumption, and the preparation of the food. The nurse should consider these factors when teaching parents concerning the nutritional needs of their child. The child's appetite should be respected, and changing caloric needs based upon varying rates of growth at

TABLE 13–4. Food and Nutrition Board, National Academy of Sciences— National Research Council Recommended Daily Dietary Allowances,[a] Revised 1974

Designed for the maintenance of good nutrition of practically all healthy people in the U.S.A.

	Age (years)	Weight (kg)	Weight (lbs)	Height (cm)	Height (in)	Energy (kcal)[b]	Protein (g)	Vitamin A Activity (RE)[c]	Vitamin A Activity (IU)	Vitamin D (IU)	Vitamin E Activity[e] (IU)	Ascorbic Acid (mg)	Folacin[f] (µg)	Niacin (mg)	Riboflavin (mg)	Thiamin (mg)	Vitamin B6 (mg)	Vitamin B12 (µg)	Calcium (mg)	Phosphorus (mg)	Iodine (µg)	Iron (mg)	Magnesium (mg)	Zinc (mg)
Infants	0.0–0.5	6	14	60	24	kg × 117	kg × 2.2	420[d]	1,400	400	4	35	50	5	0.4	0.3	0.3	0.3	360	240	35	10	60	3
	0.5–1.0	9	20	71	28	kg × 108	kg × 2.0	400	2,000	400	5	35	50	8	0.6	0.5	0.4	0.3	540	400	45	15	70	5
Children	1–3	13	28	86	34	1,300	23	400	2,000	400	7	40	100	9	0.8	0.7	0.6	1.0	800	800	60	15	150	10
	4–6	20	44	110	44	1,800	30	500	2,500	400	9	40	200	12	1.1	0.9	0.9	1.5	800	800	80	10	200	10
	7–10	30	66	135	54	2,400	36	700	3,300	400	10	40	300	16	1.2	1.2	1.2	2.0	800	800	110	10	250	10
Males	11–14	44	97	158	63	2,800	44	1,000	5,000	400	12	45	400	18	1.5	1.4	1.6	3.0	1,200	1,200	130	18	350	15
	15–18	61	134	172	69	3,000	54	1,000	5,000	400	15	45	400	20	1.8	1.5	2.0	3.0	1,200	1,200	150	18	400	15
	19–22	67	147	172	69	3,000	54	1,000	5,000	400	15	45	400	20	1.8	1.5	2.0	3.0	800	800	140	10	350	15
	23–50	70	154	172	69	2,700	56	1,000	5,000		15	45	400	18	1.6	1.4	2.0	3.0	800	800	130	10	350	15
	51+	70	154	172	69	2,400	56	1,000	5,000		15	45	400	16	1.5	1.2	2.0	3.0	800	800	110	10	350	15
Females	11–14	44	97	155	62	2,400	44	800	4,000	400	12	45	400	16	1.3	1.2	1.6	3.0	1,200	1,200	115	18	300	15
	15–18	54	119	162	65	2,100	48	800	4,000	400	12	45	400	14	1.4	1.1	2.0	3.0	1,200	1,200	115	18	300	15
	19–22	58	128	162	65	2,100	46	800	4,000	400	12	45	400	14	1.4	1.1	2.0	3.0	800	800	100	18	300	15
	23–50	58	128	162	65	2,000	46	800	4,000		12	45	400	13	1.2	1.0	2.0	3.0	800	800	100	18	300	15
	51+	58	128	162	65	1,800	46	800	4,000		12	45	400	12	1.1	1.0	2.0	3.0	800	800	80	10	300	15
Pregnant						+300	+30	1,000	5,000	400	15	60	800	+2	+0.3	+0.3	2.5	4.0	1,200	1,200	125	18+[h]	450	20
Lactating						+500	+20	1,200	6,000	400	15	80	600	+4	+0.5	+0.3	2.5	4.0	1,200	1,200	150	18	450	25

[a] The allowances are intended to provide for individual variations among most normal persons as they live in the United States under usual environmental stresses. Diets should be based on a variety of common foods in order to provide other nutrients for which human requirements have been less well defined. See text for more detailed discussion of allowances and of nutrients not tabulated. See Table I (p. 6) for weights and heights by individual year of age.

[b] Kilojoules (kJ) = 4.2 × kcal.

[c] Retinol equivalents.

[d] Assumed to be all as retinol in milk during the first six months of life. All subsequent intakes are assumed to be half as retinol and half as β-carotene when calculated from international units. As retinol equivalents, three fourths are as retinol and one fourth as β-carotene.

[e] Total vitamin E activity, estimated to be 80 percent as α-tocopherol and 20 percent other tocopherols. See text for variation in allowances.

[f] The folacin allowances refer to dietary sources as determined by *Lactobacillus casei* assay. Pure forms of folacin may be effective in doses less than one fourth of the recommended dietary allowance.

[g] Although allowances are expressed as niacin, it is recognized that on the average 1 mg of niacin is derived from each 60 mg of dietary tryptophan.

[h] This increased requirement cannot be met by ordinary diets; therefore, the use of supplemental iron is recommended.

different age levels must be understood. The general dietary allowances recommended for growing children are as follows:

Milk — 1½ pints to 1 quart

Eggs — 1 daily

Meat — 1 serving daily (liver, one serving per week)

Vegetables — 1 serving daily of potato, green leafy, and others

Fruits — 1 serving daily

Bread — 1 slice at each meal

Cereal — 1 serving daily of whole grain or enriched cereal

Butter — 1 to 2 tbsp. daily

Desserts — as needed for calories

More specific daily dietary allowances are given in Table 13–4.

The recommendations in the table do not take into consideration economic status, social needs, religious custom, food availability, or specific needs of disease processes. The chart is designed as a *guide* to evaluating the diet. It should be noted that Canada, the United Kingdom, and other countries have different recommended dietary allowances as there is no current universal standard. This must be taken into consideration when working with people from other countries.

XIX.   Feeding Infants with a Cleft Palate

A fissure between the oral and nasal cavities, resulting from a failure of the maxillary and premaxillary processes to fuse, is known as a cleft palate. Aspiration of the fluid formula and the swallowing of air are the major feeding problems encountered with an infant who has a cleft palate. A vacuum in the mouth is necessary for successful sucking. The infant with a cleft palate is unable to suck because the fissure present in the upper palate prevents the formation of a vacuum in the mouth. Since a cleft palate is not usually repaired before two years of age, the nurse must initiate early parent teaching concerning the techniques of feeding. The nurse should be familiar with the cleft-palate nipple, dropper feeding, cup feeding, and gavage feeding.

Since adequate nutrition is essential for the infant, accurate evaluation of the infant's feeding capabilities is essential. The technique best suited to the individual child must be selected. The nurse must observe the infant for choking, cyanosis, and abdominal distention during feedings.

The infant must be held in an upright position in order to aid swallowing and prevent aspiration. Frequent burping is necessary because large amounts of air are usually swallowed with the formula.

Special cleft-palate nipples are available. The rubber flange on one side of the cleft-palate nipple is designed to fit over the fissure area, preventing aspiration and making it possible for a vacuum to be created in the mouth. The nipple may be placed on the formula bottle and sterilized in the conventional manner or separately wrapped, sterilized, and affixed to the standard formula bottle.

When a medicine dropper is used for feeding purposes, a rubber tip should be attached to the glass dropper in order to prevent trauma to the infant's gums. The rubber tip should be placed on top and to the side of the tongue. Fluid should flow from the dropper slowly and in small amounts. Allow enough time for swallowing before placing more formula in the infant's mouth.

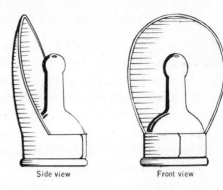

FIGURE 13–4. The Cleft-Palate Nipple The nipple is inserted in the infant's mouth with the rubber flange toward the upper palate. The flange should be cut to the size of the cleft in the palate.

Side view   Front view

Occasionally the doctor will order a thick formula. The principle involved in thick-formula feeding is flow via gravity to prevent aspiration through the fissure at the upper portion of the palate. Thick formulas are prepared by mixing a baby cereal (Pablum) with the milk and feeding through a regular nipple with a large hole. See the following section for the principles and techniques of gavage feedings.

XX. The Gavage Feeding

Ingesting food through a tube passed through the nares, pharynx, and esophagus into the stomach is known as a gavage feeding. When infants or children cannot be fed orally, a gavage tube feeding may be ordered by the doctor. The gavage tube may be passed via the oral or nasal route. Equipment necessary for gavage-tube insertion includes:

1. Small catheter or polyethylene gavage tube (silicone tubing is less irritating than rubber tubing)
2. A 30 cc. or 50 cc. syringe
3. A cup of water

Insertion of the Gavage Tube

The infant is placed in a mummy restraint (see p. 64) and his neck slightly hyperextended by placing a small towel or sheet roll under his shoulders. Using a number 5 to 12 Fr. catheter, measure the distance from the bridge of the nose to a point midway between the xiphoid process and the umbilicus. (This will allow the tip of the catheter to enter the stomach.) The catheter will be inserted to this preselected point. Stabilize the infant's head with one hand and gently pass the catheter through the nose. If the infant coughs, chokes, or becomes cyanotic, the catheter should be removed and reinserted.

After the tube is inserted it should be secured with adhesive tape to the face of the infant. The end of the tubing should be affixed above the level of the stomach to prevent seepage of stomach content through the tube. If a clamp is applied to the end of the gavage tube *between* feedings, air will not enter the stomach. If a clamp is *not* applied to the tubing *following* a feeding and vomiting occurs, aspiration is unlikely.

The tube may be left in place 3 to 7 days before replacement through the alternate nostril. In some cases the catheter may be inserted via the mouth and removed after each feeding.

Ways to Test Gavage-Tube Position

If the gavage tube is in the respiratory tract, drowning could occur as a result of tube feeding. The nurse must test the position of the gavage tube before *each* feeding. This may be done in one of the following three ways.

1. Attach a syringe to the gavage tube. The withdrawal of stomach contents assures that the tube is in the stomach.

2. Invert the gavage tube in a glass of water. If bubbles appear simultaneous with breathing, the tube is *not* in the stomach.

3. Place a stethoscope over the epigastric region. Insert 0.5 cc. of air through the gavage tube with a syringe. Listen for the sound of air as it enters the stomach.

Technique of Gavage Feeding

1. Obtain the formula.

2. Attach a syringe barrel to the tubing after checking the position of the tube.

3. Aspirate the contents of the stomach prior to feeding. (If any of the previous feeding is obtained it may be a signal to reduce the amount of feeding, and should be reported to the doctor.)

4. Pour a small amount of formula into the syringe barrel.

5. Raise the syringe barrel 6 to 8 inches above the mattress and allow the fluid to flow *slowly* with the aid of gravity. Force should not be necessary if the tube is in the correct position.

6. Just before the syringe is empty, pinch the tubing with the fingers (to prevent air from entering the stomach) and add formula to the syringe barrel.

7. Follow the feeding with a small amount of sterile water to cleanse the tubing.

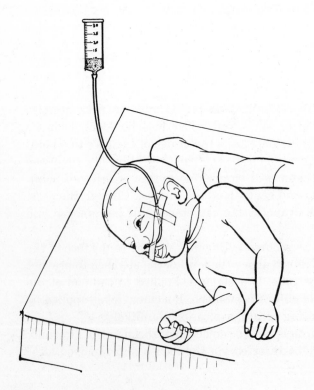

FIGURE 13–5. The Gavage Feeding The infant should be on his right side, propped with a blanket roll. Note the adhesive tape securing the gavage tube to the infant's face.

Note: Overfeeding will result in vomiting.

Charting should be descriptive and accurate and should include the time of feeding, the type of gavage, the amount given, and the amount retained. To remove the gavage tube, clamp it, remove the adhesive, and withdraw the tube quickly.

XXI.   Nasojejunal Feedings

A nasojejunal feeding, using a polyvinyl tube, may be prescribed instead of a traditional nasogastric or gavage feeding. In the nasojejunal feeding the tubing *bypasses the pylorus* of the stomach and enters the *jejunum.* This type of feeding reduces complications such as regurgitation, aspiration, and gastric distention in long-term tube feedings of infants.

In a nasojejunal feeding, a special, soft 24-inch vinyl tubing is used. This tubing is threaded into a 10 Fr. nasotracheal tube and introduced in the traditional manner into the stomach. The nasotracheal tube is then gently withdrawn over the feeding tube and the feeding tube is advanced through the pylorus. Oral insertion of the tube for jejunal feedings is not advisable because the oral stimulation results in increased salivation, air-swallowing, and regurgitation. The feeding technique is the same as in conventional gavage feedings. (See p. 100.)

Specific Nursing Responsibilities

1. The infant is kept on his right side with the hips slightly elevated for 4 hours after the tube is initially inserted. The infant may then be turned to his back or abdomen but should *not* be turned on his *left* side.

2. Feedings of low solute milk (usually SMA) are given frequently in small amounts. The infant should remain in a recumbent position during and following jejunal feedings to prevent symptoms of the "dumping syndrome."

3. The tube should be adequately rinsed with distilled water after each feeding to prevent blockage.

4. The nurse should check and record the rate of feeding, osmolarity, and the type and concentration of fluid given and should immediately report any signs of hypovolemic shock and diarrhea in the infant.

XXII.   Vomiting

Regurgitation or "spitting up" small amounts following feedings in the first 6 months of life is considered within normal limits. Regurgitation can be minimized by:

1. Burping during and after feedings.
2. Gentle handling and a happy environment during feedings.
3. Placing infant on right side for nap after feedings.
4. Being sure infant's head is not lower than its body after feedings.

Vomiting is the ejection of gastric contents through the mouth. In small children, vomitus usually comes through both the nose and the mouth. To prevent aspiration, the infant should be placed on his side and suctioned as necessary. The nurse must observe and accurately report and record:

1. The time of vomiting in relation to feeding.
2. The nature of vomiting (projectile or nonprojectile).
3. The type of vomitus.

A verbal complaint of nausea is seldom made by a child under five years of age. Nausea in infants may be evidenced by excessive salivation, restlessness, pallor, and a refusal to eat.

Evaluation of Types of Vomiting

The types of vomiting which the nurse should observe are:

Projectile.   An explosive emesis. The vomitus may travel 3 to 5 feet. This type of vomiting is usually indicative of pyloric stenosis or brain injury.

Nonprojectile.   A mild type of emesis, *accompanied by abdominal contractions.* This type of vomiting usually occurs with systemic disease processes.

Regurgitation.   A nonforceful expelling of food from the stomach *without* abdominal contractions. It is a form of "splitting up." This type of vomiting usually occurs as a result of overfeeding or improper burping.

Types of Vomitus

The nurse should observe the type of vomitus which may show the presence of:

Undigested food.   It may contain uncurdled milk. This type of vomitus may indicate atresia of the esophagus or G. I. tract obstruction.

Milk curds.   This type of vomitus usually indicates that the formula does not agree with the infant.

Bile.   Bile is present in the vomitus if the vomitus turns green upon exposure to the air. This is a nonpathological occurrence.

Fecal material.   This usually indicates bowel obstruction and is of a serious nature.

Blood.   Blood or blood streaks in the vomitus must always be reported immediately. The condition may be nonpathological in the newborn who has swallowed blood during delivery or in the child who vomits repeatedly. Coffee-ground vomitus may be indicative of internal bleeding and should be promptly reported.

XXIII.   The Use of Coffee in the Newborn Nursery

The newborn premature and term infant who is prone to apnea spells may benefit from small doses of coffee given regularly. Many hospitals use the following schedule:

Mix: 1 teaspoon coffee in 3 ounces of water. Give 2 to 3 cc. every other feeding P.O.

Preliminary reports show a significant decrease in apnea spells in infants fed the coffee mixture.

BIBLIOGRAPHY

Armstrong, I. L., and Browder, J. J.: *The Nursing Care of Children.* 3rd Edition, F. A. Davis Co., Philadelphia, 1970.

Andersen, C. F., Nelson, R. A., Margie, J. D., Johnson, W. J., and Hunt, J. C.: Nutritional Therapy for Adults in Renal Disease. *Journal of the American Medical Association, 223*:68, 1973.

Berenberg, W., Mandell, F., and Fellers, F.: Excessive Sodium Concentration From Skimmed Milk. *Modern Medicine,* Mar. 9, 1970, p. 137.

Chan, J. C.: Dietary Management of Renal Failure in Infants and Children. *Clinical Pediatrics,* Philadelphia, *12:*707, 1973.

Coodin, F., Gabrielson, I., and Addigo, J., Jr.: Formula Fatality. *Pediatrics, 47:*438, 1971.

Erhard, D.: A Starved Child of the New Vegetarians. *Nutrition Today, 8:*16:10, 1970.

Feingold, B. F.: Food Additives and Child Development, *Hospital Practice, 8:*11, 1973.

Gellis, S.: PKU Mental Development, Behavior and Termination of Low Phenylalanine Diet. *Yearbook of Pediatrics,* 1969, p. 44–46.

Harper, A. E.: Those Pesky Recommended Dietary Allowances. *Nutrition Today; 9:*2:1974.

Hill, L.: Infant Feeding, Historical and Current. *Pediatric Clinics of North America, 14:*255, 1967.

Kang, E., Solleen, N., and Gerald, P.: Results of Treatment and Termination of Diet in PKU. *Pediatrics, 46:*881, 1970.

Menkes, J., Welcher, D., Levi, H., Dallas, J., and Gretsky, N.: Relationship of Blood Tyrosine to Ultimate Intellectual Performance of Premature Infants. Paper presented at 13th International Congress of Pediatrics, Vienna, Austria, Sept., 1971.

Michaelsson, G., Petterson, L., and Juhlin, L.: Purpura Caused by Food and Drug Additivies. *Archives of Dermatology, 109:*49, 1974.

Noid, H. E., Schulze, T. W., and Winkelmann, R. K.: Diet for Patients with Salicylate Induced Urticaria. *Archives of Dermatology, 109:*866, 1974.

Rhea, J., and Kilby, J.: A Nasojejunal Tube for Infant Feeding. *Pediatrics, 46:*36, 1970.

Vaughn, V. C., III, and McKay, R. J.: *Nelson Textbook of Pediatrics.* 10th Edition, W. B. Saunders Co., Philadelphia, 1975.

Clues for Newborn in Breast Milk. *Medical World News 16:*21:1, 1975.

New Evidence Favors Breast Feeding. *Medical World News, 16:*3:26, 1975.

Proceedings of Annual Medical Symposium on Current Pediatric Therapy. Variety Children's Hospital, Miami, Florida, 1976.

PRODUCT REFERENCES

Gerber Products Co., Fremont, Michigan: "Recipes for Toddlers," and "Making Meals Appealing for Special Diets."

Davol Rubber Co., Providence, Rhode Island: Cleft-Palate Nipple.

Mead Johnson Laboratories, Evansville, Indiana: Lofenalac.

Chapter Fourteen

THE INTENSIVE CARE UNIT

CARE OF AN INFANT IN AN INCUBATOR

PRINCIPLES

NURSING RESPONSIBILITIES

I. General Use

The doctor prescribes the use of an incubator for each infant as needed. His order should indicate the amount of humidity desired, the liter flow of oxygen, and the oxygen concentration desired.

The nurse should observe and record the infant's responses to extrauterine life. (See Chapter 3.) The doctor should be notified if deviations such as cyanosis, retraction, grunting respiration, or subnormal temperature are observed.

The nurse may use her judgment in placing a newborn infant who weighs less than 5 pounds 8 ounces in an incubator until the doctor arrives.

The incubator is designed to provide optimal conditions of temperature, humidity, and oxygen for the infant's survival.

At least one vacant incubator should be kept ready for use at all times. An incubator should not be placed in direct sunlight or near a radiator.

Since the objective of applying external heat is to maintain the infant's temperature within the normal range, it is necessary to take his body temperature in

The nurse should take and record the body temperature of an infant in an incubator every hour until it is stabilized, and then every 4 hours. If the infant's

104

order to determine the amount of external heat required.

Abrupt changes in the incubator temperature can cause untoward metabolic responses in the newborn that can result in apnea.

When one is using an incubator that does not need to be opened during routine care, the atmospheric conditions within the incubator remain constant.

Exposing the chest facilitates effective observation for respiratory difficulties.

temperature is elevated or subnormal, the temperature dial of the incubator should be adjusted. The normal range of body temperature for a newborn infant is between 96° and 98° F. (35.4° and 36.3° C.), rather than an exact reading of 98.6° F. (37° C.).

Special gowns and masks are not necessary when caring for an infant in an incubator.

When one is using an incubator that provides stable atmospheric conditions during routine care, the infant need not be fully clothed.

II. Oxygen

Oxygen therapy is most effective when interruptions in the oxygen administration are kept to a minimum.

High oxygen concentrations are harmful to the newborn infant.

When the oxygen supply is not centrally located, the oxygen tank must be changed at intervals in order to insure continuous therapy. When the pressure gauge reading falls below 100 lb. the oxygen technician should be notified.

The oxygen concentration within the incubator should be checked every 4 hours (see p. 112).

III.   Weaning the Infant from the Incubator

The removal of an infant from an incubator should be a gradual process to avoid chilling due to the change from the incubator temperature to room temperature.

Dress and wrap the infant warmly and open all the incubator portholes. After the incubator gradually cools, the infant may be removed and placed in a regular bassinet.

IV.   Terminal Cleaning

Stagnant water harbors virulent pathogens. Thorough cleansing of the unit and removal of the water will prevent the spread of infection.

Alcohol, ether, or acetone will dissolve plastic.

When an infant is removed from an incubator, the unit should be thoroughly cleaned before reuse. All water should be removed from the reservoirs.

Alcohol, ether, or acetone should not be used to clean plastic parts.

TECHNIQUES

I. Recommendations Concerning Oxygen Administration

Oxygen may be administered to young infants in an incubator (see Chapter 16) and to older infants via Croupettes, masks, or endotracheal tubes. Regardless of the method used, the nurse should be aware of and be prepared to carry out the principles involved in oxygen administration.

The recommendations of authorities include:

1. Oxygen tension of arterial blood should not exceed 100 mm. Hg and should be maintained between 60 and 80 mm. Hg. The nurse should prepare for blood sampling and call the attention of the doctor to the lab results.

2. The concentration of inspired oxygen should be at a level necessary to maintain the proper arterial oxygen range.

3. Oxygen may be given in a concentration just high enough to abolish cyanosis. Immature infants must have regular blood gas sampling.

4. Radial or temporal arteries are the best site for blood sampling for oxygen arterial tension studies.

5. When an infant is placed in an oxygen enriched environment, the concentration of oxygen should be measured q. 2 h. with an oxygen analyzer. (See p. 112 for use of oxygen analyzers.)

6. Oxygen administered by endotracheal tubes, masks, funnels, hoods, or incubators should be warmed and humidified.

7. Immature infants who have received oxygen should return for periodic eye examinations.

II. The Isolette Infant Incubator

The Isolette is an example of an incubator that can control temperature, humidity, and oxygen concentration while providing a high degree of isolation through the slight positive pressure maintained by the air circulation system. The Servo-Control model shown in Figure 14–1 uses a patient probe to the abdominal skin as a guide in controlling the heater output of the unit.

Indicator lights (A). One of the two white lights on the control panel will light to indicate that power is on and the air circulation system is operating. If this light goes off, the plug and outlet should be checked, and the hospital electrician should be notified. The white Infant Servo-Control light (ISC) will remain on continuously when the Servo-Control is in operation. The heater light will go on when the heating unit is elevating the temperature of the incubator and will automatically go off when the desired temperature is reached. The "high temperature" alarm is a safety device that lights only if the incubator overheats.

Temperature indicator meter (B). Provides continuous readings of the infant's temperature when the probe is affixed to his skin.

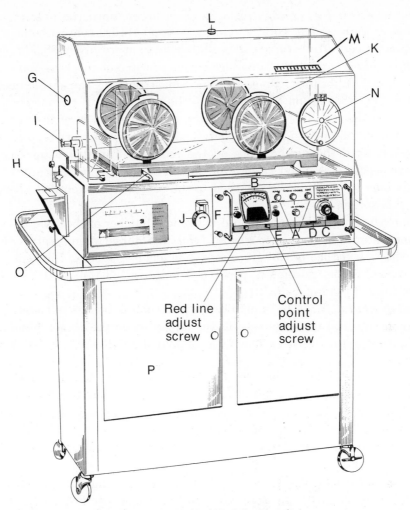

FIGURE 14-1.   The Isolette Infant Incubator.

Thermostat knob (C).   Turn thermostat knob fully clockwise until black arrow points to "ISC control." The white Servo-Control indicator light will remain on continuously. The unit will heat according to the reading of the *infant's skin temperature.* To obtain thermostat control of the *incubator air temperature,* turn this knob counterclockwise to the position that will maintain the incubator temperature at the desired level. The thermostat control indicator light will remain on when the knob is in this position. Refer to the thermometer on the hood of the incubator for an accurate reading of the temperature in the incubator.

Patient probe (D).   Insert the plug of the patient probe fully into this socket to ensure good electrical contact. Use a nonirritating opaque tape to secure the probe to the midline of the abdomen, halfway between the umbilicus and the xiphoid. Be sure the entire tip is covered by the tape.

Control point adjust button (E).   The temperature control point of the ISC unit is factory preset at 97° F. (36.1° C.). The temperature control point may be adjusted by pressing this control point adjust button and waiting until the meter stops. While the button is depressed turn the control point adjust screw (located on the underside of the panel) clockwise to raise, or counterclockwise to lower, until the needle stops at the desired temperature control point. (Usually, a temperature control point of 97° F. or 36.1° C. skin temperature is correlated with a body temperature of 98.5° F. or 36.9° C.).

Red line adjust button (F).   Provides a quick means of checking the temperature meter for proper calibration. Press red line adjust button. The meter needle should slowly swing up, stopping on the red line on the meter face. If the meter needle stops above or below the red line, keep the button depressed and turn the red line adjust screw (located on the underside of the control panel) clockwise to raise, or counterclockwise to lower, until the needle stops on the red line. Tap the meter face gently to stabilize the needle. The meter calibration should be checked periodically.

Oxygen inlet (G).   The tube attached to the source of oxygen flow should be connected at this oxygen inlet.

Ice chamber (H).   Ice may be placed in the ice chamber of the Isolette incubator to cool the incubator temperature to a point *below* the nursery temperature. Fill the ice chamber with cracked ice (about 10 pounds) and add one quart of cold water. Turn the humidity control to the "minimum" position. The ice will last about three hours. Check the temperature of the incubator frequently.

Humidity control (I).   The humidity control knob is on the left end of the hood. Push the knob in until the arm engages the projection on the sliding humidity control plate and turn it to the desired humidity level. High humidity aids in relieving respiratory difficulties.

Humidity chamber (J).   The humidity chamber should be filled with *sterile* distilled water at all times. The addition of 0.8 to 2.5 ml. of a 1:10,000 solution of silver nitrate or 2.5 g. of 99 per cent glacial acid per liter of water will help inhibit growth of microorganisms. The water should be drained and replenished daily to the level indicated by a black line. To drain the humidity reservoir, turn the fill pipe counterclockwise.

Portholes and plastic sleeves (K).   The complete handling and care of the infant is accomplished through any of the four entry portholes (see also Fig. 14–2).

Weighing facility (L).   The vent at the top portion of the plexiglass hood is used to facilitate weighing the infant while he is in the Isolette incubator (see also Fig. 14–3).

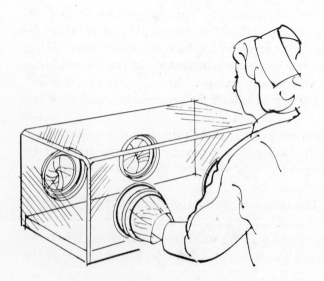

FIGURE 14–2. Placing the Hand Through the Porthole The porthole is opened by turning the metal ring that surrounds the plastic sleeve counterclockwise. After removing your hands, the portholes should be closed securely by turning the outer metal ring clockwise.

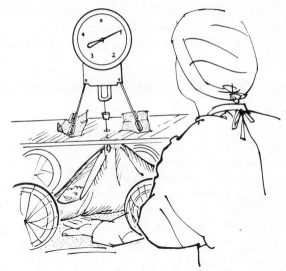

FIGURE 14-3. Weighing an Infant in an Incubator Place the scale on top of the incubator hood. (Note the paper barrier between the legs of the scale and the hood of the incubator.) Attach the hook to the scale and push the rubber stopper up so that the hook hangs free in the hole. Place the infant in the cloth sling and then place the metal rings of the sling on the hook that is attached to the scale. Read and record the weight.

Thermometer (M).   The thermometer inside the incubator accurately registers the temperature over the mattress area and is calibrated in Fahrenheit degrees. The optimum temperature of the incubator is that temperature which stabilizes the infant's body temperature within the normal range.

Plexiglass porthole (N).   The plexiglass porthole is a hinged plexiglass door through which contaminated linen and other articles may be removed from the incubator. The porthole is located at the foot of the incubator, enabling the nurse to adhere to the principles of microbiology involved in preventing contamination of clean areas.

Plastic bar (O).   Plastic bars, located at the head and at the foot of the incubator, are used to support the mattress in the Fowler or the Trendelenburg position. Hook the raised end of the mattress board over the plastic bar to achieve the desired position. For reasons of safety, the mattress *must* be flat when the plexiglass hood is lifted to open the incubator.

Storage cabinet (P).   The base of the incubator provides a storage area for individual linen and supplies. The weighing scale may also be stored in this space.

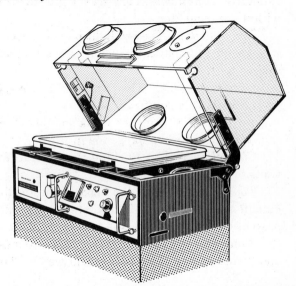

FIGURE 14-4. Opening the hood of the Incubator The Isolette incubator hood tilts open for increased access. The hood will lock open. A release lever on the outboard hinge disengages the lock for closing.

Note: 1. The microfilter pad of the air filter at the rear of the incubator should be changed every 3 months.

2. Alcohol should never be used to wipe the plexiglass hood.

III. The Ohio-Armstrong Incubator

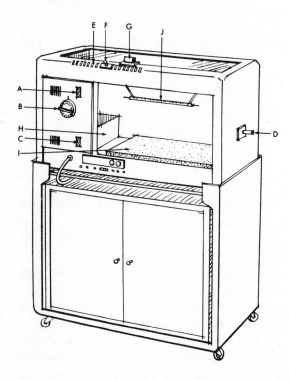

FIGURE 14–5.   The Ohio-Armstrong Incubator.

Green light (A).   The green light indicates that the unit is working. If the light goes off, check the plug and outlet and notify the hospital electrician.

Heater dial (B).   This dial controls the temperature within the incubator and is calibrated in numbers. Turning the dial to a higher number increases the temperature within the incubator.

Red light (C).   The red light indicates that the heater unit is functioning. The light will go off automatically when the temperature within the incubator reaches the desired level.

Oxygen inlet (D).   The tube from the oxygen source should be connected to the oxygen inlet at this point.

Air vents (E).   The air vents should remain open when oxygen is not in use and should be closed when oxygen is in use.

Control knob (F).   Pushing the knob to the left or right opens and closes the air vents.

Top hood (G).   The top hood of the incubator is opened for the routine care and handling of the infant. It is therefore desirable for an infant to be fully clothed to prevent chilling while in this type of incubator.

Water basket (H).   The water basket inside the incubator is the source of humidity and should be half-filled with warm water. The basket lifts out for cleaning and filling.

Mattress (I).   The mattress inside the incubator may be positioned in Fowler's or the Trendelenburg position by means of wooden blocks or sheet rolls placed under the mattress board.

Incubator thermometer and humidity indicator (J).   This instrument indicates the temperature and humidity within the incubator. It fits into a groove in the posterior wall of the incubator. Water to keep the humidity wick moistened is put in the container provided.

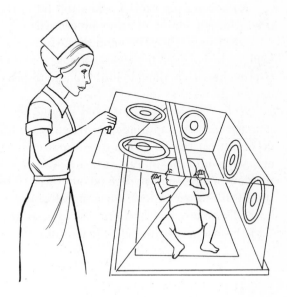

FIGURE 14–6.   Ohio Care-ette Incubator   This incubator opens by pulling on the handle between the portholes on the front of the unit. The mattress can then be pulled forward to gain complete access to the infant.

IV.   The Oxyhood

The Oxyhood is used to provide a chamber for controlled administration of high oxygen concentrations. It may be used on infants under a radiant warmer, or in a 40 per cent oxygen incubator when a concentration over 97 per cent is prescribed. When the head of the bassinet is elevated, a sling restraint may be used to prevent the infant from sliding down (see p. 69).

Inlet for I.V.'s (A).   The openings on each side of the hood are used to place I.V. tubing that is attached to a scalp vein.

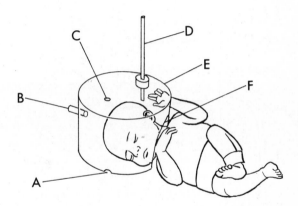

FIGURE 14–7.   Oxyhood.

Inlet for oxygen (B).   This is an oxygen inlet with a deflector to avoid direct blowing on the infant's head. The oxygen source is connected here.

Inlet for monitoring (C).   The probe from the oxygen analyzer is placed in this opening to monitor oxygen concentration within the hood. (See oxygen analyzer, below.)

Temperature monitor (D).   A thermometer mounted in a safety shield provides constant temperature monitoring within the hood. The temperature should be recorded on the chart with the vital signs of the infant.

Removable top lid (E).   The top lid is removable to provide complete access to the infant for suctioning or other procedures.

Open neck (F).   The open neck (in 6, 8, or 10 inch diameters to fit infants up to 18 pounds) is designed to fit close enough to retain oxygen concentration, but loose enough to prevent carbon dioxide buildup and to provide a safety factor in case of failure of the oxygen delivery system.

Note: The oxygen delivered should be warmed, or chilling will occur and further increase oxygen requirements. When humidified oxygen is delivered through a porthole, do not direct the flow onto the infant, or hypothermia can occur. Do not direct the flow of oxygen onto the analyzer sensor, or false readings can be obtained. In an oxygen hood, the flow of oxygen should be no less than 10 liters per minute for a large infant or no less than 6 liters per minute for a small infant to avoid carbon dioxide buildup within the hood. Therefore, a combination of oxygen and compressed air may be required to maintain the necessary liter flow per minute while avoiding high oxygen concentrations.

V. The Oxygen Analyzer

When using the oxygen analyzer, place a paper barrier on the incubator hood and place the oxygen analyzer on top of the barrier. Place the long tubing (A) inside the incubator through one of the open vents. Pump the bulb (B) 10 to 15 times; then press the button (C) and read the meter (D). The meter reading should not exceed the 40 per cent level. *Note:* The oxygen analyzer will not function properly in the presence of anesthesia gases.

The accuracy of the machine can be tested by performing this procedure in the environmental air and checking for approximately a 20 per cent reading.

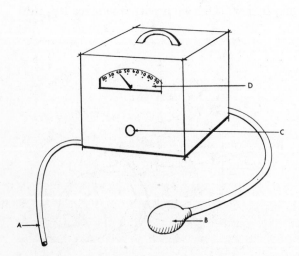

FIGURE 14–8.   The Oxygen Analyzer.

VI. Bathing the Infant in an Incubator

Daily skin care usually involves the use of clear water only, although a cleanser may be used for soiled areas such as the buttocks. Place the soft cloths and the paper cup with the bath water in the incubator, between the plastic hood and the mattress, and proceed to gently cleanse soiled areas of the skin.

Special attention should be given to the folds of the skin. Turn the infant on his abdomen to wash his back. Dry him thoroughly. Diaper the infant and place him on his side to allow the greatest amount of air to enter his lungs. The use of disposable plastic diapers should be avoided on infants in incubators or radiant warmers to promote safety and prevent heat rashes. A sheet roll may be used to prop the infant in position, and it should extend from the head to the buttock area. Soiled linen should be stripped from the mattress starting at the top and working toward the foot of the bed; it may be removed via the porthole at the foot of the incubator. Soiled articles should not be passed over a clean area or come in contact with the infant's face. Clean linen should be tucked well under the mattress to avoid occluding the open air vents.

Premature infants should be provided with tactile, visual, and auditory stimuli in order to humanize the unnatural environment of the incubator.

Studies have shown that the interiors of most incubators have high noise levels, which may affect the hearing of young infants, especially those receiving ototoxic drugs such as neomycin or kanamycin. Follow-up care concerning hearing development should be provided for all incubator babies. Studies have also shown that newborn infants will relax and sleep with environmental sounds similar to those in the uterus. Some nurseries provide records or tape recordings of heart and circulatory noises to conserve the energy of small infants by reducing crying time.

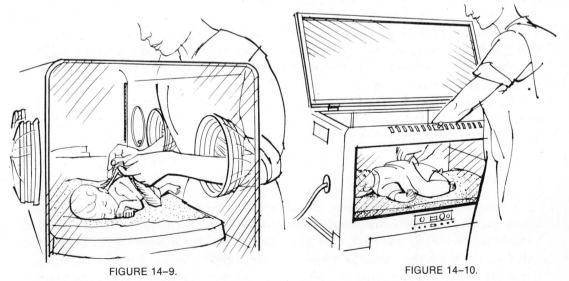

FIGURE 14–9.   FIGURE 14–10.

FIGURES 14–9 and 14–10. Caring for an Infant in an Incubator Portholes in the hood of an incubator facilitate bathing and routine infant care without disturbing the atmospheric conditions within the incubator (Fig. 14–9). Some incubators require opening of the top hood to facilitate routine infant care. Infants in this type of incubator should be fully clothed to prevent chilling (Fig. 14–10).

VII.   Feeding an Infant in an Incubator

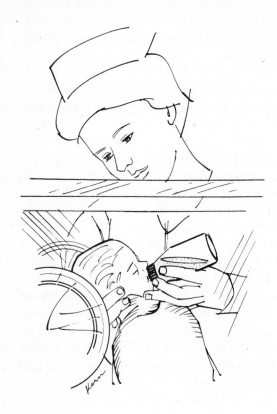

FIGURE 14–11.   Feeding an Infant in an Incubator.

The nurse lifts the child in an incubator into a semi-Fowler's position for feeding. Note that the level of milk in the bottle covers the nipple area to prevent ingestion of air. The mattress may be left slightly elevated after the infant has been fed and burped.

The incubator should always be turned so that the face of the infant is visible through the plastic hood. The position of the infant should be changed frequently. The nurse should record the temperature and humidity of the incubator and the responses of the infant on the chart.

When the infant is removed from the incubator for feedings, the Servo-Control should be placed at the "manual control" zone, or the incubator temperature will drop. The infant should be warmly wrapped when removed from the incubator.

Prewarming the Incubator

A thermal-neutral environment is one in which the infant's temperature is maintained at a level where the least oxygen consumption is required for metabolism (usually between 97.7° and 98.6° F. or 36.5° and 37° C.). For infants weighing less than 3 lb. 5 oz. (1500 g.), the incubator should be prewarmed to 94° to 97° F. (34° to 36.1° C.). For infants weighing more than 3 lb. 5 oz., the incubator should be prewarmed to 93° to 95° F. (33.9° to 35° C.).

After the infant is placed in the incubator, a correlation between incubator temperature and the infant's temperature may help to identify nonenvironmental causes of temperature instability. The skin temperature of an infant weighing less than 3 lb. 5 oz. should be maintained at 98° F. (36.6° C.). The skin temperature for an infant weighing more than 3 lb. 5 oz. should be maintained at 97° F. (36.1° C.). (The skin temperature is approximately one degree cooler than the rectal temperature.) The infant should be warmed gradually to prevent apnea.

PHOTOTHERAPY FOR HYPERBILIRUBINEMIA

Phototherapy changes indirect bilirubin into a water-soluble substance that can be eliminated by the kidney. This type of therapy, when used before bilirubin reaches toxic levels, often eliminates the need for exchange transfusions in the newborn.

PRINCIPLES

A high concentration of bilirubin in the blood of newborns can cause kernicterus and irreversible brain damage. Bilirubin can reach dangerous levels as a result of physiological jaundice in Rh positive premature infants as well as in Rh negative newborns who may have a hemolytic disorder.

The skin of the infant should be exposed to the light in order to gain maximum effect of phototherapy.

Delicate eye tissues can be injured by exposure to intense light.

Light therapy requires several hours to take effect. Light augments the clearance of bilirubin by altering the route of excretion. However, a very rapid rise of bilirubin that may occur in hemolytic disease may not be helped by phototherapy.

Any *cool,* bright, white or blue light can be used for phototherapy. A fluorescent light with a spectrum of 420–500 mu is ideal.

NURSING RESPONSIBILITIES

All newborn infants should be checked for signs of increasing bilirubin levels, such as jaundice. Reports of blood levels of bilirubin exceeding 10 mg. per 100 ml. should be reported to the doctor immediately.

All clothing should be removed and the infant placed in an incubator during treatment. The infant should be turned frequently to expose different areas of the body to the light.

It is essential that eyes be protected by means of sterile eye patches worn at all times when exposed to phototherapy.

Close observation of jaundice levels and blood reports of bilirubin and hemoglobin should be maintained. The nurse should be aware that light bleaches the skin, removing external signs of jaundice before systemic effects are achieved.

Two or three days of exposure may be required for maximum effect. Proper insertion of bulbs and safety precautions to prevent injury by burns or bulb breakage are essential.

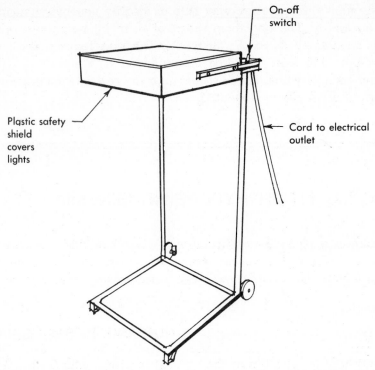

On-off
switch

Plastic safety
shield
covers
lights

Cord to electrical
outlet

FIGURE 14–12. A Bilirubin Reduction Lamp   This single unit lamp fits over any type of incubator and affords easy access to the infant.

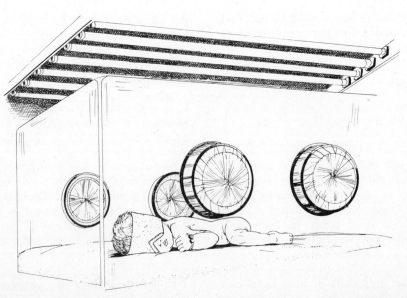

FIGURE 14–13. Phototherapy for Hyperbilirubinemia   Note that the infant receiving light therapy is completely naked in the incubator to provide maximum skin exposure. Sterile eye patches prevent eye injury from the light. The infant is turned frequently to expose different areas of the skin. The lamp does not significantly increase the incubator temperature.

Nursing Care of Infant Receiving Phototherapy

1. Remove clothing to maintain proper skin exposure.
2. Turn infant frequently to expose all skin areas.
3. Record and report jaundice and reports of blood levels of bilirubin.
4. Record and report changes in body temperature.
5. Check and maintain eye patches in place to prevent eye injury from the intense light. Be sure the eyes are closed before applying the eye patch, to prevent corneal irritation. The eye patch should be loose enough to avoid excessive pressure, but firm enough to prevent eyes from opening. Eye patches should be changed every 8 hours and eye care given.
6. The nurse should expect the infant's stools to be green and loose and the urine dark, because of photodegradation products.
7. Serum bilirubin and hematocrit should be monitored during therapy and for 24 hours following therapy.
8. Mother should not breast feed infant, as hormones keep bilirubin level high.

Common Side Effects of Phototherapy

1. *Loose, greenish stools* caused by the photodegradation products. The frequency of stools is not increased, nor is a water loss excessive.
2. *Transient skin rash* similar to flea bite dermatitis can occur and is self-limiting. No treatment is advocated, and no adverse effects have been noted.
3. *Bronze discoloration of the skin* occurs in infants with liver disease and elevated direct-reacting bilirubin levels.
4. *Late anemia* may occur in infants with Coombs' positive red blood cells who receive phototherapy and who have not had exchange transfusions. Follow-up care and checks should be arranged to detect this occurrence.
5. *Hyperpigmentation* can occur in black infants because of reoxidation of preformed melanin. This coloring will fade gradually over a period of months after phototherapy ceases.

RADIANT WARMER

Maintaining the body temperature in the newborn plays an essential role in influencing oxygen consumption, apnea, and acid-base balance. Although an incubator is the best means of assisting the newborn to maintain optimum body temperature, there are occasions when the newborn needs to be more accessible for procedures such as an exchange transfusion, minor surgical procedures, resuscitation, and burn therapy. A radiant warmer may be required in the delivery room, the nursery, or the intensive care unit to enable such procedures to be carried out without heat loss in the infant.

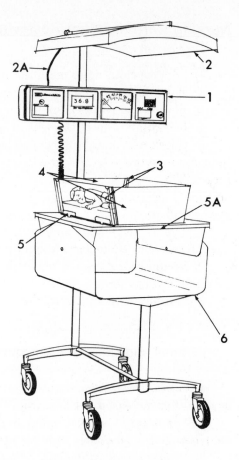

FIGURE 14–14. The IMI Infant Care Center This radiant warmer employs a 22 × 35 inch radiant panel providing infrared energy to produce penetrating as well as surface heat. The thermometer probe should be attached to the infant with the shiny side of the disc in direct contact with the skin.

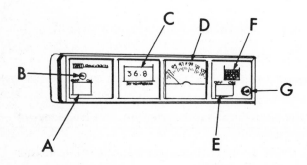

Control Panel

Off-on switch (A).   Turns power on or off.

Power light (B).   Amber light illuminated when power is on. If light is out, check plug or call electrician to check unit.

Set temperature (C).   When thermistor is in place, radiant energy is maintained at a level which will heat the child to desired control temperature.

Temperature (D).   Displays temperature of infant as measured by the thermistor probe.

Audio off-on (E).   Turns audible alarm on or off.

Audible alarm speaker (F).   Emits audible alarm when temperature measured by thermistor falls below 34° C. (93.2° F.) or exceeds 38° C. (100.4° F.). If alarm sounds, check connection of thermometer probe to infant before resetting.

Visible alarm light (G).   Red light flashes when temperature measured by thermistor falls below 34° C. or exceeds 38° C. If light flashes, check position of thermistor probe attached to infant and adjust heat control as necessary.

Hood

The hood (2) contains the radiant heat panel. To raise or lower the hood, loosen the adjusting knob at the rear of the hood and apply pressure to place hood at desired level.

The radiant heat panel will automatically turn on and off to maintain the infant's temperature as desired by temperature control and thermistor attached to infant. *Caution:* Do not allow hood to come within 5 inches of the control panel.

Power cord (2a).   Cord connects hood to (L) on rear of control panel.

Retaining clips (3).   These clips hold the glass sides of the bassinette in place. Raise these clips and the side will swing down to lie flush with the procedure table to allow easy access to baby. The sides can then be removed if desired by keeping a firm upward pressure with fingers and pulling gently on the glass.

Head and foot panels (4).   The head and foot panels may be lowered or removed by pulling the tab on the slide fastener on each end until a disengaging click is heard.

Bassinette procedure table (5).   The bassinette may be placed in varying levels of Fowler or Trendelenburg position by squeezing the handle under the table top. (See 5a.)

Squeeze handle (5a).   Squeeze to adjust table to Trendelenburg or Fowler position.

Storage area (6).   Linens and equipment necessary for the individual care of the infant may be stored here.

Rear of Control Panel

Power cord (H).   Connect to 120 volt AC outlet.

Control reset: Circuit breaker (I).   Depress button to restart after temporary power failure. If power is not restored, call electrician.

Element reset: Circuit breaker (J).   Depress button to restore heating panel power after temporary failure. If power is not restored, call electrician.

Thermistor connection (K).   The thermistor which measures the child's temperature and controls the radiant output of the warmer is connected here. The shiny side of the disc should be attached securely to the infant's skin.

Radiant heat panel connection (L).   (The controller output to the radiant heat panel.) The power cord from the hood is plugged in at this point.

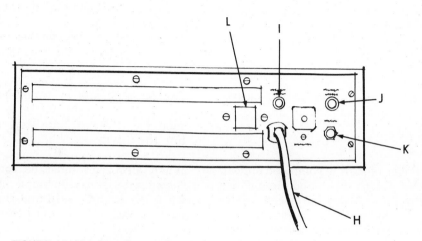

FIGURE 14-15.   Rear Control Panel of Radiant Warmer Shown in Figure 14-14.

Nursing Responsibilities in Using a Radiant Warmer

1. Do not use a rectal temperature probe, as the skin can burn before internal temperature reaches normal.

2. Secure the probe to the skin surface that faces the heater. Reposition the probe whenever the infant is turned. Never place a probe *under* the infant.

3. Place the probe over the liver area when possible for most accurate temperature reading.

4. Record the temperature and check the probe attachment every 30 minutes.

5. Do not interchange probes from different makes of machines.

6. Radiant warmers cause more insensible water loss than incubators. Check for signs of dehydration.

7. Change eye pads every 8 hours and check blinking reflex to avoid excessive drying of the eyes.

APNEA ALARM MACHINES

PRINCIPLES

A newborn sustaining an apneic period of 30 seconds or less can be stimulated to breathe again with little effort. A longer apneic time causes more difficult resuscitation.

The apnea machine is sensitive to respiratory movements of the infant and will sound an audible and visible alarm when respirations cease for a preselected period of time.

Premature babies need to be closely watched for apnea to prevent brain damage and death.

The top layer of skin is composed of dead skin cells, skin oils, and impurities which insulate passage of electrical signals to electrodes. These layers must be removed to permit proper contact of electrodes.

NURSING RESPONSIBILITIES

Some type of apnea alarm should be used for infants when there is a high risk of apnea attacks. Some indications for use include premature infants, cesarean section newborns, infants born of traumatic deliveries, postoperative periods, or during any procedure requiring extensive draping.

Care should be taken to preserve effective functioning of the apnea alarm by:
1. Insuring proper and secure attachment of all leads to the infant and to the machine.
2. Insuring proper maintenance of the machine by an electrician at regular intervals.

The nurse should immediately check to see why the apnea alarm sounded and should take appropriate steps to resuscitate the infant.

When electrodes must be connected to the infant's skin, the nurse should first wash the infant's skin and then wipe it with alcohol or a prepared cleaner swab.

Apnea Alarm Mattress

Air mattress (A).   Remove the plug from the spare tube and inflate the mattress to 4 mm. Hg using a sphygmomanometer. Insert the plug. Do not overinflate. The mattress should be inflated sufficiently to support the baby comfortably and clear the bottom of the incubator. Too much air will reduce sensitivity of the mattress and may damage the mattress. The mattress may be placed in an incubator with the lead protruding from a slot in the incubator or through a porthole. Be sure tubes are not kinked. A thin sterile sheet or diaper may be used to cover the mattress if desired. The mattress and manifold may be cleaned with a mild disinfectant daily.

Thermistor sensor (B).   One end is connected to the manifold and the other plugged into the "detector" outlet of the machine.

Delay switch (C).   Set delay switch to 10 seconds. This switch will emit short click sounds in response to the infant's movements, verifying that the machine is operating correctly.

Loud-soft alarm (D).   After setting delay time to 10, 15, or 20 seconds, set "loud-soft switch" to LOUD position. (After 10 seconds, alarm should sound if mattress is undisturbed. This is the method of *testing* the alarm prior to use.)

Sensitivity control (E).   First set this control to MAXIMUM and test-check alarm as described in (D). Then operate all electrical appliances near crib or incubator and decrease sensitivity control until alarm is not affected by appliances. Record the sensitivity level to be maintained. Use the minimum sensitivity setting that allows proper functioning.

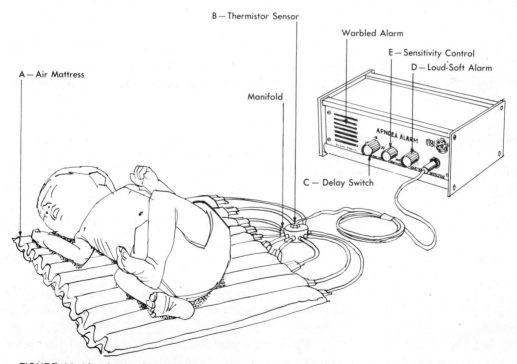

FIGURE 14–16. **Apnea Alarm Mattress** This apnea monitor requires no direct connection to the baby. The baby lies on the air mattress which can be placed in the bassinette or incubator, and the displacement of air caused by respiratory movements is detected by the machine. The alarm sounds when respiratory movements cease for a preselected period of time.

Nursing Care of Infant on an Apnea Alarm Machine

1. Use only a thin diaper to cover infant to prevent any cushioning of respiratory movements. A sterile sheet or diaper may be used over the mattress. Be sure diaper does not extend above waist level.

2. Check:
   a. *Position of baby:* Baby must lie *lengthwise* on mattress for proper functioning of machine.
   b. *Mattress inflation:* An overinflated or deflated mattress will cause the alarm to sound.
   c. *Connection of electrical leads:* All leads must be secure to insure effective functioning of machine.

3. Test machine daily by removing infant from mattress for 10 seconds while machine is on. The alarm should sound.

4. Request the electrician to check the batteries every 2 months.

INFALARM (RESPIRATORY AND HEART RATE MONITOR)

Power light (1).   Light is on when machine is working.

Off-on-test switch (2).   Turns power on or off. In "test" position it will activate aural alarm to test operational status and battery charge. If battery is fully charged the meter indicator will move to the green colored zone labeled "test" (6).

High heart rate selector (3).   The selector sets the higher limit of the heart rate desired. If infant's heart rate exceeds this level the alarm will sound.

High heart rate alarm (4).   Light flashes when infant's heart rate exceeds level selected by (3).

Heart rate indicator (5).   This displays the average heart rate of infant in beats per minute.

Meter test zone (6) (Green zone).   Meter indicator will come to this zone if battery is fully charged when switch is in "test" position (see 2).

Low heart rate alarm (7).   The light flashes when the infant's heart rate falls below the preset limit.

Low heart rate selector (8).   Set this knob to minimum heart rate allowable for individual infant.

Apnea alarm indicator (9).   The light flashes when respiratory rate ceases for preselected period of time.

Respiratory rate indicator (10).   This indicates the average respiratory rate of the individual infant. This rate may not be accurate in infants with irregular breathing patterns.

Impedance meter scale (11).   When impedance switch (14) is pressed the impedance will increase if electrode contact with the infant's skin is inadequate. A reading in the red area indicates alarm will not be effectively activated. The electrodes should be re-applied. Readings of 0–1K indicate electrode contact with infant is good.

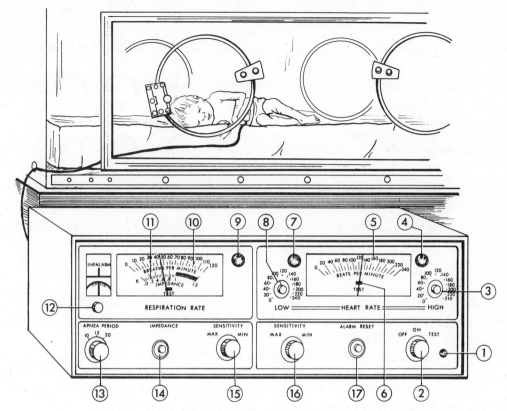

FIGURE 14–17. **Infalarm** This infalarm monitors respiratory and heart rate through two electrodes placed on the infant's skin. Both visual and audible alarms are activated if the heart rate exceeds or drops below pre-selected levels or if respirations cease for a preselected period of time.

Visual breathing indicator (12).   The yellow light flashes with each inspiratory phase of respiration.

Apnea period switch (13).   The apnea period switch selects length of time that will elapse from the time the baby stops breathing to the time the alarm will sound.

Impedance switch (14).   (See 11.) The impedance switch is used to see if the machine is functioning properly. Impedance readings should be taken and recorded at least once each shift.

Respiratory sensitivity (15).   Select minimum or maximum detection of levels of air intake by infant. Rotate knob clockwise while observing the visual breathing indicator until light flashes synchronously with infant's respiration. Always use minimum sensitivity required.

Heart rate sensitivity (16).   Detects minimum to maximum heart signals. Rotate clockwise while listening for QRS beep. Advance slightly after hearing beep. Always use minimum required sensitivity.

Alarm reset (17).   Press this button to reset machine after alarm has been set off. (Alarm may sound during adjustment of machine to desired heart-respiratory rates. Press this button to cancel and reset alarm.)

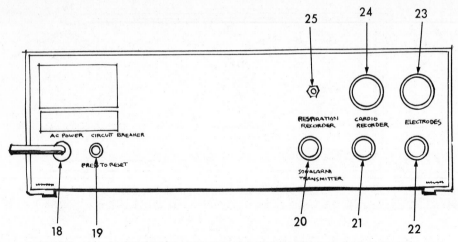

FIGURE 14–18.   Rear Panel of Infalarm.

Rear Panel

AC power cord (18).   Plug into standard 120 volt outlet.

Circuit breaker (19).   Press to return power to unit after momentary power failure.

Respiration recorder (20).   Outlet provides records of respiration and apnea or displays rate on oscilloscope when connected to optional equipment.

Cardio-recorder (21).   Provides records of heart rate and ECG or displays rate on oscilloscope when such optional equipment is used.

Electrode receptacle (22).   The electrode cable plugs into this receptacle.

Audible alarm speaker (23).   Produces audible tone when dual alarms are activated.

Heart rate indicator (24).   Emits a beep each time a QRS complex is detected in heart rate.

QRS on-off (25).   Turns QRS audio on or off.

Application of Electrodes

Cleanse skin thoroughly to remove skin oils and impurities. Remove an adhesive washer from the strip, exposing one adhesive side (Fig. 14–19 *A*). Center the washer over the electrode cavity and press firmly together.

Fill the electrode cavity completely with electrode jelly, so the gel surface extends slightly above the electrode (Fig. 14–19 *B*).

Remove the remaining paper cover and firmly press and smooth out the exposed edges of the adhesive washer to the skin (Fig. 14–19 *C*). (Do *not* press on the back of the electrode as this will result in the gel being forced out of the cavity causing poor electrical contact.)

The electrodes may be placed just below or to the side of the nipples, one on each side, or one electrode over the fifth or sixth rib at the midline and the other high up on the left side of the chest. Nursing responsibilities include checking the impedance once each shift. If higher than 1K, remove, clean, and reapply electrode. This machine should *not* be used when a defibrillator is being used on the infant.

When using intradermal electrodes:

1. Use steam autoclaved needles; cleanse sites with Betadine.
2. Insert in area of low muscle activity:
   Under clavicle
   Under lower sternum
3. The points of all the needles should face in the same direction.
4. Place cotton under the hub of the needle and tape with micropore tape.
5. Change electrodes every 3 days.

When using standard topical electrodes:

1. Cleanse sites with Betadine.
2. Apply self-stick electrodes to leads.
3. Place negative electrode under right clavicle or right arm.
4. Place positive electrode under lower sternum or left arm.
5. Place ground electrode under left clavicle, or on leg or abdomen.
6. Replace and reposition electrodes every 3 days or as needed if loosened.

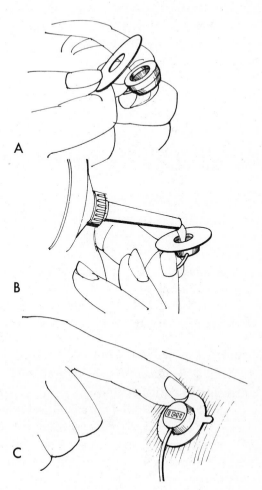

FIGURE 14–19. Application of Electrodes of Infalarm.

THE INFANT SENTRY APNEA ALARM

This apnea monitor does not require attachment of wires to the infant. A small magnet transensor is taped to the infant's stomach, a pickup antenna is placed under the infant, and the receiver alarm is set up by the crib.

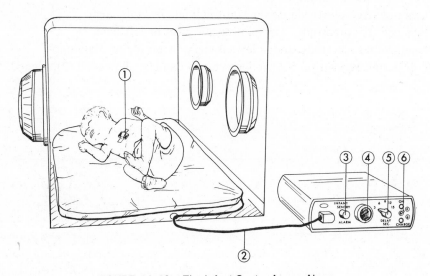

FIGURE 14–20.   The Infant Sentry Apnea Alarm.

Transensor (1).   This is taped to the infant near the diaphram so that normal respirations will provide the movement required for monitoring.

Antenna (2).   The antenna pad is placed under the bassinette or incubator mattress and the wire firmly attached to the "antenna" outlet on the machine.

Visual alarm (3).   This visual alarm indicator will light when respirations cease for a preselected period of time. A blinking light indicates normal respiratory movements.

Audible alarm (4).   A high-pitched alarm will sound when respirations cease for a preselected period of time.

Delay timer (5).   This switch sets the delay (apnea) time in seconds. If respirations cease for a period of time exceeding the delay time selected, the alarm will sound.

Power switch (6).   This switch should remain in the "on" position when the Infant Sentry Monitor is in use. It may be left in the "charge" position when the machine is not in use.

TRANSCUTANEOUS MONITORING OF BLOOD OXYGEN TENSION LEVELS

An electrode has been developed to monitor the blood oxygen tension levels via the skin in neonates, children, and adults. Use of this electrode will make frequent blood sampling for oxygen tension levels unnecessary. Such noninvasive measures for continuously monitoring vital functions in the critically ill child are valuable aids in determining care and prognosis.

At present, a disposable in-dwelling catheter electrode is being used to monitor arterial PO_2 continuously for up to 3 days. However, later development of the "Marburg" electrode and one modified by Hutch enables a continuous noninvasive *transcutaneous* monitoring of arterial PO_2 levels, making frequent blood sampling unnecessary. Careful PO_2 monitoring is essential with any infant or child receiving any type of inhalation therapy.

NURSING CARE OF INFANTS WITH TRANSCUTANEOUS ELECTRODES

1. *Placement of electrodes:* A drop of water is first put on the skin; the electrode is placed on top of it and is held in place by an adhesive electrode ring. The heated electrode may be placed on the infant's sternum, or on the back a few centimeters lateral to the spine if the infant is in the prone position. In adolescents, the electrode may be placed on a shaven area of the forearm. The area selected should have minimal subcutaneous fat to enhance accuracy of function.

2. Calibration:

A. When used on one infant for a long period of time, the electrode should be removed, recalibrated in a water bath, and replaced at the same site, every 3 hours.

B. When one electrode is used to take consecutive readings on several infants in an intensive care unit, recalibration immediately before application to each infant is essential.

3. Local hyperthermia directly under the electrode can cause redness of the skin. The nurse should be alert to the development of blisters and should record and report her findings. Overheating of the electrode surface (above 113° F. or 45° C.) should be avoided. Alarm systems to prevent this problem may be available with some electrodes.

4. Check for proper contact between electrode and skin to maintain accurate readings.

5. A blood pressure cuff should not be applied to the same arm to which a transcutaneous electrode is attached.

6. Infants less than 3 days old usually have a marked reduction of transcutaneous PO_2 levels during vigorous crying. More accurate PO_2 levels are obtained when the infant is at rest. The rate of $tcPO_2$ decrease during total apnea is about 30 mm. Hg per minute. A sudden significant drop in transcutaneous PO_2 levels should alert the nurse to an imminent need for resuscitative measures.

7. Record arterial PO_2 levels on the chart of the infant every half hour or as ordered by the doctor, and report findings that deviate from normal or reveal a sudden change in the status of the infant.

NURSING CARE OF A CHILD WHO IS ON A LIFE-SUSTAINING DEVICE

Many patients react to modern life-sustaining devices by means of denial, isolation, avoidance, or terror, even when a detailed explanation of each machine is offered to them. The more independent personality will usually fear the dependence forced by the intricate machine. Suspicious and distrustful personalities may fear machine failure. Children who have basic trust and confidence in others usually adapt easily.

The nursing approach should be geared to meet the individual responses. Often, nurses are so busy checking and tending to the machine they forget to communicate with the patient who is attached to the machine. A simple but essential requisite in the nursing care of a child on a life-sustaining device is to initiate communication appropriate for the patient's age level. Perhaps just touching him gently with the hand, or calling to him by name, or offering frequent explanations of his environment may be helpful. It is equally important to look and listen for individual responses to the immobilization, the dependence, and the effects of the general environment. The nursing care approach should be based upon the individual responses noted.

PREVENTING ELECTRICAL HAZARDS

The electric and electronic equipment in an intensive care unit can create a hazardous environment. Therefore, special precautions are essential to provide and maintain basic safety standards. For example, if an electrical ventilator being used on a tracheotomy patient is not properly grounded, an electrical charge can build up on the patient's body via the wet tubing and tracheotomy tube and can, if associated with cardiac or respiratory monitors, cause fatal electrocution of the patient. A nurse, touching the metal part of an electric bed can cause a lethal leakage of current to the patient who is on a cardiac monitor.

Essential aspects of a safe electrical environment include:

1. All equipment must be properly grounded.

2. Long-line cords should not be used. (They usually produce leakage of current.)

3. A cheater-adaptor (3- to 2-prong) should never be used to connect a 3-prong plug to a 2-hole wall outlet.

4. All lamps and portable electric equipment should have the metal grounded through a 3-wire cord.

5. Extension cords or multiple outlet plugs should never be used.

6. The hospital electrician should check groundings and outlets of all electrical equipment on a regular basis.

HEELSTICK FOR HYPOGLYCEMIA

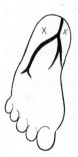

FIGURE 14–21.   The X's show the sites for heelstick (to obtain capillary blood) in relation to the lateral and medial plantar artery.

1. Swab skin with antiseptic.
2. Quickly pierce skin at appropriate site (see Figure 14–21) with lancet.
3. Place drop of blood on reactive tip of Dextrostix. Leave for one minute.
4. Place bandage on heelstick site.
5. After 1 minute, rinse Dextrostix with water and read, using color code on Dextrostix bottle.
6. Report values less than 45 mg. per 100 ml.

NURSING RESPONSIBILITIES IN THE CARE OF ARTERIAL CATHETERS

1. Keep a Kelly clamp in a conspicuous place (tape inside Isolette).
2. Place a conspicuous sign "I.V. via arterial catheter" at infant's unit to alert personnel.
3. Use IVAC (see p. 200) for infusion rate control.
4. Have heparin on hand.
5. Observe:
    A. For clots in tubing.
    B. Color of legs. Blanching, mottling, cyanosis, or coolness should be reported immediately.
6. When changing stopcock q8h, or if contaminated, clamp arterial catheter with a Kelly clamp first.
7. Secure stopcock to tongueblade using plastic tape, and check for secure connections. Infant can hemorrhage from a loosened connection.
8. Do not place infant on abdomen or cover stopcock with diaper or sheet.

AVOIDING COMPLICATIONS OF GENERAL INTENSIVE CARE

COMPLICATION	NURSING RESPONSIBILITIES
Intubation	
Ulceration of nares due to pressure of tube; narrowing of nostril due to tissue damage and scarring.	Only polyvinyl tubes that do not contain tin (which is toxic to cells) should be used.
Irritation of vocal cords; persistent hoarseness; stridor; edema of larynx.	The use of an endotracheal tube of the smallest practicable size will reduce local tissue ischemia. Frequent changes of the tube should be avoided and movement of the tube in the site should be avoided. Suctioning should not be too vigorous. Maintaining aseptic technique is essential.
Umbilical Catheterization	
Arteriospasm is a frequent complication of umbilical catheterization.	Any blanching of the leg during the procedure should be reported. The smallest size catheter possible should be used for this procedure.
Blockage of circulation can cause necrosis.	The nurse should be prepared to warm the leg if spasm is persistent and should have parenteral Priscoline available for use.
Heparin is often used during the procedure to avoid formation of a thrombus.	The catheter should not be removed for six hours after infusing heparin to avoid hemorrhage.
Oxygen Therapy	
Concentration of oxygen above 40 per cent can be toxic to eye tissues.	Arterial blood samples should be monitored.
	The nurse must report O_2 tension levels on lab reports that are above 80 mm. Hg or below 50 mm. Hg.
	The oxygen concentration within a Portahood, incubator, or oxygen tent should be analyzed frequently and recorded (see p. 112).

Oxygen can be toxic to the lung when administered by a positive pressure respirator. Oxygen may also be toxic to cerebral blood vessels.

As little oxygen as possible for the shortest possible time is an essential rule in pediatric intensive care. The nurse should observe and record the infant's response to therapy so that adjustments according to the individual need of the patient may be prescribed.

Pneumonia can be caused by Pseudomonas contamination.

Stagnant water in the reservoir of an incubator or mist tent should be drained, the reservoir washed and then refilled. Any water reservoir should never just be refilled, or bacterial contaminants will thrive. Oxygen tubing should also be changed daily.

Blood Sample Monitoring

Anemia can be caused by frequent withdrawals of blood samples.

The cumulative amount of blood withdrawn must be accurately recorded. (If more than a 10 per cent estimated blood volume is removed, replacement therapy may be indicated.)

BIBLIOGRAPHY

Behrman, R. E. (Ed.): *Neonatology.* The C. V. Mosby Co., St. Louis, 1973.

Cordero, L., and Hon, E. H.: Neonatal Bradycardia Following Nasopharyngeal Stimulation. *Journal of Pediatrics,* 78:446, 1971.

Elder, R. L.: Ultraviolet Light Hazards From Phototherapy. *Journal of the American Medical Association,* 227:203, 1974.

Gellis, S. S., and Kagan, B. M. (Eds.): *Current Pediatric Therapy,* 7th Edition, W. B. Saunders Co., Philadelphia, 1976.

Gluck, L.: Design of a Perinatal Center. *Pediatric Clinics of North America, 17*:777, 1970.

Johnson, D. G.: Shock and its Management in Pediatrics. *Hospital Medicine, 11*:8:22, 1975.

Lewin, J.: An Apnea-alarm Mattress. *Lancet,* 2:667, 1969.

Lucey, J. F.: Neonatal Jaundice and Phototherapy. *Pediatric Clinics of North America, 19*:827, 1972.

Lucey, J., Ferreiro, M., and Hewitt, J.: Prevention of Hyperbilirubinemia in Prematurity by Phototherapy. *Pediatrics, 41*:1047–54, 1968.

Marlow, D.: *Textbook of Pediatric Nursing.* 3rd Edition, W. B. Saunders Co., Philadelphia, 1969.

Maurer, H. M., Shumway, C. N., Draper, D. A., and Hossaini, A.: Controlled Trial Comparing Intermittent Phototherapy and Continuous Phototherapy for Reducing Neonatal Hyperbilirubinemia. *Journal of Pediatrics, 82*:73, 1973.

Sackner, M. A., Landa, J. F., Greeneltch, N., and Morton, J. R.: Pathogenesis and Prevention of Tracheobronchial damage with Suction. *Chest, 64*:284–90, 1973.

Segal, S., and Pirie, G.: Equipment and Personnel for Neonatal Special Care. *Pediatric Clinics of North America, 17*:793, 1970.

Shirkey, H. C. (Ed.): *Pediatric Therapy.* 5th Edition, The C. V. Mosby Co., St. Louis, 1975.

Sinclair, J.: Heat Production and Thermoregulation in the Small-for-date Infant. *Pediatric Clinics of North America, 17*:147, 1970.

Vaughn, V. C., III, and McKay, R. J.: *Nelson Textbook of Pediatrics.* 10th Edition, W. B. Saunders Co., Philadelphia, 1975.

Von Der Mosel, H.: Is Your CCU Electrically Safe? *Medical-Surgical Review, 6*:28, 1970.

Walter, C.: Electrical Hazards in Hospitals, *Hospital Practice, 5*:53, 1970.

Woody, N., and Brodkey, M.: Tanning from Phototherapy for Neonatal Jaundice. *Journal of Pediatrics, 82*:1042, 1973.

Both Drugs and Environment Affect Hearing of Little People. *Infectious Diseases,* 5:22, 1975.
Pediatric Group Gives Rules on Oxygen Use for Newborns. *Medical Tribune.* p. 8, Apr. 7, 1971.
Potential Harm of Kernicterus is Said to Offset Risk of Therapy. *Pediatric News, 9*:10, 1975.
Proceedings of Annual Pediatric Symposium on Current Pediatric Therapy, Variety Children's Hospital, Miami, Florida, 1976.
Proceedings of XIII International Congress of Pediatrics. Vienna, Austria, 1971.

PRODUCT REFERENCES

Air-Shields, Inc. (A Division of National Aeronautical Corp.), Hatboro, Pa.: The Isolette incubator.
American Electronic Lab Inc., Lansdale, Pa.: Infant Sentry Apnea Monitor.
Beckman Instruments Inc., Fullerton, Cal.: Oxygen analyzer.
Dr. H. Frankenberger, Lübeck, Germany: Transcutaneous arterial oxygen tension monitor.
IMI, Division of Becton Dickinson Corp., Newport Beach, California: IMI infant Care Center, Infalarm.
Medical and Biological Instrumentation Ltd., Kent, England: Apnea Alarm Mattress (Available in the U.S. from Codman & Shurtleff, Inc., Randolph, Mass.)
National Biological Corp., Cleveland, Ohio: Bilirubin reduction lamp.
Ohio Chemical & Surgical Equipment Co. (A Division of Air Reduction Co. Inc.), Madison Wisconsin: The Ohio-Armstrong incubator; Hope resuscitator.
Olympic Medical Corp., Seattle, Washington: Oxyhood.

Chapter Fifteen

RESUSCITATION OF INFANTS AND CHILDREN

PRINCIPLES

Effective breathing is essential for the preservation of life and the prevention of permanent brain damage.

A resuscitator should be available in the admitting unit, the delivery room, the newborn nursery, and the pediatric unit.

Resuscitators provide intermittent positive pressure, with or without a negative phase, to force air in and out of the lungs.

If resuscitation measures are initiated before obstructive materials are removed from the airway, the goal of the therapy will be thwarted.

The pharynx is widened by the extension of the cervical vertebrae.

During cardiopulmonary resuscitation the lungs should be inflated rapidly with one breath to each 4 to 5 cardiac compressions.

NURSING RESPONSIBILITIES

The nurse must be alert to the need for resuscitation in the newborn infant. Children suffering from asphyxia, electrical accidents, drowning, or smoke inhalation may require resuscitation. The respiratory rate should be taken during the resuscitation procedure and afterward until respiration becomes stable.

Positive pressure should be used with caution to prevent rupture of the alveoli. The doctor should prescribe the amount of positive pressure desired.

Before any efforts at resuscitation are initiated, a clear airway should be established. (See suctioning, p. 152.) The neck should be slightly hyperextended to facilitate optimum positioning of the trachea.

Hyperextension of the neck and forward displacement of the mandible can overcome soft tissue obstruction caused by a short, fat neck in infants.

The nurse may initiate therapy using bag and mask devices (see p. 142) or she may employ mouth to mouth resuscitation techniques (see p. 139).

The usual rate for cardiac compression for infants is 80 per minute; for older children, 60 per minute. For closed chest cardiac massage to be effective a firm vertebral support is essential. A small rigid board can be used for this purpose. If the compression is held for a fraction of a second, a larger stroke volume will be ejected.

Maintenance of effective cardiac output in infants can be provided by applying maximum pressure with the tips of two fingers over the middle third of the sternum while the vertebral column is firmly supported. In young children, the heel of the hand applies pressure over the sternum opposite the fourth interspace. In larger children, the heel of the left hand is placed over the right hand to increase pressure effectiveness.

Sodium bicarbonate compensates for metabolic acidosis that rapidly occurs in infants and children with severely impaired circulation. Epinephrine increases myocardial contraction force without lowering systemic pressure.

Drugs such as epinephrine and sodium bicarbonate must be on hand. Charts showing, average doses for various age levels should be posted on the emergency cart at all times.

Chilling causes pulmonary vasoconstriction and increases the metabolic need for oxygen.

Abdominal skin temperature should be kept between 96.8° to 98.6° F. (36° to 37° C.). Thermoregulating equipment controlled by a thermistor taped to the skin of the abdomen, or an incubator heated to 89.6° to 93.2° F. (32° to 34° C.) with 80 to 90 per cent humidity should be available to minimize heat loss during handling.

Debilitated infants and children are highly susceptible to infections.

After the resuscitator has been used, all parts should be disassembled and thoroughly cleaned.

TECHNIQUES

I. Respiratory Arrest

Principal factors in the emergency care of a child with respiratory arrest include:
1. Prepare for such emergencies.
2. Respond immediately to the incident and delegate appropriate duties as needed.
3. Assess the cause of respiratory arrest. (Be aware of the diagnosis for the child.)
For example, positive pressure may be used with success in respiratory distress syndromes but can be fatal in diaphragmatic hernias.

II. Emergency Procedure
   in Cardiorespiratory Arrest

1. Suction to clear the trachea.
2. Apply 5-second external cardiac massage.

3. Use bag and mask resuscitation. Watch for chest expansion.

4. Add oxygen to the system.

5. Prepare for intubation.

6. If gastric distention occurs, express manually or pass a nasogastric tube. *Note:* Continue cardiac massage until a palpable pulse is observed and provide ventilation after every fourth cardiac compression.

7. Prepare medications such as narcotic antagonists (Lorfan, Nalline), cardiac stimulants (epinephrine, calcium gluconate), and hypertonic glucose solution.

8. Call for EKG.

9. Have information for doctor concerning time of last oral intake, medications, seizures, respiratory problem, and fever.

10. Prepare for blood sampling as ordered by the doctor.

11. Preserve body temperature during resuscitation.

Note: When spontaneous respiration starts, it is often inadequate, and marked hypoxic damage and respiratory acidosis can result. Respirations must be assisted until the doctor determines if respiratory exchange is adequate.

External Cardiac Massage for Infants and Children

External cardiac massage is the simple compression of the heart, trapped in the mediastinum, between the sternum and the vertebrae. The size of the patient determines the technique to be selected. In all cases, external cardiac massage should be provided in a 1:5 ratio with artificial ventilation.

Infants

1. A finger or thumb compressing the *midsternum* at a rate of 100 or more per minute.

2. Depth of compression should be equal to approximately 1/5 of the anterior-posterior diameter of the chest. (Midsternum pressure is used because the ventricles lie higher in the infant's chest than in that of older children and adults.)

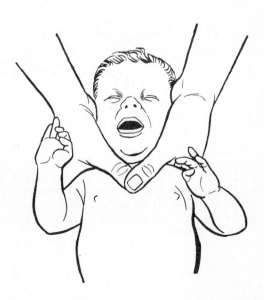

FIGURE 15–1. External Cardiac Massage for Infants Firm local support may be provided by placing one hand under the infant's back, or by encircling the entire chest, with the hands resting on the vertebral area, and using thumbs for compression.

Young children

1. The heel of the hand is placed over the midsternum and compresses the sternum about 60 or more times per minute.

2. The child must be on a firm surface, either on the floor or on a cardiac arrest board.

3. The entire weight of the nurse should not be used on children during compression of the chest.

Older child or adolescent

1. The heel of one hand is placed over the sternum of the older child.

2. The heel of the other hand is placed over the first hand.

3. The entire weight of the nurse may be placed on the sternum for compression (depending on the size of the patient). The rate of compression should be about 60 per minute.

4. The child must be lying on a firm surface.

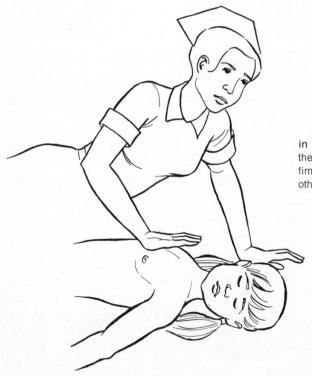

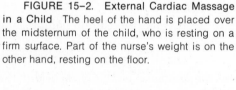

FIGURE 15–2. External Cardiac Massage in a Child   The heel of the hand is placed over the midsternum of the child, who is resting on a firm surface. Part of the nurse's weight is on the other hand, resting on the floor.

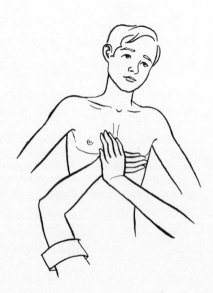

FIGURE 15–3. External Cardiac Massage in Older Children   The heel of the left hand is placed over the right hand to increase pressure effectiveness. The rate of compression should be about 60 per minute.

Management of Airway Obstruction

Obstruction of the airway is a common problem in infants and young children who may inhale a foreign body, or in older children or adolescents who may choke on a particle of food. Before effective resuscitation measures can be initiated, the airway must be cleared.

Some hospitals and ambulance services use equipment specifically designed for removal of food from the airway. One such type of device is the Throat-E-Vac.

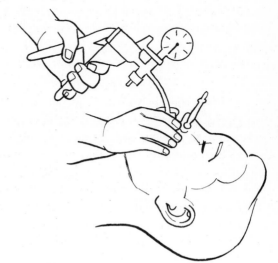

FIGURE 15-4.   Use of Throat-E-Vac.

Using the Throat-E-Vac

The patient is positioned with the head slightly hyperextended. The correct size mouthpiece from the Throat-E-Vac kit is placed on the end of the tube on the pump and inserted into the child's mouth, over the tongue. The nurse uses her hand to seal the mouthpiece. The nose is closed with a nose clip. The nurse pumps with quick strokes and watches the gauge for any rise in vacuum. When the blockage is dislodged, the vacuum gauge will suddenly drop to zero. Resuscitation measures can then be initiated.

This unit is designed for use in complete airway obstruction. If pumping fails to produce a rise in the level of the vacuum gauge, then the airway is not completely obstructed and other resuscitative measures may be initiated until a physician is available.

The Heimlich technique

When special equipment is not available, the Heimlich technique has been recommended to dislodge food or foreign bodies from the airway. This technique works on the principle that forcing the diaphragm up causes residual air in the lung to be forcefully exhaled, "popping" the obstruction out of the airway. When the airway is cleared, conventional cardiopulmonary resuscitation can be initiated. This technique may also have value in removing some water from the lungs in cases of drowning, thus permitting more effective resuscitation.

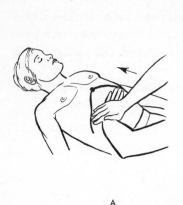
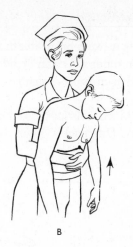

FIGURE 15–5.   Heimlich Technique.

A   B

1. Press the heel of the hand against the abdomen just below the rib cage, providing a *quick upward thrust* against the diaphragm. Should vomiting occur, turn the head to the side to prevent aspiration (A).

2. Stand behind the child and press the thumb side of the fist with a *quick upward thrust* into the abdomen below the rib cage. This forces the diaphragm up, increasing air pressure in the tracheobronchial tree, forcing the foreign particle out of the trachea (B).

Another method of dislodging foreign particles is to invert the child over your arm and offer a blow between the shoulder blades with the heel of your hand (see Figure 15–6).

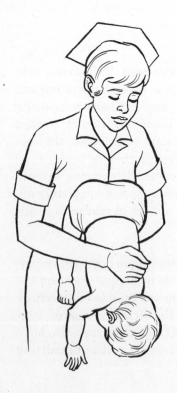

FIGURE 15–6.   The nurse is administering a blow between the child's shoulder blades with the heel of her hand to dislodge any foreign particles present.

Mouth to Mouth Resuscitation in Infants and Children

Mouth to mouth resuscitation provides more ventilatory volume than the bag-valve-mask technique because of the difficulty in providing a leakproof seal while maintaining an open airway. The technique of mouth to mouth resuscitation is the same as for adults with these exceptions:

1. For infants and small children the nurse covers both the nose and the mouth of the child with her mouth, and uses small breaths with less volume to inflate the lungs once every three seconds (or one breath to every three to four cardiac compressions when given together with cardiac resuscitation).

2. The tilt of the child's head should only be slight to prevent obstruction of the breathing passages.

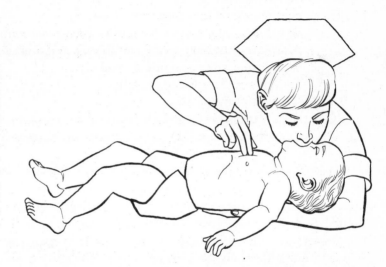

FIGURE 15–7. Cardiopulmonary Resuscitation of an Infant   The nurse uses the tips of her index and middle fingers to apply chest compression over the midsternum area at about 80–100 per minute. The back of the infant is well supported or counterpressure may be applied with the nurse's other hand and arm. The nurse's mouth covers both the nose and mouth of the infant and the head tilt is modified. The nurse removes her mouth to permit the child to exhale.

III.   Complications of Resuscitative Techniques

Fractured ribs, compression injury to internal abdominal organs, and ruptured stomach are some complications that might occur with vigorous resuscitative measures. The nurse must be alert to these complications and closely observe the patient following resuscitation. However, fear of such complications should not deter anyone from initiating lifesaving measures in an emergency.

Suggested Measures to Prevent Complications During Resuscitation

1. To avoid liver damage, do not press on xiphoid process.
2. To avoid lung damage, do not perform external cardiac massage on children with open chest wounds.
3. Gastric distention can cause upward pressure on the diaphragm and reduce

ventilatory capacity of the lungs, resulting in vomiting and aspiration. Gastric distention should be relieved before resuscitation is continued.

4. Do not press on epigastrium to relieve gastric distention *during* external cardiac resuscitation, to avoid injury to internal organs.

IV.   Postanoxic Care

After the acute phase, when respiratory exchange is adequate, the nurse should observe and report:
1. Signs and symptoms of pneumothorax
2. Hyperexcitability
3. Fever
4. Incoordination (in older children)
5. Renal shutdown

If an endotracheal tube is inserted:
1. Maintain strict aseptic technique during suctioning.
2. Maintain humidity to prevent drying and occluding of endotracheal tube.
3. Maintain accurate record of vital signs.
4. Record results of blood sampling.
5. Turn child frequently.

If ventilator care is prolonged, the inspiratory pressure should be less than 40 mm. Hg, PO_2 less than 125 mm. Hg, and oxygen concentration less than 40 per cent to prevent lung and other complications.

The type of ventilator selected depends upon the size of the patient and the type of problem. Usually, when muscular weakness is the chief problem and the lungs are normal, a pressure limited ventilator is selected. However, in pulmonary disease, volume limited devices are preferred. The doctor selects the type of respirator and must specify the proper rate, tidal volume, pressure, inspiratory-expiratory ratio, oxygen concentration, and humidification for each child and determine if assisted or controlled ventilation is desired.

V.   Assisted Ventilation — Inhalation Therapy for Infants and Children

If a patent airway and an increased oxygen environment do not provide adequate gas exchange then mechanical respiratory aids will be ordered by the doctor. Oxygen may be administered by bag, respirator, wall outlets, and tanks. Oxygen from wall outlets or tanks should *not* be directly connected to an endotracheal tube or tracheotomy tube, to avoid rupture of the alveoli.

Continuous Positive Pressure Breathing (CPPB) and synonymous terms — *Continuous Positive Pressure Ventilation* (CPPV); *Positive End-Expiratory Pressure* (PEEP), and *Continuous Residual Airway Pressure* (CRAP) — are designed to prevent atelectasis and allow for greater oxygen and carbon dioxide exchange at the alveolar-capillary level.

The apparatus to achieve continuous positive pressure breathing therapy is available as an optional accessory attachment to many mechanical ventilators.

Factors Influencing Inhalation Therapy

Size.   The smaller size of the respiratory passageways and the immaturity of the lung influence the size and type of equipment required and best suited for the purpose.

Cooperativeness.   Special techniques to gain cooperation of the pediatric patient and maintain effectiveness of therapy is essential.

Disease entity and sites of affliction peculiar to pediatrics.   Some diseases such as croup involve upper respiratory obstruction, while bronchiolitis involves lower respiratory obstruction. Asthma involves expiratory problems; cystic fibrosis is a combination of respiratory obstruction, areas of collapse, and infection. Each ailment requires a different type of respiratory assistance.

The Kreiselman Resuscitator

A Kreiselman resuscitator is a mobile, explosion-proof infant resuscitator.

On-off switch (A).   This switch controls the heating unit of the resuscitator which provides body warmth during the resuscitation procedure.

Suction switch (B).   This switch controls the electric suction apparatus that is attached to the unit.

Oxygen cylinders (C).   Two oxygen cylinders fit into a special groove at the foot of the unit. The nurse should check the oxygen supply in the cylinders daily.

Oxygen gauge (D).   The oxygen gauge indicates the pressure in the cylinder connected to the regular oxygen mask (I). When the handle is turned clockwise, oxygen will flow steadily from the mask.

Manometer (E).   The manometer indicates the mask pressure used when administering positive pressure oxygen. The pressure should not rise above the 12 mm. level indicated by the red line; otherwise alveolar rupture is possible.

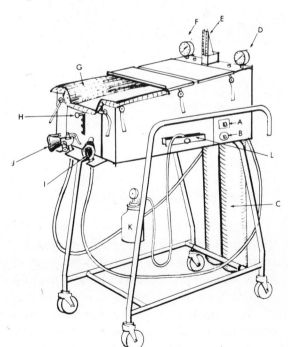

FIGURE 15–8.   The Kreiselman Resuscitator.

Positive pressure gauge (F).   Oxygen pressure in the cylinder attached to the positive pressure mask (J) is indicated by this gauge. Oxygen flows only when the handle of the mask is depressed.

Quilted lining and mattress (G).   The infant is placed on the quilted, fitted lining and mattress. The lining should be changed and the unit cleaned after each use.

Mattress adjustor (H).   The handle fits into grooves to adjust the mattress to the Trendelenburg position.

Regular oxygen mask (I).   Oxygen flows steadily when the handle on (F) is turned.

Positive pressure mask (J).   Oxygen flows intermittently as the handle of the mask is depressed. This mask is used only when other methods of resuscitation fail.

Suction apparatus (K).   The suction apparatus is controlled by a switch (B). The meter on top of the suction jar indicates the amount of pressure used during suction. The jar unscrews for cleaning.

Drawer (L).   This drawer contains suction catheters and intubation equipment.

The Hope Pediatric Bag

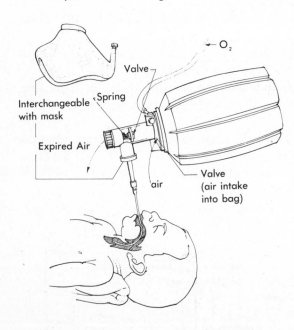

FIGURE 15-9.   The "Hope Pediatric Bag"
This provides a means of administering oxygen through a bag connected to the endotracheal tube.

The Portable Resuscitator

The portable resuscitator, used for older children, involves principles similar to those for using positive-pressure resuscitation. Apply the mask to the child's face and intermittently deflate the bag with your fingers to force air into the lungs. An automatic valve prevents rebreathing of expired air. The mask may be used with air or oxygen. When regular breathing is established, the resuscitator is removed.

Intermittent use for 5 of every 20 minutes or a similar time schedule is one method of providing assisted ventilation. This is often referred to as "bagging the patient," and a portable resuscitator or the Hope pediatric bag is frequently used for this procedure.

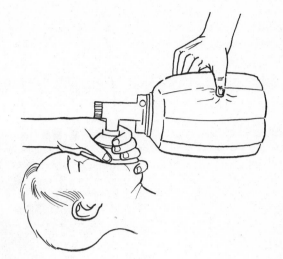

FIGURE 15–10.   "Bagging" an Infant.

"Bagging" the Infant

Nursing responsibilities

1. Suction each nostril briefly. Clear mouth and stomach as needed.

2. Put feeding tube in infant's stomach and tape in place if bagging is to be done for more than 2 minutes (to prevent gastric distention).

3. Try to coordinate rhythm of bagging with voluntary efforts of infant's respiration.

4. Never bag an infant after a feeding unless the stomach is aspirated first.

5. Never bag with dry oxygen.

Examples of oxygen concentrations delivered when "bagging" infants

Liter flow per minute	"Bagging" rate	Concentration (per cent) of oxygen delivered
5	60 per minute	28
10	60 per minute	38
15	60 per minute	45
10	30 per minute	53
15	30 per minute	62

Note: Do not use flow rate exceeding 15 liters per minute or valve lock will occur in bagging apparatus.

VI.   Positive Pressure—Assisted Breathing Ventilation

Bennett MA-1 Respiratory Unit

Spirometer alarm (1).   Audible alarm sounds if a set tidal volume is not reached within approximately 20 seconds. To silence the alarm, the switch must be turned off and then back on. Check for power or machine failure when this alarm sounds.

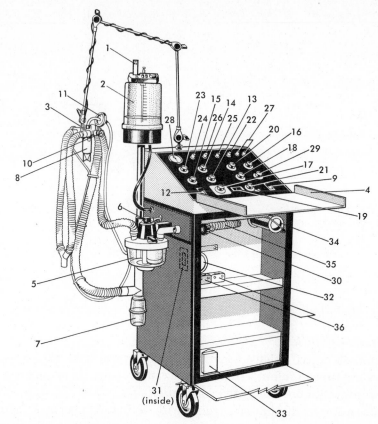

FIGURE 15–11.   The Bennett MA I Respirator   The MA I Respiration unit, sometimes called the "Mary-Ann," may be used with room air or oxygen, as a respiratory:

1. *Controller.*   Inspiration is begun by a timer, providing a constant number of breaths per minute and a constant volume per breath.

2. *Assistor.*   Inspiration is begun by patient effort and is monitored by adjustable sensitivity control.

3. *Assistor-controller.*   Inspiration is patient-triggered with timed starting assured if patient does not exert sufficient effort.

Spirometer (2).   Indicates expired tidal volume in ml. after correction for tubing compliance. Marked in 100 ml. increments from 0 to 2200 ml.

Tubing and manifold system (3).   Held by an adjustable support arm.

Cover (4).   Dust cover to protect controls and indicators when unit is not in use.

Humidifier module (5).   An adjustable heated humidifier. Fill jar with distilled water to the full mark.

Humidifier temperature (6).   An adjustable thermostat, which controls water temperature and relative humidity so the temperature of the saturated inspired gas is at body temperature. The control is not calibrated, but is numbered and color coded for guidance. Blue—room temperature to body temperature; white—body temperature; red—above body temperature.

Water trap (7).   Collects condensation from tubing and spirometer. Do not allow container to fill up.

Nebulizer (8).   Place medication or additive liquid desired in the nebulizer vial.

Nebulizer control (9).   Controls gas flow to the nebulizer. Nebulization is in inspiration only.

Thermometer (10).   Indicates the temperature in the tube system near the patient, and so approximates the temperature of the inspired gas.

Nebulizer tubing and bacteria filter (11).   Main bacteria filter for the nebulizer. Replace every 1000 hours.

Power switch (12).   Controls all electrical power to the unit. Turn the power switch off before connecting the cord to power supply.

Normal volume (13).   Sets the volume of gas delivered in normal inspiration. When the volume limit is reached, inspiration ends. Adjustable and calibrated.

Normal pressure limit (14).   Limits the pressure that may be developed in the tube system in a normal inspiration. If the pressure limit is reached, inspiration ends. Adjustable and calibrated, 20 to 80 cm. H_2O.

Peak flow (15).   Limits the rate of flow from the unit to the patient. Adjustable and calibrated.

Oxygen percentage (16).   Sets oxygen concentration in the delivered gas. Infinitely adjustable and calibrated, 21 per cent (air) to 100 per cent.

Rate (17).   Sets rate of controlled cycling. Adjustable and calibrated, off, and 6 to 60 cycles per minute. Adjustable, not calibrated, 60 to 100 or more cycles per minute.

Sigh Volume (18).   Sets the volume of gas to be delivered in a sigh inspiration. When the volume limit is reached, inspiration ends. Adjustable and calibrated.

Manual normal or sigh inspiration start (19).   Used to start a single normal or a single sigh inspiration. Rate rephases itself when the switch is pressed.

Sigh pressure limit (20).   Limits the pressure which may be developed in the tube system in a sigh inspiration. If the pressure limit is reached, inspiration ends. Adjustable and calibrated.

Sigh intervals per hour (21).   Sets frequency of the sigh, which is triggered by normal rate or assist. Adjustable and calibrated, off, and 4–6–8–10–15 times per hour with a choice of 1–2–3 sighs per interval.

Sigh indicator (22).   Lights during the sigh breathing cycle.

Sensitivity (23).   Set degree of patient effort required to trigger unit into inspiration. Not calibrated.

Assist indicator (24).   Lights when patient effort triggers inspiration. Also lights if the sensitivity control is set so that the unit self-cycles. Used to establish a very sensitive assist response.

Inspiration-expiration ratio warner (25).   Operates only when ventilation is controlled. Lights when inspiration is longer than the following expiration. Indicates that the combination of control setting and patient condition has created an inspiration/expiration ratio of less than 1:1.

Pressure limit warner (26).   Lights if normal or sigh pressure limit is reached.

Oxygen signals (27).   A green light indicates that oxygen percentage has been set to enrichment. A red light and an audible alarm warn if oxygen percentage is less than the setting because of inadequate source pressure.

System pressure gauge (28).   Indicates pressure in the tube system in cm. H_2O.

Expiratory resistance (29).   Used to retard expiratory flow. Adjustable, not calibrated. Effects are observable on the gauge and spirometer.

Main-flow filter (30).   The main bacteria filter for the unit. Replace every 1000 hours.

Pressure limit warning buzzer (31).   A three-position switch, loud, soft, or off, which controls the buzzer.

Elapsed time indicator (32).   A nonresettable 100,000 hour time meter.

Cooling fan and filter (33).   A washable filter which screens lint from room air drawn into the motor/pump chamber. Wash every 200 hours.

Air inlet filter (34).   A washable filter, which intercepts air drawn into the bellows system for delivery to the patient. Wash every 500 hours.

Flexible tube (35).   Connects the main-flow filtering system to the humidifier.

Circuit breakers (36).   The right hand circuit breaker protects the low voltage components from overload. The left hand circuit breaker protects the high voltage components (off-on switches).

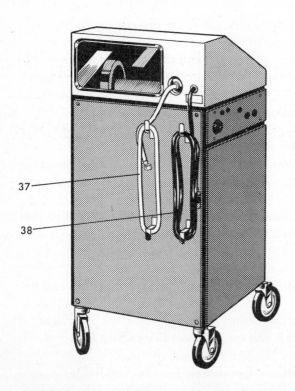

FIGURE 15-12. Back view of Bennett MA I Respirator.

Oxygen inlet and pressure hose (37).   High pressure hose, connect to the oxygen supply.

Power cord (38).   Plug into standard 120 volt outlet.

The BABYbird Ventilator

Oxygen blender (1).   Provides precise control of oxygen concentration from 21 per cent (air) to 100 per cent. An audible low pressure alarm system detects failure in the supply of gas or when pressures fall below 45 p.s.i. Sources of air and oxygen under about 50 p.s.i. of pressure are required.

Pressure manometer (2).   Provides constant monitoring of the pressure of the air/oxygen mixture being delivered to the ventilator. A green wedge on the manometer dial indicates mandatory operational pressure range between 45 and 55 p.s.i.

Respiratory gas flow control (3).   Regulates the flow of gas mixtures delivered to the system.

Respiratory gas flow gauge (4).   A visual readout of respiratory gas flow mixture, calibrated in liters per minute (LPM).

Nebulizer control (5).   Controls the aerosol density of the inspired gases. The usual setting is in the 12 o'clock position with 5 LPM or more. Maximum position is used for flows below 5 LPM and topical pulmonary chemotherapy.

Proximal airway pressures (6).   Provides monitoring of actual proximal physiological airway pressures. Calibrated in mm. Hg and cm. H_2O.

Inspiratory time (7).   Controls the inspiratory time. Adjustable in a time range of 0.4 or less to 2.5 seconds.

Expiratory time (8).   Controls the expiratory time. Adjustable in a time range of 0.4 or less to 10 seconds.

Inspiratory relief pressure (9).   Controls peak inspiratory pressures during mechanical ventilation.

Mode selection control (10).   Provides for spontaneous respiration or mandatory ventilation.

Expiratory flow gradient (11).   Controls expiratory jet flow.

Inspiratory time limit and reset (12).   Adjustable. Nominally set at three seconds. Audible alarm signals when inspiratory time exceeds 3 seconds. Push to reset. It is mandatory that inspiratory time (7) be readjusted.

Mechanical testing controls (13).   Provides a method of checking the function of the ventilator before making the final airway connection to the patient.

Outflow valve (14).   Adjustable. Maintains a constant positive breathing pressure and positive end expiratory pressure.

AIRbird compression bulb (15).   Manual ventilation can be accomplished by squeezing the bulb. May serve as a back-up system. Can be used to sigh the patient. Changing the unit over to manual operation is not necessary.

Nebulizer (16).   500 ml. inline micronebulizer for continuous nebulization.

Therapy micronebulizer nebulizer (17).   Provides humidification and topical pulmonary chemotherapy.

Extension arm (18).   Supports the breathing circuit tubing in desired position. Easily adjusted.

Connector (19).   Connect to patient.

Breathing circuit tubing (20).   Provides a circle system of five (A, B, C, D, E) connections attached to the base of the ventilator. Fully labeled and indexed to provide easy change of tubing for resterilization.

Water traps (21).   Collects condensation from tubing.

Utility tray (22).   Attached to a castered base, vertical pole type of stand. Provides an area for extra equipment.

High pressure oxygen hose (23).   Connect to oxygen supply outlet.

High pressure air hose (24).   Connect to compressed air supply outlet.

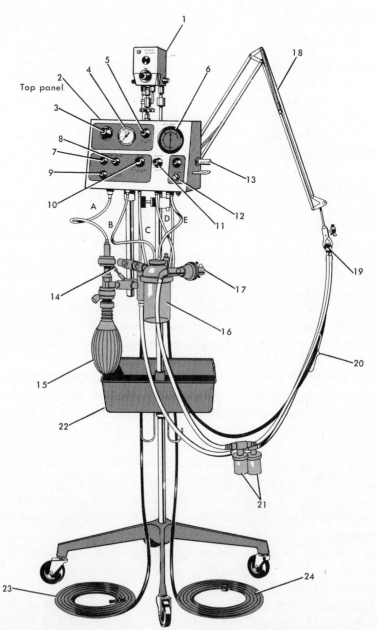

FIGURE 15–13.   The BABYbird Ventilator   *A*, A pneumatically powered ventilator, which operates from a mixture of oxygen and compressed air. It can be used as a pressure preset or a tidal volume preset ventilator.

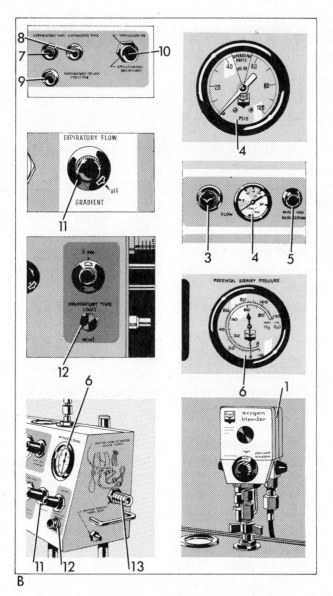

FIGURE 15–13. *Continued. B,* Details of ventilator.

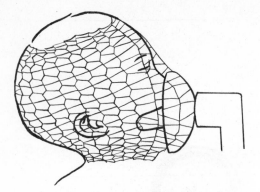

FIGURE 15–14. A tubular elastic netting, such as Dressinet, can be used to keep continuous positive airway pressure (C-PAP) face masks in place without harming the infant. This eliminates the use of a strap with the mask that often causes facial edema, molding of the skull and cerebellar hemorrhage.

VII. Monitoring Children on Mechanical Ventilators: Points to Observe and Record

1. Accurately recording all gauge settings is of utmost importance when the ventilator is first put into operation. These include: pressure, flow rate, sensitivity, oxygen concentration, tidal volume setting and temperatures.

2. The best indicator of effective alveolar ventilation is arterial blood gas determinations. Accurately recording amounts of blood removal is vital to prevent cardiac decompensation from hypovolemia. It is important to record the time the sample is drawn and the patient's status.

3. Auscultation and configuration of chest to assure ventilation of both lungs. Observe for hyperexpansion, and degree and location of retractions. Rate and depth of ventilation. Early detection of pneumothorax.

4. Periodic sighing to prevent atelectasis caused from continuously breathing a constant tidal volume. Sigh approximately every third inspiration, consisting of about two times the normal tidal volume which is determined by the physician.

5. Monitor the spirometer to determine if preset tidal volume is being delivered.

6. Observe the inspiratory/expiratory ratio warning light which indicates a ratio of less than 1:1 (normal is usually 1:1.5 to 1:2).

7. Observe for abdominal distention, which can cause undue pressure on the diaphragm and prevent full lung expansion.

8. Observe and record temperature of inspired gas; it should approximate body temperature.

9. All water volumes of the humidifying systems are important. Low volumes increase ventilator compliance. Condensation in tubing must be removed and discarded so as not to alter air flow through tubing.

10. Strict aseptic techniques must be observed to prevent infection. These include: periodic filter changes (see Section VIII); culture humidifying containers for bacterial growth; use of sterile suctioning equipment; removal of accumulated tracheobronchial secretions to reduce recurrent infections (see sections on Chest Physiotherapy and Suctioning).

11. Hypotension from alterations in intrathoracic pressure is a hazard. Observe pulse quality and rate, blood pressure, and urinary output.

12. An "Ambu" or similar bag should be available at all times for emergency ventilation in case of any ventilator malfunctioning. Any leaks in the ventilator-patient circuit will render the ventilator ineffective. Alarm systems should be tested periodically.

VIII. Complications of Assisted Ventilation

COMPLICATION	NURSING RESPONSIBILITIES
Nasotracheal Tube Placement	
Excess angulation of tube against nasal cartilage can cause necrosis.	Watch for redness in nasal area, and report. Prepare to assist with replacement tube to opposite side.
The tube can obstruct the sinus duct causing sinusitis, a problem in an unconscious patient.	Report complaints of facial or ear pain and fever. Check closely for signs of these complications.
The tube can obstruct the eustachian tube and cause acute otitis media.	
Ventilator Defects or Malfunctions	
Alarm may be turned off for suction or treatment and not turned on again.	Be sure alarm is turned on. Test alarm periodically.
When the humidifier malfunctions, the air may be underhumidified and the patient's secretions become more difficult to remove, or the air may be overhumidified and water particles may enter the lung. It may overheat the oxygen and cause lung burn.	The nurse should touch the inspirating tube at its connection to the endotracheal tube and estimate its warmth. If it is too hot to touch, it is too hot for the patient. Check ventilatory rate and cycling with doctor's order.
Medical Problems	
Respiratory acidosis can occur if there is insufficient tidal volume or respiratory rate, or improper cycling is delivered to the patient, or if there is a leak in the ventilator.	Arterial blood gas analysis should be made 15 minutes after initiating assisted ventilation and each time a major adjustment of oxygen concentration, tidal volume, or rate is made. The nurse should test the alarm system of the ventilator to be sure it is functioning.
Sedatives and narcotics decrease the respiratory rate, and alveolar hypoventilation can occur if the cycling rate is set far below the rate at which the patient will trigger the mechanism.	Use sedatives and narcotics sparingly when patient is on assisted ventilation. Carefully measure respiratory rate of ventilator and recheck automatic cycling rate.
Respiratory alkalosis or hyperventilation can occur and can cause cardiac problems.	Frequent blood gas analysis is essential. The nurse should also check the ventilatory rate with the vital signs of the patient.
Pneumothorax can occur with PEEP therapy when tidal volumes are excessively large.	Know and observe for signs of pneumothorax in all patients on assisted ventilation: 1. Sudden change in vital signs. 2. Sudden change in inspiratory pressure requirements.

3. Sudden change in blood gas analysis results.

Atelectasis can occur from endobronchial mucous obstruction and can cause hypoxemia.

Check and maintain adequate humidification and endotracheal suction. Turn patient frequently and use postural drainage techniques when possible (see p. 153).

Contaminated Equipment

Nosocomial infection can occur from use of contaminated equipment and can be fatal to a patient with impaired lung function.

Prevent equipment contamination. Replace all potentially contaminated parts after each patient use and every 24 hours. Use only sterile water to fill cannisters and nebulizers.

Cannisters should be emptied, washed and dried regularly. Maintain sterile technique for endotracheal suctioning.

Bronchopulmonary Dysplasia

Immature lungs, when exposed to inspired oxygen concentrations over 40 per cent for more than 24 hours, via positive pressure ventilation, may develop bronchopulmonary dysplasia.

Long-term follow-up care must be provided for every newborn receiving inhalation therapy longer than 24 hours. Accurate recording of time on or off inhalation therapy is essential.

IX. *Endotracheal Suctioning*

If patient is on a respirator:

1. Set suction gauge for 60 to 80 mm. Hg depending on the size of the patient and the viscosity of mucus.

2. Remove the respirator and instill 1/4 cc. normal saline into the nasotracheal tube. (Cover the trachea adapter with a needle holder to prevent contamination.)

3. Using sterile gloves, moisten the tip of a 5-8 Fr. catheter with sterile water.

4. With the infant's head turned to the right, insert the catheter gently until you meet an obstruction, then withdraw about 1/2 cm. Apply suction and continue to withdraw catheter with a rotating motion. Suctioning should last 5 to 10 seconds.

5. Reconnect respirator and allow infant to breathe.

6. Repeat with infant's head turned to the left.

7. Rinse catheter with sterile water and suction the mouth.

8. Reconnect endotracheal tube to the respirator.

Note: Each time endotracheal suction is attempted, a new sterile catheter should be used.

If patient is not on a respirator:

1. See general procedure described here.

2. Suction oropharynx first, allow infant to breathe.

3. Insert catheter *upward* into the nares gently, then continue *downward*, progressing catheter on inspiration only.

4. Apply intermittent suction and withdraw within 5 to 10 seconds.

5. Repeat with infant's head turned to opposite direction.
6. Stimulate infant to cry at end of procedure.
7. Provide "T.L.C."

CHEST PHYSIOTHERAPY

This therapeutic measure is employed in treating acute or chronic obstructive or restrictive pulmonary conditions to effect removal of secretions from lung segments and prevent atelectasis by purposeful positioning, percussing (clapping) and vibrating over the involved lung area, combined with breathing exercises and coughing. Chest physiotherapy can be combined with topical pulmonary chemotherapy delivered by inspiratory positive pressure.

PRINCIPLES

The physician prescribes chest physiotherapy for each individual as needed. The order should include: chest segment to which treatment should be directed, duration and frequency of treatment, medication and pressure to be used if combined with positive pressure therapy.

Adequate systemic hydration is essential to liquefy pulmonary secretions.

Recording of observations should be ongoing and accurate.

NURSING RESPONSIBILITIES

Gaining the child's confidence and cooperation by use of therapeutic play and age-appropriate games and toys. Treatments should be coordinated not to conflict with meal times and other medications which have synergistic actions if pulmonary chemotherapy is employed.

Maintaining adequate age-appropriate oral fluid intake or accurate monitoring of intravenous fluids. Maintain a highly humidified atmosphere and proper oxygen concentration if ordered.

The nurse should record response to treatment, tolerance of treatment, pulse, rate and depth of respiration, amount and type of secretions, length and duration of treatment, medications used, and lung segments involved.

TECHNIQUES

I. Postural Drainage and Percussion for Children

Positioning may vary from an upright position to a 45° Trendelenburg position. The involved lung segment is positioned uppermost and the upper segments are drained first, working downward. The sequence is: (1) positioning (Fig. 15–15), (2) clapping (Fig. 15–16), (3) vibration (Fig. 15–17), (4) coughing, and (5) removal of secretions, using suction if necessary.

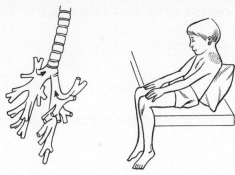

1. To drain upper lobes, apical segments. Bed or drainage table flat. Patient leans back on pillow at 30° angle against therapist. Therapist claps with markedly cupped hand over area between clavicle (collarbone) and top of scapula (shoulder blade) on each side.

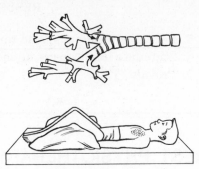

2. To drain upper lobes, anterior segments. Bed or drainage table flat. Patient lies on back with pillow under knees. Therapist claps between clavicle (collarbone) and nipple on each side.

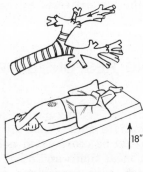

5. To drain lower lobes, anterior basal segment. Foot of table or bed elevated 18 inches (about 30°). Patient lies on side, head down, pillow under knees. Therapist claps with slightly cupped hand over lower ribs. (Position shown is for drainage of left anterior basal segment. To drain the right anterior basal segment, patient should lie on his left side in the same posture.)

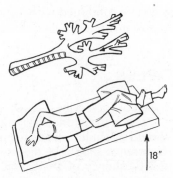

6. To drain lower lobes, lateral basal segments. Foot of table or bed elevated 18 inches (about 30°). Patient lies on abdomen, head down, then rotates 1/4 turn upward. Upper leg is flexed over a pillow for support. Therapist claps over uppermost portion of lower ribs. (Position shown is for drainage of right lateral basal segment. To drain the left lateral basal segment, patient should lie on his right side in the same position.)

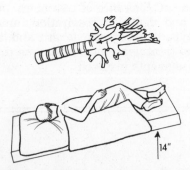

9. To drain right middle lobe. Foot of table or bed elevated 14 inches (about 15°). Patient lies head down on left side and rotates 1/4 turn backward. Pillow may be placed behind from shoulder to hip. Knees should be flexed. Therapist claps over right nipple area. In females with breast development or tenderness, use cupped hand with heel of hand under armpit and fingers extending forward beneath the breast.

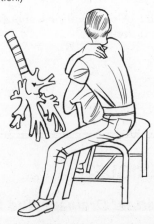

10. To drain upper lobe, posterior segment. A position in which the individual can perform self-therapy. Lean forward over back of chair on folded pillow at about 30° angle. Clap with cupped hand and vibrate over upper back extending fingers forward and upward.

FIGURE 15–15. Positioning for Postural (Bronchial) Drainage for Children (From *Guide to Diagnosis and Management of Cystic Fibrosis*, 1974. Courtesy of Cystic Fibrosis Foundation, Atlanta, Georgia.)

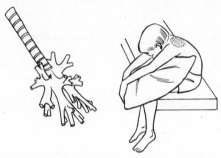

3. To drain upper lobes, posterior segments. Bed or drainage table flat. Patient leans over folded pillow at 30° angle. Therapist stands behind and claps over upper back on both sides.

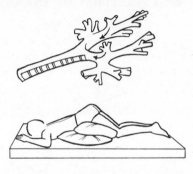

4. To drain lower lobes, superior segments. Bed or table flat. Patient lies on abdomen with two pillows under hips. Therapist claps middle of back at tip of scapula (shoulder blade), on either side of spine.

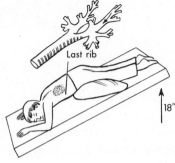

7. To drain lower lobes, posterior basal segments. Foot of table or bed elevated 18 inches (about 30°). Patient lies on abdomen, head down, with pillow under hips. Therapist claps over lower ribs close to spine on each side. Never clap or vibrate directly over the spine.

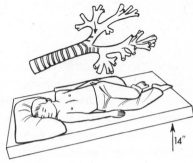

8. To drain left upper lobe, lingular segments. Foot of table or bed elevated 14 inches (about 15°). Patient lies head down on right side and rotates ¼ turn backward. Pillow may be placed behind from shoulder to hip. Knees should be flexed. Therapist claps with moderately cupped hand over left nipple area. In females with breast development or tenderness, use cupped hand with heel of hand under armpit and fingers extending forward beneath the breast.

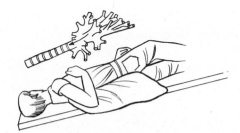

11. To drain right middle lobe. A position in which the individual can perform self-therapy. Foot of bed elevated 10 to 14 inches, about 15° angle. Lie on left side ¼ turn, head down (pillow behind from shoulder to hip), knees flexed. Clap and vibrate over right nipple.

FIGURE 15–15. *Continued.*

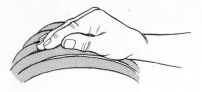

FIGURE 15–16. Clapping Cupping position of the hand for clapping. The wrist movement involves a brisk relaxed flexion and extension. Be very careful not to use *only* the fingers or *only* the heel of the hand. Clapping is usually done for 1 to 2 minutes.

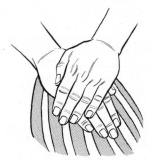

FIGURE 15–17. Vibrating Position of the hands for vibrating. Vibration is most effective following clapping and it is done only during expiration, usually three or four times, after which coughing is encouraged.

Very young children will cooperate if therapy is approached as being a game simulating a trip to outer space. Puppets are most effective in working with nonverbal children. Breathing exercises can be effected by blowing tissue paper mobiles or blowing bubbles. Counting games facilitate slow expirations by counting 1, 2, 3, and clapping hands raised over the head to provide for expansion of chest.

When chronic pulmonary conditions make it necessary to perform postural drainage and chest physiotherapy in the home, the positioning may be achieved by improvising with home furnishings: stacks of newspapers or telephone directories padded with pillows and covered with the child's favorite blanket; a chair placed upside down and appropriate for size, also padded with pillows and the favorite blanket; an ironing board over the end of the bed can be converted to an adjustable tiltlike table; triangular lounging pillows can also be used. A pillowed lap may be best for infants.

II. Postural Drainage and Percussion in the Neonate

The purpose is to promote drainage to the main stem bronchi and to enable effective suctioning.

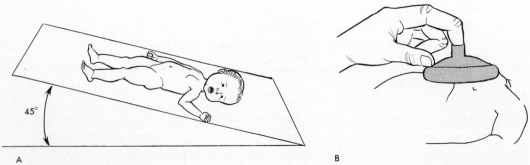

A

B

FIGURE 15–18. *A* shows newborn infant lying—face turned to side, on table with 45° angle. *B* shows finger stuck in resuscitation mask.

1. Position infant in Trendelenburg for 5 minutes (Fig. 15–18 *A*).

2. Percuss for 2 to 3 minutes, using a resuscitation mask on the finger (see Fig. 15–18 *B*). Percuss anterior, posterior, and lateral chest. Do not percuss sternum, vertebrae, kidney, or abdominal area.

3. Then place two fingers over the area and gently vibrate.

4. Support the side opposite the percussion with a rolled diaper.

5. Suction as needed.

BIBLIOGRAPHY

American Academy of Pediatrics: *Care of Children in Hospital.* Committee on Hospital Care, 1971.

American Heart Association: National Academy of Sciences; National Research Council: Standards for Cardiopulmonary Resuscitation and Emergency Cardiac Care. May 1973.

Barach, A. L., and Segal, M. S.: The Indiscriminate Use of IPPB. *Journal of the American Medical Association, 231*:1141, 1975.

Burgin, W. W. J.: Respirator Therapy: What it Can and Cannot Do. *Consultant, 15*:50, 1975.

Chernick, V.: Continuous Negative Chest Wall Pressure Therapy for Hyaline Membrane Disease. *Pediatric Clinics of North America, 20*:407, 1973.

Daily, W. J. R., and Smith, P. C.: Mechanical Ventilation of Newborn Infants. Part I. *Anesthesiology, 34*:132–138, 1971.

Davis, N. J.: In Consultation: Seconds to Clear a Blocked Trachea. *Medical World News, 16*:21: 45–54, 1975.

Downs, J. J., Fulgencio, T., Raphaely, R. D.: Acute Respiratory Failure in Infants and Children. *Pediatric Clinics of North America, 19*:423, 1972.

Gellis, S. S., and Kagan, B. M. (Eds.): *Current Pediatric Therapy.* 7th Edition, W. B. Saunders Co., Philadelphia, 1976.

Goddard, R. F.: *Inhalation Therapy for Infants and Children.* Lovelace Foundation for Medical Education and Research, Albuquerque, New Mexico, 1968.

Heimlich, H. J.: Lifesaving Maneuver to Prevent Food Choking. *Journal of the American Medical Association, 234*:415, 1975.

Heimlich, H. J., Hoffman, K. A., and Canestri, F. R.: Food Choking and Drowning Deaths Prevented by External Subdiaphragmatic Compression: Physiological Basis. *Annals Thoracic Surgery.* In press.

Hodson, A., and Chernick, V.: Respiratory Emergency in Infants. *Hospital Medicine, 5*:18, 1969.

Husinger, D., Lisnerski, K., Maurizi, J., and Phillips, M.: *Respiratory Technology: A Procedure Manual.* Reston Publishing Co., Reston, Virginia, 1973.

Kempe, H., Silver, H., and O'Brien, D.: *Current Pediatric Diagnosis and Treatment.* 3rd Edition, Lange Medical Publishing Co., Los Altos, California, 1974.

Klaus, M. H., and Fanaroff, A. A.: *Care of High-Risk Neonate.* W. B. Saunders Co., Philadelphia, 1973.

Marlow, D.: *Textbook of Pediatric Nursing.* 4th Edition, W. B. Saunders Co., Philadelphia, 1973.

Marvin, J., Teefy, I., and Johnson, J.: The Integumentary System. *In* Scipien, G., et al. (Eds.): *Comprehensive Pediatric Nursing,* McGraw-Hill, New York, 1975.

Northway, W. H., Jr., Rosan, R. C., and Porter, D. Y.: Pulmonary Disease Following Respirator Therapy for Hyaline Membrane Disease: Bronchopulmonary Dysplasia. *New England Journal of Medicine, 276*:347, 1967.

Shapter, R. K. (Ed.): Cardio-Pulmonary Resuscitation: Basic Life Support. CIBA *Clinical Symposia, 26*:5, 1974.

Slonim, N., Schneider, S., Weng, T., and Fields, L.: *Pediatric Respiratory Therapy.* McGraw-Hill, New York, 1975.

Vaughn, V. C., III, and McKay, R. J.: *Nelson Textbook of Pediatrics.* 10th Edition, W. B. Saunders Co., Philadelphia, 1975.

Visintine, R. E., and Baick, C. H.: Ruptured Stomach after Heimlich Maneuver. *Journal of the American Medical Association, 234*:415, 1975.

Zwillich, C. W., Petty, T. L., Nett, L. M., and Schatz, M. E.: How to Reduce The Complications of Assisted Ventilation. *Modern Medicine, 3*:52, 1975.

Conference on Pediatric Research. *Problems of Neonatal Intensive Care Units.* Ross Laboratories, Columbus, Ohio, 1969.

Debate Over First-Aid For Food Choking: Squeeze or Tweeze. *Medical World News, 15*:14–15, 1974.

Guide to Diagnosis and Management of Cystic Fibrosis. National Cystic Fibrosis Research Foundation, Atlanta, Georgia, 1971.

Proceedings, Annual Medical Symposium on Current Pediatric Therapy, Variety Children's Hospital, Miami, Florida, 1976.

Proceedings, XIII International Congress of Pediatrics, Vienna, Austria, 1971.

PRODUCT REFERENCES

Bennett Respirator Products (A Subsidiary of Puritan-Bennett), Lenexa, Kansas: MA-I respirator.
Bird Corporation, Palm Springs, California: BABYbird ventilator.
Diffusan Dressinet Bandage System, Woodmere, New York: Dressinet.
Neward Enterprises, Inc., Cucamonga, California: Throat-E-Vac.
Ohio Chemical & Surgical Equipment Co. (A Division of Air Reduction Co., Inc.), Madison, Wisconsin: Kreiselman resuscitator, portable resuscitator.

Chapter Sixteen

OXYGEN THERAPY FOR INFANTS AND CHILDREN

PRINCIPLES

If the oxygen supply to the cerebrum is diminished, irreversible brain damage may result.

Oxygen supports combustion. Oils ignite readily in the presence of high oxygen concentrations. Blankets made from wool and some synthetic fibers are not desirable when oxygen therapy is used because of the hazards resulting from static electricity.

Interruption of oxygen therapy may result in the return of the symptoms of anoxia, defeating the goals of therapy.

The specific dosage and concentration of oxygen must be ordered by the doctor. The concentration of oxygen administered is of more importance than the liter flow per minute.

NURSING RESPONSIBILITIES

The nurse must be alert for symptoms of anoxia which include:
1. Increased pulse rate
2. Rapid, shallow respiration
3. Flaring of the nares
4. Cyanosis
5. Restlessness
6. Substernal or intercostal retraction

Electrical equipment must not be used when oxygen therapy is in progress. Alcohol or oil must not be used on a child in an oxygen tent. The nurse's hands must be free of oil when she is adjusting the oxygen regulator. Cotton blankets should be used to provide warmth for a child in an oxygen tent.

The source of the oxygen supply must be checked and replaced as necessary. Canopies should be tucked securely under the mattress, and all zippers kept closed. Nursing care should be provided in such a way that interruption of therapy is minimal.

The nurse must accurately record the concentration of oxygen, the duration of therapy, and the response of the child. (The analysis of oxygen concentration is discussed on page 112.)

159

An increased carbon dioxide content in the inspired air will stimulate the respiratory center in the medulla and cause harmful effects. Exhaled air contains a high concentration of carbon dioxide.

Since most oxygen tent canopies are permeable to carbon dioxide, tucking the canopy under the mattress prevents oxygen loss but allows the escape of carbon dioxide. The force of the oxygen entering the tent also aids in the dissipation of carbon dioxide. Most oxygen masks have built-in valves to assure the release of carbon dioxide in exhaled air. Carbon dioxide analyzers are available in some hospitals.

A cooled, supersaturated, aerated mist provides relief and comfort in respiratory ailments. The humidity tent provides a mist of the proper particle size to hydrate the entire respiratory tract.

When a high humidity is used, condensation within the tent may be anticipated. Proper use of the damper valve will reduce the condensation. The infant's clothing and bed linen must be changed frequently to prevent chilling.

Routine care including suctioning to maintain a patent airway is essential when caring for an infant who is receiving oxygen and humidity therapy.

The response to therapy, including the vital signs, evidence of respiratory distress, or a cough should be noted, reported, and recorded.

Proper cleaning and storage of the humidity tent after use will prevent cross-contamination and preserve the unit.

The ice tank, atomizer assembly, and drain hose may be sterilized in the autoclave after use. The canopy should be washed with soap and water and stored in a cool location.

TECHNIQUES

The nurse must be familiar with the mechanics of oxygen tanks, regulators, canopies, and tents. She should know how to analyze the oxygen concentration within the tent (see page 112) and how to clean and store the equipment so that the parts may be preserved. The nurse is responsible for maintaining the desired oxygen concentration, temperature, and humidity level within the oxygen tent.

I. The Croupette Humidity Tent

The Croupette humidity tent provides an atmosphere of increased oxygen and humidity, and is often used for infants and young children. It is a portable unit that may be assembled quickly in cases of emergency. The clear plastic canopy facilitates the nursing observations that are essential when caring for an infant or young child with respiratory problems.

Note that all working parts of this unit (illustrated in Fig. 16–2) are *outside* the canopy, out of the child's reach. Pillows or bed linen at the top of the bed should not occlude the air vents of the humidity tent. The parts are indicated as follows:

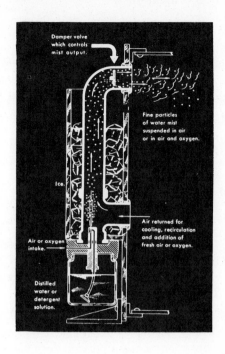

FIGURE 16–1. How the Croupette Humidity Tent Works (Courtesy of Air-Shields, Inc.) The diagram at right illustrates the mechanical principles of the Croupette humidity test. This unit provides 45 to 60 per cent oxygen concentrations and a high humidity level.

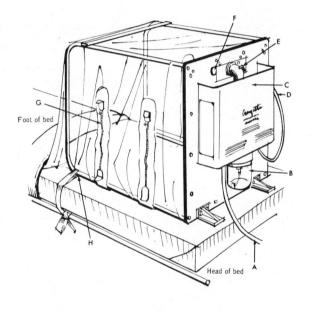

FIGURE 16–2. The Croupette Humidity Tent.

Tubing (A).   This tubing is connected to the primary oxygen source.

Jar (B).   This jar, containing distilled water, is filled to the level indicated by a black line. It requires refilling every 8 hours. To refill, remove the jar by rotating it to unscrew it from the cap. Empty the jar and wash before refilling to prevent growth of organisms.

Trough (C).   The trough is filled with cracked ice and water to a depth of 10 inches. (The level is indicated by a line.)

Drainage tubing (D).   This tubing, which is connected to the trough, should be kept elevated in the notch provided unless drainage from the trough is desired. To drain the trough, lower the tubing into a sink or receptacle.

Damper valve (E).   The damper valve should be turned one fourth open, left open for a few minutes, and then closed to minimize condensation.

Nebulizer outlet (F).   The glass nebulizer containing Alevaire or an antibiotic aerosol may be attached to this outlet, with the tubing connected to a *second* oxygen source.

Canopy zipper (G).   There are two zippers on each side of the canopy to facilitate the care of the infant with minimal interruption of therapy.

Metal frame (H).   The metal frame on which the canopy rests may be tied to the bedspring to prevent the collapse of the unit.

II. The Nebulizer

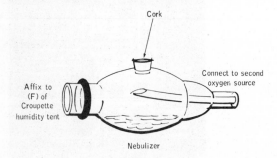

FIGURE 16–3.   The Nebulizer.

The nebulizer may be filled with Alevaire or another prescribed aerosol and attached to the Croupette humidity tent as shown in Figure 16–4. The nurse inserts the neubulizer into the neubulizer outlet of the humidity tent. Oxygen flowing through it will produce a fine mist within the tent. The nebulizer may be refilled when necessary by removing the cork at the top of the glass section.(See. Fig. 16–3.)

When a humidity tent is prescribed, the nurse should check the tent and the accessories. A plastic canopy with cracks or tears should not be used. The unit may be assembled and placed at the head of the child's crib. A rubber sheet covered with a quilted pad may be placed at the head of the bed. The metal frame of the humidity tent is

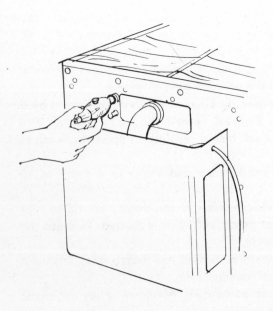

FIGURE 16–4.   Use of the Nebulizer.

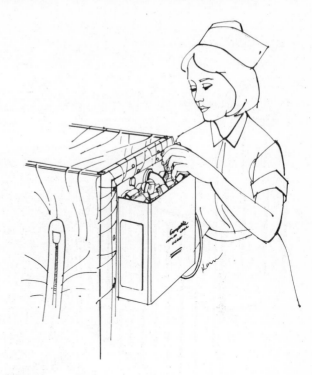

FIGURE 16–5. Placing Ice in the Trough The nurse places cracked ice in the trough of the Croupette humidity tent. The ice is replenished as needed, and water may be removed from the trough through the tubing (Fig. 16–2 D).

secured with gauze to the bedspring under the mattress to prevent the collapse of the canopy. Ice is placed in the trough to the level indicated. The tent should be flooded with oxygen before the infant is placed in the unit. An infant in an oxygen tent should be warmly covered with a cotton blanket. A small towel or a gown with a hood may be placed around his head to prevent chilling and protect the infant from condensation. When high humidity is used, his clothing and bed linen must be changed frequently to prevent chilling. The canopy is tucked under the metal frame of the humidity tent and the excess tucked loosely under the mattress and sealed with a folded drawsheet to prevent the loss of oxygen and allow the escape of carbon dioxide. The temperature within the tent should be 6 to 8 degrees below room temperature. The oxygen liter flow and the concentration of oxygen within the tent should be checked at frequent intervals (see p. 112).

When bathing the child or changing the bed linen, it may be desirable to tuck the canopy around the child's neck, securing it under the quilted pad or pillow, to prevent interruption of the therapy during nursing care.

III.   The Child-Adult-Mist (CAM) Tent

The CAM tent is designed to operate at a comfortable temperature below room temperature. The refrigeration unit may tend to cycle off and on during use; this is normal.

Position the refrigeration unit near the bedside. Make certain that the rear of the refrigeration unit is at least 6 inches from the bed or wall to allow heat from the condenser coils at the rear of the unit to dissipate. Position the semipermanent plastic canopy shown in Figure 16–6 so the vertical zipper aligns with the nebulizer for access. Tuck the plastic under the mattress on both sides and at the head.

The condensate reservoir located at the rear of the power unit should be emptied

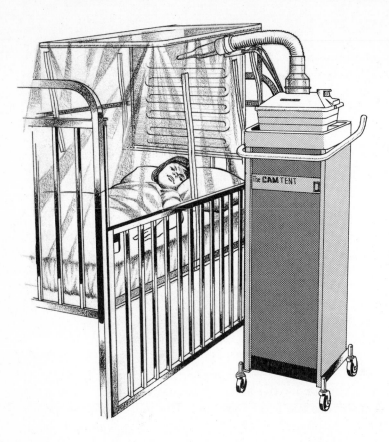

FIGURE 16–6. The CAM Tent The CAM Tent in use with electronic nebulizer. It is an automatic mist tent cooled without ice. The frame is supported by legs positioned underneath the mattress, leaving the crib unobstructed by supports. The heat generated by the patient is absorbed by the panel, maintaining a pleasant atmosphere within the tent. (CAM Tent is a trademark of the Mist-O_2-Gen Equipment Company)

every 8 to 12 hours of operation. The circulating distilled water need only be replaced if it becomes discolored or has foreign material in it. Otherwise, if the tent is in continuous use, the coolant water should be changed every 30 days.

The frame and "cool-X-changer" assemblies should be thoroughly washed after use, dried, sterilized by autoclave if desired, and placed in storage on the refrigeration unit. The residual water left in the "cool-X-changer" should be blown out with air or oxygen if the equipment is to be stored without use for more than one week.

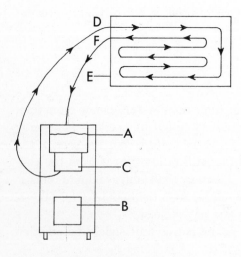

FIGURE 16–7. How CAM Operates To start operation fill tank (*A*) with approximately 1 gallon of distilled water. Plug in the electrical cord to a proper AC outlet and push the switch on the front panel "on." If the circulating fluid does not pump immediately, it indicates an air lock in the pump. This can be overcome by cycling the on-off switch three or four times at 10 second intervals. Refrigeration unit (*B*) chills this water. Pump (*C*) circulates this chilled water first through the line (*D*), through the channels of the Cool-X-Changer (*E*), and returns the water through line (*F*) back to tank (*A*) for rechilling. This is a continuous operation.

IV. Termination of Oxygen Therapy

When oxygen therapy is terminated, it is most desirable to reduce the oxygen concentration gradually. This may be accomplished by loosening the canopy or opening the side zippers for a period of time before removing the infant from the unit. The vital signs and responses of the infant must be checked frequently to observe his response to and tolerance of normal atmospheric oxygen concentrations. Deviations in vital signs should be reported to the doctor immediately.

BIBLIOGRAPHY

Gellis, S. S., and Kagan, B. M. (Eds.): *Current Pediatric Therapy.* 7th Edition, W. B. Saunders Co., Philadelphia, 1976.

Husinger, D., Lisnerski, K., Maurizi, J., and Phillips, M.: *Respiratory Technology: A Procedure Manual.* Reston Publishing Co., Reston, Virginia, 1973.

Marlow, D.: *Textbook of Pediatric Nursing.* 4th Edition, W. B. Saunders Co., Philadelphia, 1973.

Shirkey, H. C. (Ed.): *Pediatric Therapy.* 5th Edition, The C. V. Mosby Co., St. Louis, 1975.

Vaughn, V. C., and McKay, R. J.: *Nelson Textbook of Pediatrics.* 10th Edition, W. B. Saunders Co., Philadelphia, 1975.

Pediatric Group Gives Rules on Oxygen Use for Newborns. *Medical Tribune, 12*:8, 1971.

PRODUCT REFERENCES

Air-Shields, Inc. (A Division of National Aeronautical Corp.), Hatboro, Pennsylvania: Croupette humidity tent.

Mistogen Equipment Co., Oakland, California: CAM tent.

Chapter Seventeen

TRACHEOTOMY CARE FOR INFANTS AND CHILDREN

PRINCIPLES

A tracheotomy provides a patent airway via a surgical opening of the trachea.

Normally, air is filtered, warmed, and moistened in the nose and mouth. When the nose and mouth are bypassed, as in a tracheostomy, moisture and warmth must be added to the environment.

Dry gas of any composition should never be administered to a tracheotomy patient.

A continuous ultrasonic nebulizer should never be used in infants and children because of the complication of rapid water intoxication.

In pediatrics, there is no "standard size" tracheotomy tube. The size selected for use by the doctor is based upon the size of the trachea.

Small amounts of secretion or the formation of a crust can occlude the lumen of an infant tracheotomy tube. Drugs such as atropine and opiates are contraindicated, as the effects of drying secretions and depressing the cough reflex are undesirable.

NURSING RESPONSIBILITIES

The use of an artificial patent airway as a lifesaving measure depends directly upon nursing care for its success.

The room temperature should be maintained at approximately 80°F. Atomizers, masks, nebulizers, and steam are vital aids in the care of a tracheotomized child.

Inspired gas should be near body temperature and saturated with water vapor.

Water used in a nebulizer or humidifier should be sterile, and silver nitrate should be added to the reservoir.

The nurse must be aware of the diameter of the lumen of the tracheotomy tube. She must select a suction catheter of size that will leave sufficient space for breathing during the suctioning process (see Fig. 17–3 and Table 17–1).

The maintenance of high humidity of inspired air, frequent aspiration of secretions, and an adequate fluid intake are necessary to prevent the formation of a crust. "Alevaire" and Tergemist" are mucolytic agents that may be added to the oxygen mist. The tube should be drained frequently to prevent water droplets from accumulating in the tubing and drowning the patient.

There must be facilities available at the bedside to insure that:
1. Ventilation is maintained. Examples are:
   a. Oxygen
   b. Suction facilities
2. The tube is maintained in place. These include:
   a. Roller gauze bandage
   b. Dressing
3. The cannula is clean. Among the items needed are:
   a. Wire pipe cleaner (to reach inside lumen of tube)
   b. Medicine dropper and saline (to aid in loosening secretions in outer cannula)
   c. Peroxide or sodium bicarbonate (to loosen secretions in inner cannula)
   d. Emesis basin (for soaking cannula)
4. The tracheotomy tube can be replaced. Examples are:
   a. Clamp and scissors
   b. Duplicate tracheotomy tubes

The nurse must be alert to the development of symptoms of restlessness, fatigue, apathy, dyspnea, retraction, and inflammation, or bleeding around the incision. If suctioning does not relieve the symptoms, the doctor should be notified at once. Vital signs should be observed and recorded frequently.

A regular regimen of assisted coughing and postural drainage should be instituted with any child who has a tracheotomy.

The position of the child should be changed frequently.

Separate equipment should be used for nasopharyngeal suctioning.

Accidental removal of the tracheotomy tube or insertion of a foreign body into the tube will result in occlusion of the airway.

The tape around the neck that secures the outer tracheotomy tube should be tied at one side rather than at the back of the neck to avoid confusion with the tie of a bib or gown. The use of elbow restraints will prevent the child from reaching the tracheotomy tube. The nurse must prevent occlusion of the tube by linen, paper, toys, and hands.

A patent tracheotomy tube prevents the child from expressing audible sounds. The child cannot call out, and a cry cannot be heard.

Since the child is not able to express audible sounds, close observation is essential. In the case of an older child with a long-term tracheostomy, the nurse may teach the child to hold a finger over the lumen of the tube to facilitate talking.

Foods and fluids can be given by mouth. A Fowler's position is most favorable during feeding.

Any cough associated with swallowing must be reported to the doctor immediately. Care should be taken to avoid occluding the lumen of the tracheotomy tube with the bib during feeding time.

Accurate recording of all observations is essential to the evaluation of progress and therapy.

The nurse should chart the time, the amount of suctioning, the consistency of the secretions removed by the suctioning, and the effects upon respiration.

TECHNIQUES

I. The Tracheotomy Tube

The tracheotomy tube comes in three noninterchangeable parts—the outer cannula, the inner cannula and the obturator. The outer cannula is secured by means of gauze tape around the neck. The inner cannula is removed periodically for cleaning and reinserted. A duplicate set of tracheotomy tubes should be kept at the bedside for emergency use.

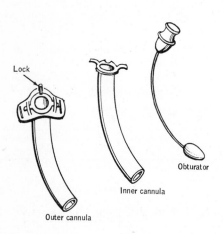

FIGURE 17–1. The Tracheotomy Tube.

The diameter of the lumen for each of the sizes of tracheotomy tubes used in pediatrics is shown in Figure 17–2. The scale shown in Table 17–1 is a guide used by the doctor in the selection of an appropriate size tracheotomy tube. The table shows the size of the suction catheter to be used for each of the different size tracheotomy tubes. Proper selection of a suction catheter will allow sufficient space for breathing during the suctioning process.

The characteristic anatomical differences between infants and adults necessitate special adaptations in the care of a tracheotomized child. For example, infants and young children have characteristically short, stubby necks. The metal lock of the tracheotomy tube can cause excoriation of the skin unless specific preventive measures

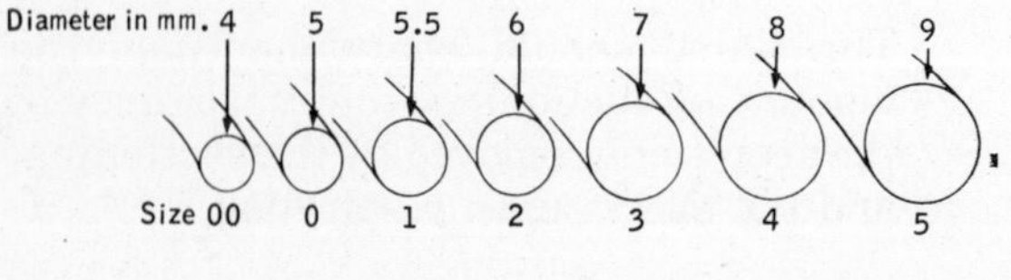

FIGURE 17–2. Diameters of Tracheotomy Tubes.

TABLE 17–1. Appropriate Sizes of Tracheotomy Tubes
and Suction Catheters

Age of Child	Size Tracheotomy Tube Selected	Maximum Size Catheter to Use for Suctioning
Newborn	00–0	8 Fr.
1 month–1 year	1	10 Fr.
1–3 years	2	12 Fr.
3–6 years	3	14 Fr.
6–12 years	4	16–18 Fr.
12 years–adult	5	18 Fr.

are taken. A small towel roll or padding placed under the shoulders of the infant will allow optimum accommodation of the trachea to the tube and prevent irritation of the skin by the metal lock. Excoriation under the chin can also be minimized by padding the chin. The use of gauze is not advisable, as loose strands of gauze may enter the tracheotomy tube and act as a foreign body.

FIGURE 17–3. The Tracheotomy Tube in Place   The dotted lines show that the tip of the tracheotomy tube lies well within the trachea. A small towel roll is in place under the shoulders. Note that the neck tape securing the outer cannula is tied at the side to prevent confusion with the ties of a gown or bib. Elbow restraints prevent the child from reaching the tracheotomy tube, and allow for minimum restriction of movements.

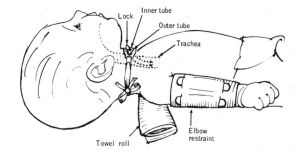

The inner cannula must be removed, inspected, and cleaned, as mucus that cannot be removed by simple suction may accumulate.

II. Removing and Reinserting the Inner Tracheotomy Tube

All equipment for cleaning the inner tracheotomy tube should be kept in readiness at the bedside.

1. Unlock the tracheotomy tube by turning the latch that holds the cannula (Fig. 17–4 *A*).

2. Grasp the inner tube and slowly remove it, using an outward and downward half-arc movement of the wrist (Fig. 17–4 *B*).

3. Clean, soak, and inspect the inner cannula.

4. Suction the outer cannula.

5. Reinsert the inner cannula while the lock is in the *unlocked* position.

6. Lock the tube in place to prevent accidental coughing out of the inner tube.

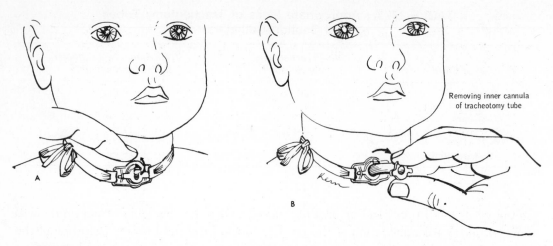

Removing inner cannula
of tracheotomy tube

FIGURE 17–4.   *A*, Unlocking Inner Cannula of Tracheotomy Tube. *B*, Removing Inner Cannula of Tracheotomy Tube.

III.   Cleaning the Inner Tracheotomy Tube

The inner tube may be soaked in a solution of peroxide or sodium bicarbonate to loosen secretions. A pipe cleaner may then be used to push the loosened secretions through the ends of the tube. The tube is then rinsed with water, soaked in Zephiran, rinsed with saline, inspected, and replaced.

IV.   Care of the Outer Cannula

While the inner cannula is soaking, the nurse may gently aspirate the outer cannula. The nurse must be sure that the size of the suction catheter is small enough to enter the lumen of the tracheotomy tube. Correct aspiration technique usually clears the airway successfully.

V.   Suction Technique

Sterile technique should be maintained during suctioning of a tracheotomized child. The use of a catheter of proper diameter relative to the lumen of the tracheotomy tube will prevent rapid aspiration of oxygen from the airway system which could cause hypoxia. (See Table 17–1, p. 169.) The ratio of the catheter size to the tube lumen should be 1:3.

1. The depth of insertion of the suction catheter should be specified by the doctor. The catheter may be inserted deep enough to stimulate coughing and suction the tracheobronchial tree.

2. Suction is applied *as the catheter is withdrawn.* Pinch the catheter as you introduce it into the outer cannula; then release and rotate the catheter as you withdraw it. The catheter must be withdrawn intermittently in order to prevent hypoxia resulting from occlusion of the airway. Repeat the procedure, allowing the child to catch his

breath in between. A drop of saline may be inserted into the outer cannula to aid in loosening secretions for more effective suctioning.

3. The catheter must be withdrawn if coughing exists, or the forced expiration against the catheter may increase the positive pressure within the chest and interfere with cardiac circulation.

It is important for the nurse to be aware that vagal stimulation can occur during suctioning and can precipitate cardiac arrest. Therefore, only nursing or medical personnel should be assigned to suction a tracheotomized child. The heart rate should be monitored during and after the suctioning procedure.

In patients who have tracheotomy tubes with inflated cuffs, the secretions accumulate above the cuff and upon deflation will descend into the lung causing atelectasis and pneumonia. To prevent this, the cuff should be deflated and positive pressure applied to the airway via the tracheostomy. This causes the secretions to be ejected over the vocal cords where they may be swallowed or suctioned from the oropharynx.

Closed Suction Technique

In the closed suction technique (Fig. 17–5) the tube is pinched off during insertion, then released, rotated, and withdrawn. The tube should be rinsed in water to remove thick, adherent secretions before reinsertion.

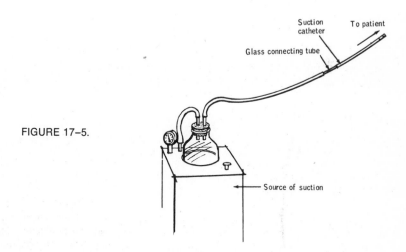

FIGURE 17–5.

Y-Tube Suction Technique

When the Y-tube suction technique (see Fig. 17–6) is used, the catheter is introduced into the tracheotomy tube, and suction is initiated by closing the Y valve with the fingertip. Gently rotate the catheter as it is withdrawn. If the catheter "grabs," intermittently release the suction by lifting the fingertip from the Y tube.

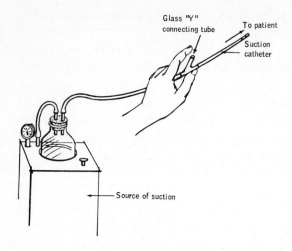

FIGURE 17–6.

Aspiration of the Tracheobronchial Tree

When deep aspiration beyond the carina is required, positioning the patient is of the utmost importance. To aspirate the left bronchus, turn the infant's head to the right and tilt the chest to the left. Reverse the patient's position for aspiration of the opposite bronchus.

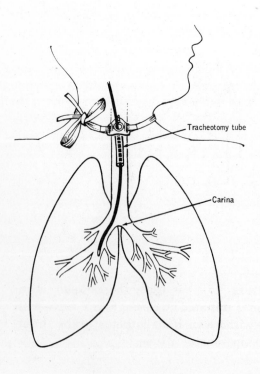

FIGURE 17–7. Suctioning the Tracheobronchial Tree When suctioning the tracheobronchial tree, the principles of general tracheotomy suctioning should be adhered to: gentle insertion, rotation, and intermittent withdrawal of the suction tube.

VI. The Tracheotomy "Nose"

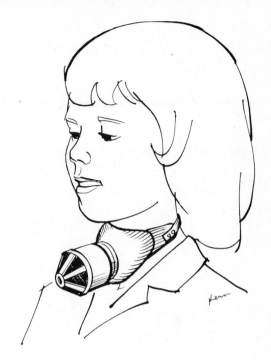

FIGURE 17–8. The Tra-Care Tracheotomy Nose (Courtesy of Oxygen Supply and Equipment Magazine) The tracheotomy nose is designed to maintain the warmth and humidity of inspired air. Mounted on a polyethylene mask, the apparatus is secured over the tracheotomy tube. It is available in infants' and children's sizes to facilitate adaptation to the contours of the throat.

VII. Weaning the Child from the Tracheotomy Tube

When the condition of the child permits, the doctor may order the tracheotomy tube to be gradually occluded. The tube is rarely removed without a test trial of oronasal respiration.

The lumen of the inner cannula is partially occluded each day until it is completely closed. Crying and anxiety may cause the child to appear to have respiratory difficulty during the adjustment or weaning phase. Psychological support is necessary. When the child tolerates a completely closed tracheotomy tube for a specified length of time, the tracheotomy tubes are removed by the doctor. A tracheotomy set should be kept available for emergency use at the bedside until the patient is ready for discharge.

BIBLIOGRAPHY

Crocker, D.: The Critically Ill Child: Management of the Tracheotomy. *Pediatrics, 46:*286–296, 1970.

Fearon, B.: Acute Obstructive Laryngitis in Infants and Children. *Hospital Medicine, 4:*51, 1968.

Gellis, S.: Factors Affecting Pediatric Endotracheal Tube Size. *Yearbook of Pediatrics,* Yearbook Medical Publishers, Chicago, 1969.

Marlow, D.: *Textbook of Pediatric Nursing.* 4th Edition, W. B. Saunders Co., Philadelphia, 1973.

Varga, C.: *Handbook of Pediatric Medical Emergencies.* 4th Edition, The C. V. Mosby Co., St. Louis, 1968.

Vaughn, V. C., and McKay, R. J.: *Nelson Textbook of Pediatrics.* 10th Edition, W. B. Saunders Co., Philadelphia, 1975.

Young, J., and Crocker, D. *Principles and Practice of Inhalation Therapy.* Yearbook Medical Publishers, Chicago, 1970.

PRODUCT REFERENCE

Oxygen Equipment Co., Chicago, Illinois: Tra-Care tracheotomy nose.

Chapter Eighteen

ADMINISTRATION OF MEDICATIONS TO INFANTS AND CHILDREN

PRINCIPLES

I. Computing Dosages

A standard dosage is nonexistent in the pediatric unit, as the dosage varies with the age, weight, and body surface area of the infant.

Most drug companies supply medications in a standard adult-dosage strength.

Since the pediatric dosage is often small, a slight mistake in the amount of a drug administered is actually a greater proportional error.

II. Identification

Accurate identification of the child is essential before a drug is administered.

The infant cannot give his name, and the

NURSING RESPONSIBILITIES

Although the doctor prescribes the dosage of a medication, it is the nurse's responsibility to know the safe dosage range of any medication she administers to children. If the dosage of a drug or infusion prescribed appears to be excessive for the individual infant, the doctor must be consulted. The nursing supervisor is also available for consultation when the nurse is in doubt.

Accuracy in computing, measuring, and administering dosage is essential in pediatric drug administration.

Before a medicine ticket is written or a drug administered, the nurse must calculate the safe dosage range for the individual child and compare it with the dosage prescribed.

The nurse should check the child's identification band and the bed card with the name on the medicine ticket before administering any medication.

child is likely to be playful and state a nickname or the name of another child he is friendly with.

III. Carrying out Orders

Clear, specific medication orders will reduce the possibility of error in drug administration.

Many medications have a cumulative effect in the body and may cause harm if administered over a prolonged period of time.

Medicine cards should be written for each individual child according to the written orders of the doctor.

The nurse should check the medicine cards daily and place those cards requiring renewal of the order in a specially designated area. The doctor should be notified when a medication must be reordered.

IV. Drug Interactions

Very often, more than one drug is administered to a child at one time. One drug may work synergistically with the other or it may diminish, abolish, or potentiate the effect of the other drug.

An understanding of mechanisms that produce drug interactions may help the nurse anticipate and prevent drug therapy problems, and therefore increase effectiveness of drug therapy to the individual child.

The nurse must be aware of all the medications the child is receiving, not only the medication she administers during her contact with the child. The nurse must be alert to drug-drug interactions, drug-food interactions, and drug-patient (allergic) interactions.

The nurse must understand the physiological reason for administering specific drugs before, during, after, or between meals and not adhere to "routine" medication hours.

V. Administering Oral Medications

The nurse should give all medications in a way that helps her establish a constructive relationship with the child.

A positive, kind, but firm approach will meet with more success than threats or bribes.

Medications should be made as palatable as possible. If medications are mixed with a food, the child may develop a dislike for that food.

A child should be praised when he cooperates in taking a medication, but he should also be allowed to express his fears.

The nurse should approach a child as if she expected him to take the medication without difficulty.

Most oral medications may be mixed with a simple syrup to make the taste more pleasant. Pills may be crushed, dissolved in water, and mixed with a simple syrup.

VI. Cultural Aspects of Pediatric Pharmacology

Prescribed as well as nonprescribed medication taken by the child must be con-

The nurse should always take a detailed history of drugs given to the child within

sidered together because they constitute a continuum, under which interaction of the drugs, toxic responses, and responses of the child will be affected.

24 to 48 hours prior to admission, including vitamins and aspirin. The nurse should check during visiting hours that parents are not bringing home medications or "cultural remedies" for their child and continuing self-medication habits in the hospital setting. Strengthening doctor-parent-nurse relationships can prevent this self-medication activity.

VII. Intramuscular Injections

The quadriceps muscle of the mid-anterior thigh is the site of choice for intramuscular injections in young infants.

The technique of injection is the same as for adults. (The needle is inserted at a 45° angle with the needle pointed down toward the knee, and care is taken to insure that the needle does not enter a vein.)

When the buttocks are used, the injection should fall in the upper outer quadrant of the buttock.

Injection sites should be rotated.

All procedures should be explained to the child whenever possible. Participation in the procedure nurtures cooperation.

Injections should be given as quickly as possible to avoid prolonging a fear-provoking experience. Older children may assist in the procedure by cleansing the area for the injection.

Adequate restraint of the infant or child is necessary in order to assure safe and correct administration of intramuscular injections.

The need for another person to assist in the restraint of the child depends upon the technique used and the size and strength of the child.

The nurse should re-establish the nurse-child relationship after painful therapy.

The nurse should hold and comfort the infant following the injection.

VIII. Instilling Nose Drops

Most nose drops act as vasoconstrictors and their excessive use may be harmful.

Nose drops should be discontinued after 72 hours unless they are reordered by the doctor.

A congested nose will impair the infant's sucking ability.

Nose drops should be instilled 20 minutes prior to feedings. The nose should be gently suctioned prior to administering nose drops.

IX. Instilling Ear Drops

The shape of the auditory canal in infants and young children differs from that in the adult.

Hold the pinna of the ear slightly down and straight back to facilitate the instillation of ear drops in children under three years of age. Hold the pinna of the ear up and back for older children and adults.

X. Intravenous Therapy

An infant depletes his extracellular fluid reserve more rapidly than an adult.

The nurse must observe and report symptoms of excessive fluid loss in infants. These include:
1. Sunken fontanels
2. Sunken eyes
3. Poor skin turgor
4. Dryness of the mouth
5. Loss of weight
6. Concentrated urine

Site of Venipuncture

Since infants do not have large veins at the antecubital fossa, a scalp vein is the site frequently chosen for infusions.

The nurse must shave the scalp at the site for injection and adequately restrain the infant's body and head. (See pages 63 to 70.)

Rate of Flow

The rate of flow of the intravenous solution should be specified by the doctor. An excessively fast infusion rate may precipitate cardiac failure.

Special pediatric scalp-vein sets and pediatric intravenous tubing should be available in the unit. The desired rate of flow should be established and checked frequently.

A patient's venous pressure is not constant. As venous pressure increases, the flow rate of a gravity infusion will decrease.

The child who coughs, sneezes, cries, rolls over, or sits up may need the I.V. flow rate adjusted.

Addition of Supplementary Medication

When a needle pierces the wall of the intravenous tubing, air may be introduced into the veins and results in an embolism.

Supplementary medication should be added:
1. Directly into the bottle
2. Using a stopcock set-up
3. Using Y-tube equipment
4. Using specially equipped intravenous tubing.

Certain medications may cause untoward reactions when added to specific intravenous solutions.

Supplementary medications should not be added to intravenous solutions containing protein.

Recording

Since intravenous therapy can cause a circulatory overload and precipitate cardiac failure, careful observation and accurate recording are essential.

A 24-hour intake and output record must be kept for all infants receiving intravenous therapy. The intake and output record may be kept at the bedside, and all personnel instructed to use it. The records should then be affixed to the infant's chart.

Terminating Infusions

Before the needle is removed from the vein, the flow should be stopped so that the fluid will not enter subcutaneous tissues.

When the infusion reaches the 100 cc. level, the nurse should check with the doctor for further orders before discontinuing intravenous therapy.

Precautions

The administration of too much or too little fluid or electrolytes will produce clinical symptoms that are observable.

The nurse should closely observe any infant receiving intravenous therapy and accurately report and record her observations in the nurse's notes on the chart.

Morphine and barbiturates stimulate the posterior pituitary gland to secrete antidiuretic hormone regardless of the body's need for water elimination. Therefore, tolerance to intravenous fluids will be altered.

The nurse should report to the doctor that an infant is receiving barbiturates or morphine preparations or both before initiating intravenous therapy.

A transfusion of whole blood will clump when it comes in contact with a solution containing calcium.

Whole blood should not be administered through tubing that has carried any solution other than normal saline.

The longer the I.V. set is in use, the greater the chances for contact with harmful bacteria. The number of bacteria contaminating I.V. solutions will increase with time.

I.V. tubing should be changed every 24 hours. For a 24-hour "keep-open" I.V., a 250 ml. bottle should be used to help assure that the bottle will not be used for longer than that period. The date the bottle was started should be noted on the bottle.

Drop size can vary between types of I.V. sets. Most regular sets deliver 15 drops per milliliter, microdrip pediatric sets deliver 60 drops per milliliter, and blood administration sets deliver 10 drops per milliliter.

The nurse should select the I.V. set most suitable for the pediatric patient with consideration of the medicinal additives and the viscosity of the fluid.

XI. Parenteral Hyperalimentation

A high rate of blood flow is necessary to dilute the highly hypertonic solution used in total parenteral nutrition.

The solution must be administered slowly and continuously into a central vein. A peristaltic pump maintains a continuous flow without risking infection.

The chemical composition of the infusate formula makes it an excellent culture medium for microorganisms.

The solution used for parenteral nutrition should be prepared by a pharmacist; it should be sterile, and test cultures should be made. The solution should be stored at 4° C. for no longer than 72 hours after preparation. The solution may be warmed one hour prior to administration.

TECHNIQUES

I. Calculating Safe Drug Dosage

The selection of the technique used to calculate the safe dosage range for the individual child is based upon available information concerning the age or weight of the child.

$$\frac{\text{Average adult dose} \times \text{weight of child in pounds}}{150} = \text{Safe dosage range for individual child}$$

> *Example:* Aspirin, gr. 1 is ordered for a 1-year-old child who weighs 21 pounds.

$$\frac{10 \text{ gr. (average adult dose)} \times 21 \text{ (weight in pounds)}}{150} = 1\tfrac{2}{5} \text{ gr.}$$

> *Conclusion:* The medication dosage prescribed cannot be considered an overdose and is in the safe dosage range for this child.

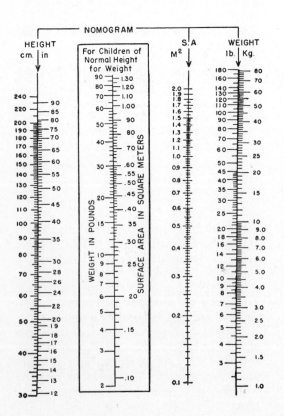

FIGURE 18–1. Nomogram for estimation of surface area. The surface area is indicated where a straight line which connects the height and weight levels intersects the surface area column; or if the patient is roughly of average size, from the weight alone (enclosed area). (Nomogram modified from data of E. Boyd by C. D. West.) Courtesy of the Commonwealth Fund and Harvard University Press.

The Nomogram

Many physiological reactions are closely related to body surface area. The "average adult dose" is prescribed for a patient weighing 140 pounds with a body surface area of 1.7 sq. meters.

Surface area rule:

$$\frac{\text{Surface area of child (in sq. meters)}}{1.7} \times \text{adult dose} = \text{safe dosage for individual child}$$

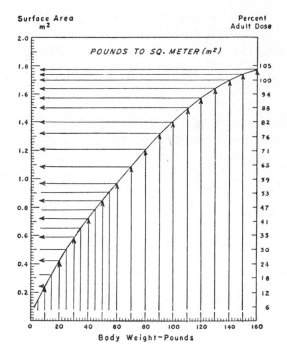

FIGURE 18–2.   Relations between body weight in pounds, body surface area, and adult dosage. The surface area values correspond to those set forth previously (Crawford et al., 1910). Note that the 100 per cent adult dose is for a patient weighing about 140 pounds and having a surface area of about 1.7 square meters. (From N. B. Talbot et al.: Metabolic Homeostasis—A Syllabus for Those Concerned with the Care of Patients. Cambridge, Harvard University Press, 1959.)

Determining drug dosage according to body size is only one aspect of pediatric pharmacology. The nurse must keep in mind some other factors affecting the response of the infant or child to drug therapy. Factors determining the pharmacological effects of a drug are the properties of the drug, the physiology of the patient, absorption, distribution, metabolism, and excretion.

Distribution of a drug in the body is somewhat dependent upon its retention. The retention of a drug in the body is dependent upon the plasma protein–binding capacity. Newborns have low concentrations of plasma proteins, and therefore, drug responses are altered. Local blood flow, integrity of membrane barriers, and the water and protein content of tissues affect distribution and excretion of a drug in the body. These factors vary in the developing newborn and infant physiology, and therefore, drug distribution and excretion will be affected. In some instances, after multiple doses of a drug, instead of reaching a plateau level in the body, levels increase to the point of toxicity owing to the immaturity of drug transport and reaction mechanisms.

The effects of a drug on infants and children can best be determined by the patient's responses. It is therefore essential for the nurse to:

1. Understand the purpose of the drug and assess changes in the patient such as lowering of body temperature in cases of hyperpyrexia.

2. Check, evaluate, and report laboratory reports promptly.

3. Know and observe for toxic effects of drugs used.

II. Carrying out the Doctor's Order

A medicine card should be written for each child. The information on the medicine card should include:

1. The unit
2. Date medication was ordered
3. Full name of child to receive medication
4. Name of medication to be administered
5. Dosage of medication prescribed by doctor
6. Amount of medication necessary to provide this dosage
7. Route of administration
8. Time and frequency of administration
9. Name of/doctor ordering drug
10. Name of nurse carrying out order

Unit Date	Ward 4N 6/1/65
Name of child	Jones, John
Medication	Atarax Suspension
Dosage	5 mg.
Amount	½ tsp.
Route of administration Hours of administration	T. I. D. 9-1-5
Doctor Nurse	Dr. Bing J. Doe

FIGURE 18–3. Sample Medicine Card.

III. Limitations and Regulations

A special box for medicine cards which require a new doctor's order should be placed at the head nurse's desk. The doctor will reorder the medications he wishes to be continued. As a general rule:

1. Narcotic medication orders should be effective for a 72-hour period only.
2. Antibiotic medication orders should be effective for a 3-day period only.
3. All other medication orders should be effective for a 1-week period only.

IV. Drug Interactions

Drug-Food Interactions

The nurse should be aware that interactions of some drugs with certain foods may create an undesirable response. The following are some examples of drug-food interactions:

Tetracycline. Tetracycline, when taken with an antacid or any calcium-containing foods, such as dairy products, can be rendered ineffective as its absorption will be blocked.

MAO inhibitors. Patients who are taking MAO inhibitors should not eat the following foods to avoid a dangerous rise in blood pressure which may result in a stroke: chicken liver, banana, yogurt, pickled herring, avocado, sour cream, canned figs, aged cheese, beer, soy sauce, raisins, cola. Some examples of MAO inhibitors include: Nardil (phenelzine dihydrogen sulfate); Parnate (tranylcypromine sulfate); Marplan (isocarboxazid); and Aventyl (nortriptyline hydrochloride).

Saccharin. A cross-reaction may occur between saccharin, which is a sulfonamide, and oral sulfonamides, oral antidiabetics, antihypertensives, and diuretics. Saccharin may be found in the diet as a sugar substitute in diet beverages, candies, and foods.

Salicylates. A high salicyclate ingestion level can result from a patient taking many of the following, each of which contains a significant amount of salicylates:

aspirin	apples	nectarines
Coricidin	apricots	oranges
chewing gum	cherries	peaches
lozenges	currants	raisins
almonds	grapes	prunes
wines	strawberries	wine vinegars

Vitamin C. Vitamin C is taken by a number of patients at home to prevent and treat the common cold. Often, parents purchase large bottles for family use. The nurse should discuss this practice with the parents, keeping in mind:

1. Vitamin C destroys the vitamin B_{12} content in foods when taken within an hour of meals. Large doses of vitamin C can inhibit body utilization of vitamin B_{12}.

2. Vitamin C decomposes upon exposure to air into a product that can cause urinary infections. Therefore, the larger the bottle purchased, the more air contact each time the bottle is opened and the greater the chance of producing illness in a family member.

Drug-Drug Interactions

The following is a selected list of drugs commonly used in pediatrics that may interact with other drugs or may have specific precautions or nursing responsibilities involved in their use. The nurse should be alert to the interactions of any drugs she may administer to a patient.

Caffeine sodium benzoate. This drug, injected into a jaundiced infant, can uncouple the bilirubin-albumin, causing kernicterus.

Piperazine. This drug is contraindicated in children with epilepsy.

Povan. This drug is contraindicated in the aspirin-sensitive patient.

Clindamycin. This drug should not be administered with erythromycins.

Kanamycin.   This drug should not be used with potent diuretics.

Neomycin.   Do not administer with potent diuretics; discontinue for tinnitus; perform audiometry twice a week during use.

Ampicillin.   When given parenterally, use within one hour of reconstitution. Do not use in prolonged I.V. drip, as it loses at least 10 per cent potency within four hours. Reconstitute in normal saline, never with 5 per cent dextrose in water.

Penicillin G.   Each million units of potassium penicillin G yields 1.68 mEq. potassium (65.8 mg.). Each million units of sodium penicillin G yields 1.68 mEq. sodium (38.7 mg.). Children with renal or cardiac problems need these electrolytes monitored.

Polymyxin E, colistin sulfate.   Use with care in children with renal impairment. Facilities for treatment of respiratory arrest must be available.

Tetracycline.   Use of this drug during the last half of pregnancy, or in the child up to 8 years of age can cause permanent discoloration of teeth.

Griseofulvin.   Barbiturates depress the potency of this drug. Patients receiving this drug should avoid direct and prolonged exposure to sunlight.

Romilar (Dextromethorphan).   Do not mix with penicillins, tetracyclines, salicylates, or sodium phenobarbital.

Dulcolax.   Caution patients not to chew tablets—they must be swallowed whole.

Magnesium sulfate (Epsom salts).   Keep calcium gluconate ready for use. Monitor blood pressure of patients receiving this drug.

Paraldehyde.   Discard bottles open more than 24 hours. Avoid plastic containers; use glass. The oral route is irritating. This drug should be diluted and flavored.

Digoxin preparations.   Interaction with potassium diuretics such as Hygroton or Lasix may cause digoxin toxicity. Electrolytes should be monitored. Barbiturates, Tanderil, or Dilantin may decrease potency of digoxin. Calcium salts, Isuprel, Adrenalin, or ephedrine, when given with digoxin, can cause problems in cardiac rhythm.

Antidiarrheal mixtures.   This type of medication is meant to adsorb toxic substances responsible for diarrhea. It can also adsorb medications administered concurrently and render them ineffective.

Antacids.   They raise the pH of the stomach and may interfere with the absorption of acidic drugs such as aspirin, penicillin, sulfonamides, and phenobarbital. They may also disintegrate the enteric coating of an irritating drug such as Dulcolax and cause nausea and vomiting.

Cathartics.   These drugs increase gastric motility and thus decrease the passage time of drugs through the G.I. tract. This can result in decreased absorption of drugs, and render ineffective the enteric coated tablet or timed-release capsules, which are designed to release chemicals slowly during normal travel time through the G.I. tract. Mineral oil will flush fat-soluble vitamins from the body.

Sulfonamides and salicylates.   These drugs have high protein affinity and can displace bilirubin from its albumin binding sites in newborns, causing jaundice. These drugs should not be used with premature or newborn infants.

Phenobarbital.   This drug is an enzyme inducer; it reduces the anticoagulant effect of coumarin and warfarin. It also increases corticosteroid metabolism and can complicate emergency treatment with steroids.

Probenecid.   Increases the blood level of penicillin by decreasing the volume of distribution as well as decreasing renal excretion.

Guanethidine and reserpine.   These drugs stimulate gastric acid secretion and may enhance the absorption of acidic drugs such as aspirin, penicillin, sulfonamides, and phenobarbital.

Allopurinol (Zyloprim).   This is a xanthine oxidase inhibitor and decreases the metabolism of 6-mercaptopurine and azathioprine. It also blocks control of iron absorption, causing hemosiderosis.

Gentamycin.   It inactivates carbenicillin in an intravenous bottle.

Polymyxin B (Aerosporin).   If given rapidly, it can cause respiratory paralysis.

Atropine or epinephrine.   These drugs can cause hyperthermia. They are neutralized in the presence of sodium bicarbonate.

Valium or phenobarbital.   These will precipitate if mixed in aqueous I.V. solution. They should be administered undiluted. They can cause respiratory arrest.

Dilantin.   This drug is not effective given intramuscularly. It will precipitate if diluted in aqueous I.V. solution and therefore should be administered undiluted.

Calcium gluconate.   This can cause sterile abscess if given intramuscularly. It precipitates if mixed with sodium bicarbonate.

Ingestion of Drugs Via Breast Milk

The following drugs, if taken by the mother while she is nursing, can affect the infant. It is a nursing responsibility to take an accurate drug history from nursing mothers.

Selected drugs and their effects on nursing infants

Drug taken by mother	*Effect on nursing infant*
Atropine	Atropine intoxication, dilated pupils, tachycardia, constipation, urinary retention.
Anticoagulants	Bleeding
Antithyroid drugs	Hypothyroidism
Antimetabolites (usually for cancer treatment)	Bone marrow depression
Cathartics	Loose stools
Radioactive preparations	Thyroid problems (nursing should be avoided for 10 days following x-ray study of mother, such as G.I. or G.B. series)
Bromides	Rash, drowsiness
Tetracycline	Discoloration of teeth
Flagyl	Anorexia, vomiting, blood dyscrasia
Steroids	Retardation of growth
Reserpine	Nasal stuffiness, lethargy, diarrhea
Sulfonamides	Kernicterus

Dilantin   Vomiting, methemoglobinemia, tremors

Aspirin   Can cause bleeding in infant
Antacids (in large doses)

Orinase   Can cause brain damage

Drug-Environment Interactions (Phototoxic Drugs)

The following list of commonly used drugs can cause skin reactions, such as severe sunburn, or allergic reactions, such as eczematous papules, when the child is exposed to the sun. Parents should be counseled accordingly, especially in warm climates or seasons when extensive exposure to the sun is likely.

Dilantin	Tetracyclines	Estrogen
Orinase	NegGram	Progesterones
Benadryl	Diuril	Librium
Phenergan	Hydrodiuril	Tofranil
Griseofulvin	Iron	Phenothiazines
Sulfonamides		Smallpox vaccine

V. Administering Oral Medications

Oral medications may be administered by the dropper method or the cup method. Older children may be capable of swallowing a pill without having it crushed and dissolved in water.

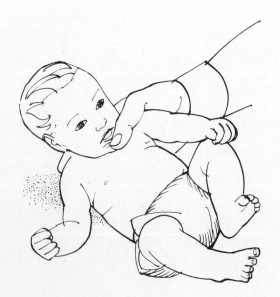

FIGURE 18-4. The Dropper Method   Depress the infant's chin with the thumb to open his mouth. The head of the infant must be elevated when oral medications are administered.

Dropper Method

The dropper method is used for infants.

1. Elevate the infant's head and depress his chin with your thumb to open his mouth.

2. Using an eyedropper, slowly drop the liquid medication on the middle of the tongue, avoiding contact between the glass of the eyedropper and the lips. Release his chin and allow the child to swallow.

3. If a rubber-tipped dropper is used, the infant may be allowed to suck and swallow the medication as it *slowly* flows into his mouth.

4. Allow the infant to swallow all the medication before returning him to his crib.

Cup Method

This method is used for toddlers and children.

1. Place the medication in a souffle cup.

2. Elevate the child's head and put the cup to his lips.

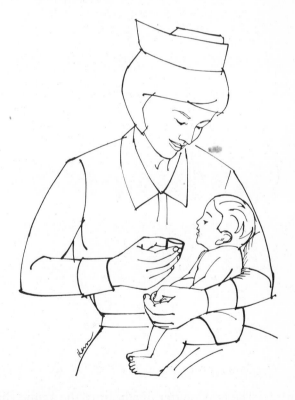

FIGURE 18–5.   The Cup Method   The nurse may hold the child on her lap and restrain his hands as shown to prevent spilling of the medication.

3. Compress the cup between your fingers and *slowly* expel the medication into the child's mouth.

4. Allow the child to competely swallow all the medication before replacing him in his crib.

5. Some toddlers and children may be able to drink from the cup independently.

VI.   Administering Intramuscular Injections

Selection of Muscle Site for Intramuscular Injection

The selection of a muscle for the site of an intramuscular injection should be based upon specific knowledge.

1. In infants and young children, the small size of the buttock and the location of the sciatic nerve lead us to avoid the gluteus muscle of the buttock and opt for the thigh or arm.

2. The nurse should also keep in mind that different muscles may significantly alter the rate of drug absorption. Studies have shown that blood flows faster through the deltoid muscle than through the gluteus, and therefore more rapid absorption of medications injected into the deltoid may be expected. Thus, the proper muscle site for injection is especially crucial in emergency settings where rapid absorption is desired. The muscle blood flow is thought to be the highest in the deltoid, medium in the vastus lateralis, and slowest in the gluteus.

Therefore, emergency drugs should be injected into the deltoid; vaccines and long acting antibiotics may be given in the thigh or gluteus muscles.

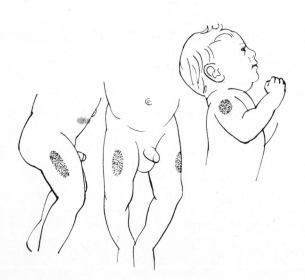

FIGURE 18–6.   Appropriate Sites for Intramuscular Injection   The blackened areas of the upper arm and thigh show appropriate sites for intramuscular injection in the young infant.

Selection of the Site When the Buttocks are Used

The upper outer quadrant of the young child's buttock is smaller in diameter than an adult's. Therefore, accuracy in determining the area comprising the upper outer quadrant in infants is essential.

1. Place your thumb on the trochanter.

2. Place your middle finger on the iliac crest.

3. Let your index finger drop at a point midway between the thumb and the middle finger and on the upper outer quadrant of the buttock.

Selection of the Site When the Thigh is Used

The anterior or lateral aspect of the thigh should be used to administer intramuscular injections to young infants.

Restraining Technique for Administering Intramuscular Injections

The technique of restraining an infant for the administration of intramuscular injections is illustrated in Figure 18–7.

1. The infant is placed on his abdomen so that he cannot use his hands to touch the needle or the injection area.

2. The nurse stands facing the foot of the crib, leans over the infant and places the *weight of her body* on her elbow *(A)*, which rests upon the *mattress (B)*. This position prevents the infant from raising the trunk of his body, but the weight of the nurse is *not* on his body.

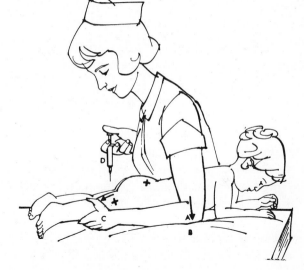

FIGURE 18–7.   Restraining a Child for the Administration of an Intramuscular Injection.

3. With the trunk of the infant now controlled, the nurse may use her free hand *(C)* to grasp the infant's knee or thigh firmly to straighten and stabilize his legs.

4. The other hand and arm is free to inject at the preselected site. The alcohol or Betadine sponge is held between the fingers of the hand holding the syringe *(D)*.

Note that the infant is close to the edge of the crib so that the nurse may gently press his hips between her forearm and her body to obtain greater stability of the hold.

VII.   The Closed Injection System

The increased use of closed injection systems has made it imperative that nurses be familiar with the basic techniques involved. One example of a closed injection system is the Tubex syringe.

The Tubex System

The Tubex system consists of two parts: (1) a disposable, sterile cartridge-needle unit, and (2) a stainless, unbreakable, reusable metal syringe. (The cartridge may be pre-filled; partly filled for mixing; or a sterile, empty unit.)

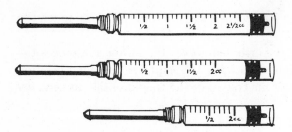

FIGURE 18-8. The Tubex Cartridge-Needle Unit The disposable, single-dose cartridge-needle units are calibrated. The needle point is imbedded in a soft gum-rubber insert within the needle sheath. The needle sheath is sealed to prevent air leakage and contamination. A popping sound will be heard when the sheath is first removed.

The nurse must read the cartridge label carefully, verify the medication order and administer the injection. Only calibrated cartridges may be used to administer fractional doses. At least two metal syringes should be available for use on each unit.

A knowledge of the basic parts is essential to the proper handling of the Tubex syringe, as it is with any precision instrument. The permanent metal syringe, illustrated in Figure 18-9, provides a comfortable weight and balance for correct injection technique.

The plunger *(A)* and rotating finger grips *(B)* are movable parts of this permanent syringe. The rotating finger grips permit one to direct the needle bevel upward for an intravenous injection. The plunger is held rigid during injections by spring tension. The cutout sides allow full visibility of calibrations on the Tubex cartridges, and the window at the needle end *(C)* shows the presence of blood during aspiration if a blood vessel has been entered. The rotating nose *(D)* of the Tubex syringe contains a slip ring which begins to turn when the cartridge is in place, preventing overtightening. The turning of the slip ring produces a clicking noise which lets the operator know the sterile cartridge-needle unit is tightened sufficiently.

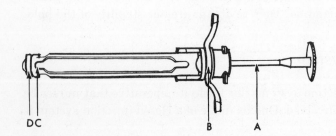

FIGURE 18-9. The Tubex Syringe.

To load the TUBEX Syringe

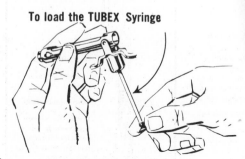

1 Grasp barrel of syringe in one hand. With the other hand, pull back firmly on plunger and swing the entire handle-section downward so that it locks at right angle to the barrel.

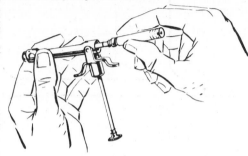

2 Insert TUBEX Sterile Cartridge-Needle Unit, needle end first, into the barrel. Engage needle ferrule by rotating it clockwise in the threads at front end of syringe.

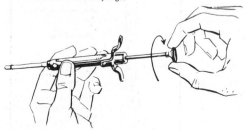

3 Swing plunger back into place and attach end to the threaded shaft of the piston. Hold the syringe barrel with one hand and rotate plunger until both ends of TUBEX Sterile Cartridge-Needle Unit are fully, but lightly, engaged. To maintain sterility, leave the rubber sheath in place until just before use. To aspirate before injecting, pull back slightly on the plunger.

To remove the empty TUBEX

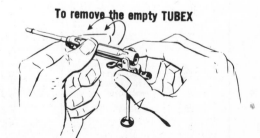

Replace sheath with a twisting motion to prevent needle from snagging. Disengage plunger from piston by rotating counterclockwise and open syringe as in step No. 1. Do not pull plunger back before disengaging or syringe will jam. Rotate TUBEX Cartridge-Needle Unit counterclockwise to disengage at front end of syringe, remove from syringe and discard.

To adapt 2-cc. syringe to 1-cc. TUBEX

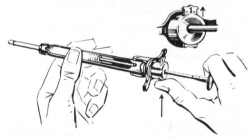

The 2-cc. syringe can be used for a 1-cc. TUBEX. Engage both ends of TUBEX and push the slide through so the number "1" appears. After use, the syringe automatically resets itself for 2-cc. TUBEX.

NOTE: Any graduated markings on TUBEX Sterile Cartridge-Needle Units are to be used as a guide in aspirating or administering measured doses.

Used TUBEX Cartridge-Needle Units should not be employed for successive injections or as multiple-dose containers. They are intended to be used only once and discarded. (Before discarding, the sheath-covered needle should be bent to seal the lumen in order to discourage pilferage or reuse.)

FIGURE 18–10. Use of the Tubex Syringe (Courtesy of Wyeth Laboratories) The method of administration is the same as with a conventional syringe. Remove the rubber sheath, introduce the needle into the patient, aspirate, and inject.

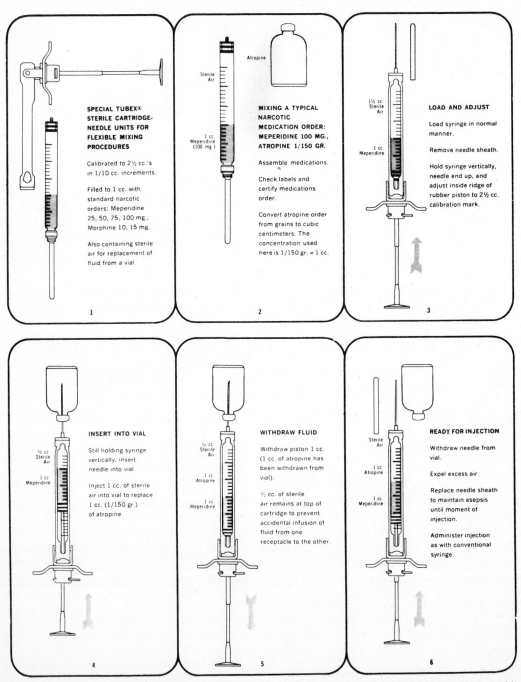

1 SPECIAL TUBEX® STERILE CARTRIDGE-NEEDLE UNITS FOR FLEXIBLE MIXING PROCEDURES

Calibrated to 2½ cc.'s in 1/10 cc. increments.

Filled to 1 cc. with standard narcotic orders: Meperidine 25, 50, 75, 100 mg.; Morphine 10, 15 mg.

Also containing sterile air for replacement of fluid from a vial.

2 MIXING A TYPICAL NARCOTIC MEDICATION ORDER: MEPERIDINE 100 MG., ATROPINE 1/150 GR.

Assemble medications.

Check labels and certify medications order.

Convert atropine order from grains to cubic centimeters. The concentration used here is 1/150 gr. = 1 cc.

Sterile Air / 1 cc Meperidine (100 mg)   Atropine

3 LOAD AND ADJUST

Load syringe in normal manner.

Remove needle sheath.

Hold syringe vertically, needle end up, and adjust inside ridge of rubber piston to 2½ cc. calibration mark.

1½ cc. Sterile Air / 1 cc. Meperidine

4 INSERT INTO VIAL

Still holding syringe vertically, insert needle into vial.

Inject 1 cc. of sterile air into vial to replace 1 cc. (1/150 gr.) of atropine.

½ cc Sterile Air / 1 cc Meperidine

5 WITHDRAW FLUID

Withdraw piston 1 cc. (1 cc. of atropine has been withdrawn from vial).

½ cc. of sterile air remains at top of cartridge to prevent accidental infusion of fluid from one receptacle to the other.

½ cc Sterile Air / 1 cc Atropine / 1 cc Meperidine

6 READY FOR INJECTION

Withdraw needle from vial.

Expel excess air.

Replace needle sheath to maintain asepsis until moment of injection.

Administer injection as with conventional syringe.

Sterile Air / 1 cc Atropine / 1 cc Meperidine

FIGURE 18–11.   Mixing Parenteral Fluids in the Tubex Syringe (Courtesy of Wyeth Laboratories)   Mixing of fluids in the Tubex syringe may be performed with two or more medications of varying dosages. The dosages of meperidine and atropine are selected arbitrarily to illustrate the mixing technique.

VIII.   Instillation of Nose Drops

The child may be placed in a mummy restraint or positioned as shown in Figure 18–12. To position the child, follow these steps:

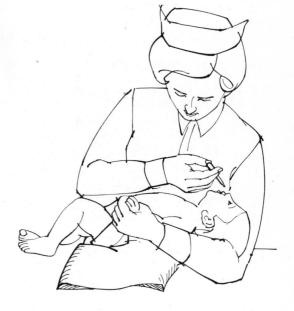

FIGURE 18–12.   Positioning a Child for the Instillation of Nose Drops.

1. Place a pillow under the infant's shoulders and allow his head to fall back over the edge of the pillow.

2. Place your elbow on the mattress above the infant's head and stabilize the head between your forearm and your body. Your hand may be used to restrain the infant's arms.

3. With your free hand, you can administer the prescribed amount of drops in the nose with minimum struggle and maximum accuracy.

Note:

A. Nose drops should be given 20 minutes before feedings.

B. Bottles of nose drops should not be used for more than one child, as they become quickly contaminated by bacteria.

C. Nose drops should not be used for more than 3 to 4 days, or irritation and chemically induced nasal congestion may be produced.

D. A child who coughs and has a profuse nasal discharge should not be given cough medicine, as it will depress the cough reflex, and aspiration from the nasopharynx is possible.

Nasal Irrigation

Place the child's head in a hyperextended position so it is lower than the body and the alae are in a horizontal plane. The prescribed solution (usually warm saline or 0.1 per cent ephedrine in saline) is dropped into one nostril while suctioning the other nostril with a nasal aspirator. This is repeated until returns are clear. The nasal chambers act like a "U" tube so the flow of a solution goes past the ostia of the sinuses. The sinuses are warmed, causing the vessels of the sinus mucosa to dilate. Nasal irrigation is most often prescribed for children with chronic purulent sinusitis.

An older child can bend his head 45° over a sink to use a special nasal irrigator tip attached to a conventional home dental Water-Pik machine to provide intermittent positive pressure nasal sinus irrigation. Holding a finger guard on the nasal tip prevents excessive pressure from being delivered.

IX.   Instillation of Ear Drops

To instill ear drops:
1. Apply a mummy restraint to the infant.
2. Turn his head so that the infant lies on the unaffected ear.
3. The drops should be warm.
4. Hold the pinna of the ear as described on page 177.
5. Allow the drops to fall on the external canal and run onto the eardrum.
6. Hold the child in position for a few minutes.

X.   Intravenous Therapy

When intravenous fluids are ordered, it is entirely the responsibility of the nurse to insure the safety of the patient.

Prior to setting up the infusion:

1. Check the label of the I.V. bottle to be sure you have the correct solution as ordered and the correct size bottle. If solutions are added or removed from the I.V. bottle, a label stating the altered contents should be immediately and securely fastened to the bottle, and the information should be accurately recorded on the patient's chart.

2. Most I.V. bottles display expiration dates on the label beyond which it is unsafe to administer the contents. The nurse must check the expiration date on the bottle prior to using it.

3. The nurse should turn the I.V. bottle upside down and hold it up to the light to inspect for obvious impurities. The solution should be clear. Cloudiness or particles floating in the fluid indicates that it may be unsafe for use. The nurse should slowly rotate the bottle against the light. Bright flashes of reflected light will help locate small cracks that may be present in the glass. Bottles containing cracks or chips should not be used.

4. The nurse should inspect the overseal of the I.V. bottle to be sure that the bottle has not been entered before. Use only bottles that have intact overseals. If a bottle has been entered and its contents altered by a pharmacist, a special label should be affixed to the bottle and its list of contents should correlate with the doctor's order for the patient.

5. Check for the presence of a vacuum in the bottle when the I.V. administration set is inserted. You will hear a hissing sound upon piercing the seal and will see bubbles rise to the surface when the bottle is inverted to hang on the I.V. stand.

6. Many hospitals use portable I.V. stands that roll to the unit. The I.V. stand should be adjusted so that the bottle is approximately 30 inches above the venipuncture site. The nurse must be sure that the telescoping section of the stand is securely locked

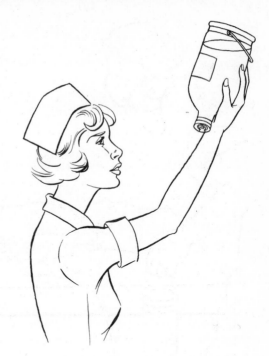

FIGURE 18-13.   Checking Infusion Fluid.

and the stand remains stable to prevent accidents to patients and personnel. The I.V. tubing should be free of kinks and strain.

7. Select the I.V. administration set that will accomplish the goals of therapy. Every set has the number of drops per milliliter delivered labeled clearly on the box. Do not *assume* the drop size of any set.

Blood Administration

The child's blood type and cross match reports must be checked with the label on the bottle containing blood for transfusion. The identification band of the child should also be checked prior to transfusion. Connect the transfusion set to the blood bottle and expel the air from the tubing. The venipuncture is performed by the doctor.

Since red cells tend to settle to the bottom, whole blood should be gently agitated to assure trouble-free flow. The rate of flow should be checked frequently, as a change in the height of the I.V. stand or the bed or repositioning of the child may alter the established rate of flow.

Infusion Therapy

An intake and output record should be attached to the bed of any child who is receiving intravenous therapy. When recording the urine output of an infant, "one wet diaper" is sufficiently accurate unless the doctor's order specifies weighing the diapers or tubing the infant. Supplementary medications containing calcium should not be added to Butler's or Darrow's solution, as crystallization will occur. The child should be closely observed for symptoms of infiltration and the development of phlebitis at the site of the venipuncture.

1. Check the positioning of the needle as follows:

A. Place the infusion bottle at a level lower than the infusion site.

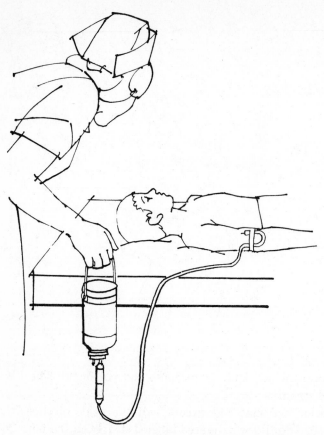

FIGURE 18–14. Checking the Position of the Needle in a Vein.

   B. Observe the tubing near the needle. If blood flows back into the intravenous tubing, the needle is positioned in the vein.

   C. Replace the bottle and allow continuation of the flow.

  2. Observe for swelling around the needle site.

If the infusion infiltrates, the flow should be stopped and the doctor notified. When a scalp-vein infusion is in progress, the infant may be picked up, cuddled, and fed without danger of causing infiltration.

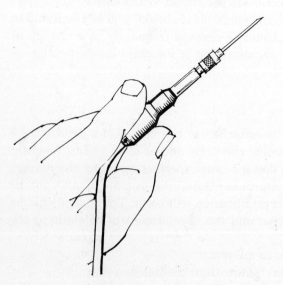

FIGURE 18–15. The Flashball Device The Flashball device, available on Plexitron administration sets, produces the same results as the usual procedure without lowering the bottle. Prior to the administration of the solution, squeeze the Flashball device, then release it. Blood will flash back into the adapter if the needle is correctly positioned in the vein.

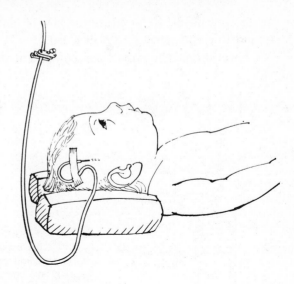

FIGURE 18–16. The Scalp-Vein Infusion
The head is immobilized with sandbags that extend from the shoulder. Note that pressure is not placed on the child's ear. The area around the venipuncture site has been shaved. The tubing is looped and secured to the head to prevent dislodgment of the needle and to avoid compressing the tubing between the sandbag and the infant's head. Clove-hitch restraints may be used to keep the child from pulling at the intravenous tubing. (See Chapter 9, Restraining and Positioning Infants and Children.)

Equipment Used for Parenteral Therapy in Pediatrics

Modern intravenous sets have increased the safety as well as the simplicity of intravenous therapy. Research concerning the medical use of electronics devices to regulate parenteral fluid administration is now in progress. In the near future a machine may, by an alarm bell or light system installed at her desk, alert the nurse to the amounts of intravenous fluids administered.

Transfusion Equipment

A blood administration set has a special drip chamber with a filter which is not present in ordinary infusion sets. Glass bottles containing blood require the insertion of

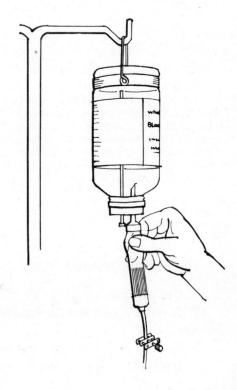

FIGURE 18–17. A Blood Administration Set
This transfusion set has a compressible drip chamber. The nurse is compressing the chamber to allow the level of the blood to cover the filter before the doctor initiates transfusion therapy. The nurse may close the clamp and compress this chamber to clear the filter of obstructions during therapy. Note the air vent needle in place. Blood should not be administered through tubing that has carried glucose in water solutions.

an air vent needle to facilitate the flow of blood. Air vent needles should not be used in conjunction with plastic bags of blood.

Several types of transfusion equipment are illustrated in Figures 18–17 to 18–21.

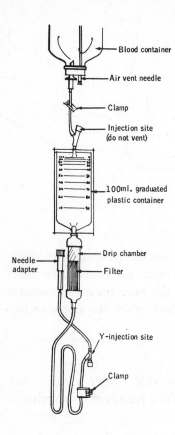

FIGURE 18–18. The Hemoset The Hemoset is designed for the controlled administration of small volumes of blood. A measured amount of blood is allowed to enter the graduated plastic container from the blood bottle. The plastic container then serves as a primary blood container from which the flow is regulated by a clamp. Ten drops from this unit is equivalent to 1 ml. of whole blood. The plastic container may be refilled to administer amounts larger than 100 ml.

FIGURE 18–19. A Scalp-Vein Set A scalp-vein set is used to administer blood or infusions to infants or young children. Flexible plastic "wings" attached at the base of the needle provide a suitable finger grip for the doctor during venipuncture. After the venipuncture, the wings are spread flat so that the unit may be firmly anchored to the head with adhesive tape. This unit may be connected to a regular blood administration set or a Hemoset.

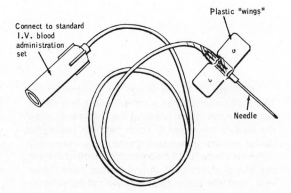

The Pediatric Metriset

1. Close clamps.

2. Invert I.V. container to moisten stopper. Remove outer cap, metal disc, and rubber disc.

3. Remove protective covering from administrative spike.

4. Insert spike through the outlet part of container stopper. Suspend I.V. container.

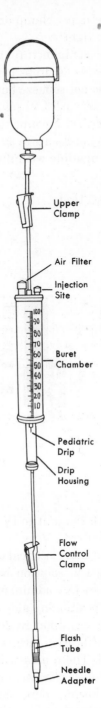

FIGURE 18–20. The Pediatric Metriset.

5. Open upper clamp, fill burette chamber with at least 20 ml. of fluid. Close upper clamp. Tap chamber gently to release any large air bubbles.

6. Squeeze drip chamber *gently* and release *slowly* until 1/3 full. This volume prevents air bubbles from entering tubing.

7. Remove protective covering from needle adapter and attach sterile I.V. needle. Open flow control clamp, fill tubing and needle with solution, expelling some solution from the needle. Close flow control clamp.

8. Open upper clamp and allow solution to fill burette chamber to desired volume. Close clamp tightly.

9. After venipuncture, adjust the rate of flow with flow control clamp. (Drip is metered to provide 60 drops per ml.). Proceed with administration.

Note: Do not squeeze burette chamber. This could force solution out through the air filter. Always expel I.V. solution through tubing and needle before filling burette chamber to prescribed amount to be administered. Supplemental medication may be added through the injection site at top of burette chamber. Gently agitate to mix. Be sure medication is compatible with fluid being administered (see p. 185).

The IVAC Unit

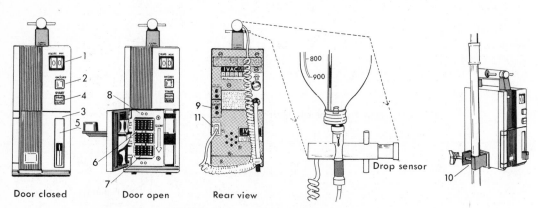

Door closed   Door open   Rear view   Drop sensor

FIGURE 18–21.   IVAC Infusion Controller.

1. Attach the unit to IVAC equipment stand or use pole adapter (10) furnished for use with standard I.V. poles. Make connection to "nurse call" receptacle (9) if applicable. Plug unit into electrical outlet. Insert sensor plug to rear of unit (11).

2. Hang I.V. solution bottle with administration set on I.V. pole hanger. Attach drop sensor to I.V. administration set drip chamber. When necessary, use one of the drop sensor positioning aids supplied with the unit. Because various brands of I.V. administration sets differ in design, this requires individually designed positioning aids. The aid identification letters are (A) for Abbott, (C) for Cutter, (M) for McGaw, and (T) for Travenol. These aids will facilitate proper placement of drop sensor on most drip chambers. *Proper placement on drop sensor is absolutely essential for correct operation of unit.* The following points should be carefully observed:

   A. Drop sensor must be positioned on drip chamber so upper surface of drop sensor is level with or slightly below point at which drops form.

   B. Level of fluid must be maintained below lower surface of drop sensor.

   C. Drip chamber must be oriented vertically. Bleed air from I.V. tubing and close administration set tubing clamp.

3. Lift door handle (5) and open door (3).

4. Prepare injection site and perform venipuncture.

5. Partially release I.V. administration set tubing clamp slowly. Check for success-

ful venipuncture. If venipuncture is in order, place I.V. tubing into white plastic tubing guides (6), between guide posts. This will center tubing over pumping mechanism (7). Be sure direction of flow is correct, from top to bottom as indicated by arrow. Close door (3) and push handle (5) down. This will stop I.V. solution flow. Fully open I.V. administration set tubing clamp. Make sure flow is completely stopped by observing if any more solution is entering drip chamber.

6. Set "drops per minute" selector (1) to prescribed infusion rate. Do not attempt to infuse more than 200 ml. per hour or alarm will sound.

7. Depress "on-off" button (2) to energize pump and push "start" button (4) to begin infusion. Verify correct operation.

8. To increase or decrease infusion drop rate, change setting of "drops per minute" selector (1). The IVAC unit will alarm and stop infusion if selected rate cannot be maintained or if bottle runs dry. It is a good practice to change position of tubing in pumping chamber every 8 hours by sliding tubing up or down two or three inches.

9. To stop or terminate an infusion, press "on-off" button (2).

Note: Make sure I.V. administration clamp is tightly closed before opening pump chamber door.

Calculation of I.V. Flow Rate:

Drops Per Minute to Milliliters Per Hour

Drops per Minute	Microdrip® Venoset® Approx. 60 drops = 1 ml.				Regular Venoset Approx. 15 drops = 1 ml.				Blood Set Approx. 10 drops = 1 ml.			
	Approx. Milliliters Infused*											
	1 hour	2 hours	4 hours	8 hours	1 hour	2 hours	4 hours	8 hours	1 hour	2 hours	4 hours	8 hours
5	5	10	20	40	20	40	80	160	30	60	120	240
10	10	20	40	80	40	80	160	320	60	120	240	480
20	20	40	80	160	80	160	320	640	120	240	480	960
30	30	60	120	240	120	240	480	960	180	360	720	1,440
40	40	80	160	320	160	320	640	1,280	240	480	960	1,920
50	50	100	200	400	200	400	800	1,600	300	600	1,200	2,400
60	60	120	240	480	240	480	960	1,920	360	720	1,440	2,880
70	70	140	280	560	280	560	1,120	2,240	420	840	1,680	3,360
80	80	160	320	640	320	640	1,280	2,560	480	960	1,920	3,840
90	90	180	360	720	360	720	1,440	2,880	540	1,080	2,160	4,320
100	100	200	400	800	400	800	1,600	3,200	600	1,200	2,400	4,800
110	110	220	440	880	440	880	1,760	3,520	660	1,320	2,640	5,280
120	120	240	480	960	480	960	1,920	3,840	720	1,440	2,880	5,760
125	125	250	500	1,000	500	1,000	2,000	4,000	750	1,500	3,000	6,000

*In actual use these factors will change slightly with variation of room temperature, bottle height, rate of infusion, viscosity of solution, and variation of size of drip orifice.

FIGURE 18–22. Calculating I.V. Flow Rates   The flow rate is calculated by counting the drops per minute falling into the drip chamber. The nurse must know the calibration (drops per milliliter) of the I.V. set being used. This usually appears on the box label containing the I.V. set. (Courtesy of Abbott Laboratories.)

When using the mini- or micro-drop intravenous administration sets, which yield approximately 60 drops per ml.:

The prescribed ml. per hour = The flow rate in drops per minute

Example: 40 ml. per hour, flow rate is 40 drops per minute.

When using other than the mini- or micro-drop intravenous administration sets:

$$\frac{\text{Drops per ml. set will yield} \times \text{Prescribed ml. per hour}}{60} = \text{Flow rate in drops per minute}$$

Example: If set yields 10 drops per ml., prescribed ml. per hour is 18.

$$\frac{10 \times 18}{60} = \text{A flow rate of 3 drops per minute}$$

XI.   *Parenteral Fluids Commonly Used in Pediatrics*

Some Solutions Which Contain Protein

Whole blood.   Citrated whole human blood is blood drawn under aseptic conditions and protected from coagulation by an anticoagulant acid-citrate-dextrose solution. Eligibility criteria for blood donors assure that the blood is free from transferable disease and contains no less than 12.5 grams of hemoglobin per 100 ml.

Blood must be stored at 4 to 10° C. and therefore should be brought from the blood bank unit of the hospital and used immediately. If blood is brought to the unit and a delay in initiating venipuncture occurs, the blood must be returned to the blood bank for storage, as most standard refrigeration facilities cannot provide the storage temperatures necessary to preserve it.

Bottled blood more than 21 days old should not be used. To avoid potassium intoxication, blood used for exchange transfusions in the newborn infant should not be more than four days old.

Epinephrine and calcium gluconate should be available for use during transfusion therapy.

If untoward symptoms occur, the blood flow should be stopped and the doctor notified.

The blood preparation used during cardiac surgery is fresh heparinized blood collected in special silicone bottles. Regular whole blood may be used postoperatively but *not* during the open-heart operative procedure.

Human packed red blood cells.   Packed cells are erythrocytes separated from citrated whole blood which has been typed and cross matched. This preparation is used to provide red blood cells without risking a circulatory overload.

Normal human plasma.   Human plasma is the pooled liquid portion of blood obtained from at least eight different blood donors. This preparation is used to restore the blood volume without causing hemoconcentration.

A type and cross match are not necessary when using pooled blood plasma. The plasma unit may be used as long as two to five years after the date of manufacture. A regular blood administration set should be used when plasma is administered.

Normal human serum albumin.   Approximately 96 per cent of the total protein contained in this preparation is albumin. Every 100 ml. contains 25 gm. of albumin, equivalent to the amount in 6 1/2 units of whole blood. This preparation is most often used to treat hypoproteinemia. Because of its highly osmotic properties, 20 ml. of albumin is capable of increasing the circulating blood volume by approximately 70 ml. within 15 minutes. Symptoms suggesting pulmonary edema and circulatory embarrassment must be watched for. It may be used within five to eight years from the date of manufacture. Typing and cross matching are not necessary.

Plasma substitutes.   Plasma substitutes are used to maintain circulatory volume in the emergency treatment of shock. The solution has a high molecular weight which is a factor in preventing rapid elimination by the kidneys and therefore maintains blood volume for a longer period of time than other parenteral solutions. Dextran is one example of a plasma substitute. Typing and cross matching are not necessary when using plasma substitutes.

Fresh frozen single donor plasma.   The liquid portion of a unit of whole blood, which has been separated from the cells and frozen within four hours after collection, is useful in the treatment of hemophilic conditions.

The preparation is stored at a temperature of 18° C. or lower and thawed in a water bath of 37° C. prior to use.

Fibrinogen.   A concentration of the fibrinogen factor that is effective in controlling severe hemorrhage caused by a deficiency of this substance in the blood. A 2 gm. unit of fibrinogen represents the quantity found in approximately 12 units of whole blood.

Fibrinogen is reconstituted with sterile distilled water no more than one hour prior to use. Fibrinogen should be administered via a blood administration set with a filter.

Amigen.   Amigen is a protein-containing solution that provides some sodium, potassium, calcium, chlorides, amino acids, and carbohydrates. Protein-containing solutions must flow at a slower rate than non-protein infusions.

Solutions Which Do Not Contain Protein

Lipomul.   Lipomul is an intravenous solution containing fat. It is most often prescribed for patients with burns, renal failure, or diseases of the central nervous system.

Lipomul must be stored in the refrigerator and should not be mixed with other parenteral solutions.

Ringer's lactate solution.   This solution contains sodium, potassium, and calcium chlorides; sodium lactate; and dextrose. The preparation is used to maintain the fluid and electrolyte balance.

Glucose.   Glucose or dextrose solutions may also contain sodium, potassium, and chlorides if they are in a saline base. They are used to provide carbohydrates.

Levugen.   This preparation contains fructose, a carbohydrate that is less dependent than most on insulin when it is metabolized in the body. It may contain sodium and chlorides if it is in a saline base.

Darrow's solution.   This preparation contains sodium, potassium, chlorides, and lactates. It is used to provide specific electrolytes.

6M sodium r-lactate.   This solution contains sodium, lactate, and water. It is used as initial emergency therapy in case of metabolic acidosis.

Homeolyte, electrolyte no. 48. This solution provides electrolyte and caloric requirements with minimal taxing of the kidneys.

Butler's solution. This solution contains sodium, potassium, chlorides, lactates, and phosphates. It is used to provide specific electrolytes.

Mixing Nonprotein-Containing Intravenous Solutions

When commercial preparations are not available in the desired concentration or composition, it may be necessary for the nurse to mix nonprotein-containing intravenous solutions. Such modification demands technical skill and *strict aseptic technique.* Calculations and measurements must be accurate. Solution modifications which may be desired are outlined in Table 18–1.

Techniques. Two different methods may be used to mix intravenous fluids to obtain the desired concentration and composition:

1. A closed method using intravenous Y-tubing. The preferred method to use when more than 50 ml. is being transferred from one bottle to the other. See Figure 18–23.

2. An open method using a 50 ml. syringe. The preferred method to use when less than 50 ml. is being transferred from one bottle to the other. See Figure 18–24.

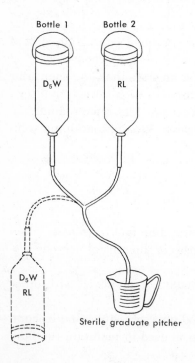

FIGURE 18–23. Closed Method for Mixing Intravenous Fluids (1) From Bottle 1, discard desired amount of solution into a sterile graduate pitcher. (2) Lower Bottle 1 and allow desired amount of solution to run into it from Bottle 2. (3) Disconnect Bottle 1 and recap tubing end. (4) Label bottle 1 and hang. D_5W is 5 per cent dextrose in water; RL is lactated Ringer's solution.

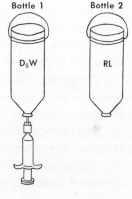

FIGURE 18–24. Open Method for Mixing Intravenous Fluids (1) Using a 50 ml. syringe, remove and discard desired amount of solution from Bottle 1. (2) Remove desired amount of solution from Bottle 2 and transfer to Bottle 1. (3) Label Bottle 1 and hang.

TABLE 18–1.   Mixing Some Nonprotein-Containing Intravenous Solutions Which May be Desired in Care of Infants and Children

Modification Desired	Combination For Each 100 ml.
2½% Dextrose in ½ Strength Lactated Ringer's (D$_{2\ 1/2}$ ½ St RL)	50 ml. 5% Dextrose in water 50 ml. Lactated Ringer's
4% Dextrose in Modified Lactated Ringer's (D$_4$ MRL)	80 ml. 5% Dextrose in water 20 ml. Lactated Ringer's
5% Dextrose in .45% Saline (D$_4$ .45% Saline)	50 ml. 10% Dextrose in water 50 ml. 0.9% Saline
5% Dextrose in ½ Strength Lactated Ringer's (D$_5$ ½ St RL)	50 ml. 10% Dextrose in water 50 ml. Lactated Ringer's
7.5% Dextrose in Modified Lactated Ringer's (D$_{7.5}$ MRL)	75 ml. 10% Dextrose in water 25 ml. Lactated Ringer's
8% Dextrose in Modified Lactated Ringer's (D$_8$ MRL)	80 ml. 10% Dextrose in water 20 ml. Lactated Ringer's
12% Dextrose in Modified Lactated Ringer's (D$_{12}$ MRL)	70 ml. 10% Dextrose in water 10 ml. 50% Dextrose 20 ml. Lactated Ringer's
15% Dextrose in Modified Lactated Ringer's (D$_{15}$ MRL)	60 ml. 10% Dextrose in water 18 ml. 50% Dextrose 22 ml. Lactated Ringer's

Selected Drug Incompatibilities with Intravenous 5 Per Cent Glucose

When using 5 per cent glucose intravenous solution:

When this drug is added:	Do not mix with these drugs:
Aminophylline	Vitamin B complex with vitamin C Tetracycline HCl Methicillin Chloramphenicol
Ampicillin	Vitamin B complex with vitamin C Tetracycline HCl Sodium phenobarbital Epinephrine chloride Chloramphenicol Atropine
Chloramphenicol or sodium succinate	Vitamin B complex with vitamin C Tetracycline Hydrocortisone phosphate

	Erythromycin
	Epinephrine
	Digitoxin
	Ampicillin
	Aminophylline
Kanamycin	Sodium bicarbonate
	Phenobarbital
	Methicillin
	Hydrocortisone
	Heparin
	Calcium gluconate
Methicillin	Vitamin B complex with vitamin C
	Tetracycline
	Sodium bicarbonate
	Potassium chloride
	Kanamycin
	Hydrocortisone
	Epinephrine
	Calcium chloride
	Atropine
	Aminophylline
Penicillin G potassium	Vitamin B complex with vitamin C
	Tetracycline
	Heparin
	Epinephrine
	Dilantin
Potassium chloride	Novobiocin
	Methicillin
Sodium bicarbonate	Vitamin B complex with vitamin C
	Tetracycline
	Phenobarbital
	Methicillin
	Kanamycin
	Hydrocortisone
	Calcium gluconate
	Calcium chloride
	Atropine

XII. Estimating the Status of Body Fluids

The nurse should be alert for symptoms of dehydration and overhydration (see Table 18–2). Her observations and recordings should include:

TABLE 18–2. Symptoms of Too Little or Too Much Fluid and
Electrolyte Therapy

Component	Too Little	Too Much
Fluid	Hemoconcentration Thirst Fever Oliguria Circulatory failure Acidosis (Sunken eyeballs, lethargy, signs of shock, dry skin, apathy, red lips)	Hemodilution Polyuria Increased intracranial pressure Headache Muscular twitching
Sodium	Loss of tissue elasticity Hypotension Circulatory failure	Edema Potassium deficiency Irritability
Potassium	Apathy Lethargy Muscular weakness Abdominal distention EKG changes Diarrhea Alkalosis (nausea; slow, shallow respiration)	EKG changes Muscular weakness Cardiac arrest
Carbohydrate	Ketosis Water losses	Hyperglycemia Glycosuria Hepatic failure
Calcium	Tetany Increased neuromuscular excitability Carpopedal spasm Laryngospasm	Hypotonia Fecal masses
Magnesium	Tetany Muscle twitching Noise sensitivity	Renal failure CNS depression Drowsiness Respiratory depression

1. *Weight determination.* Infants and children who require parenteral fluid therapy should be weighed at regular intervals. A loss of 10 per cent or more of the body weight may be indicative of a fluid deficit.

2. *Tissue turgor.* To test the tissue turgor (see Fig. 18–25) grasp the skin gently between two fingers *(A)*. When the skin is released, the tissues should return to the normal position immediately *(B)*. If the skin remains in a distorted position after release, the tissue turgor is poor.

3. *Body temperature.* An elevated body temperature can be indicative of dehydration. If it is permitted, the infant should be given water between feedings. The body temperature of an infant who is receiving intravenous therapy should be recorded every four hours.

4. *Intake and output record.* An intake and output record should be kept to facilitate a comparison of the kidney output and the total fluid intake.

5. *Palpation of fontanels.* The nurse may palpate the anterior fontanel of infants under 18 months of age. A sunken fontanel may be indicative of dehydration.

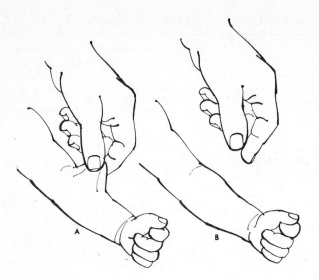

FIGURE 18–25.   Testing Tissue Turgor.

6. *Vital signs.* The vital signs may deviate from normal in cases of dehydration and electrolyte imbalance. Vital signs should be recorded on the chart, and any deviations reported to the doctor. (See Chapter 4 for the observation of vital signs.)

The daily turnover of water in the 3 kg. infant is equal to almost 25 per cent of his total body water as compared to the daily turnover of only 6 per cent of total body water in the 70 kg. adult. Therefore, fluid and electrolyte imbalance occurs readily in illness in children and is a crucial aspect of pediatric therapy.

Use of Concentrations of Dextrose Over 5 Per Cent Intravenously

The use of concentrated dextrose above 5 per cent in I.V. fluids designed to meet water requirements in infants causes loss of the dextrose in the urine. This causes a diuretic effect that in itself can increase water requirements and thwart the goal of I.V. therapy. Increased occurrence of thrombosis and infection is also a threat when high intravenous dextrose concentrations are used.

XIII.   Technique of Terminating Infusions

When terminating an infusion:

1. Clamp the tubing to stop the fluid flow so that the solution will not enter subcutaneous tissues.

2. With the needle held firmly in place, gently remove the adhesive tape by which the needle was secured.

3. With one hand, place a sterile alcohol pad over the site of the injection.

4. With the other hand, keep the hub of the needle flush with the skin and slowly withdraw the needle. (This avoids dragging the tip of the needle against the posterior wall of the vein.)

5. Hold the sterile pad over the injection site or secure the pad with a short piece of adhesive tape.

6. Record the time that the infusion was terminated.

XIV. Parenteral Hyperalimentation (Total Parenteral Nutrition)

Infants who are unable to take food by mouth for prolonged periods of time are usually started on intravenous feedings. However, intravenous feedings in which peripheral veins are used can provide only minimum nutritional requirements which are not adequate to provide for the needs of growth and development.

Parenteral hyperalimentation is the infusing of a hypertonic (30 per cent) nutrient solution directly into the superior vena cava through a jugular or subclavian vein. Venous inflammation often associated with prolonged intravenous therapy is avoided because the vena cava is a region of high blood flow and rapid dilution. This procedure maintains positive nitrogen balance and provides for nutritional needs of growth and development when prolonged parenteral therapy is required in conditions such as burns or extensive surgery. The use of nonreactive silicone tubing also decreases development of thrombotic complications.

The Hyperalimentation Solution

The infusion solution is prepared from an amino acid preparation and contains 20 per cent glucose. Sodium, potassium, calcium, magnesium, phosphorus, chlorides, and vitamins are infused at a rate of 135 ml./kg./day, providing 122 calories per kg. per day. Plasma is given twice weekly, and intramuscular vitamin K and vitamin B_{12} are also usually prescribed. The solution is delivered by a constant speed infusion pump to the superior vena cava via a long catheter. It is usually modified to meet the needs of individual patients and may vary from week to week depending upon the response of the patient and the laboratory reports. The infusion should be made up by a pharmacist in a central location under sterile conditions. Medications should *never* be added to this solution.

Insertion of Catheter at Infusion Site

Rigid sterile technique for catheter insertion is essential to prevent infection. Sterile gloves, syringes, and instruments are used.

1. The patient is positioned with the head 15 degrees lower than the feet in order to dilate the subclavian vein. (In a small infant the jugular vein may be used and then threaded to the superior vena cava.) If the jugular vein is used, a small neck incision is made and the catheter tunneled under the skin. Often the tube is subcutaneously tunneled to a scalp site exit to insure that the tubing is out of the infant's reach and away from oral and nasal flora. The infant should be restrained. (See p. 66, Fig. 9–5.)

2. Prepare the infusion site by cleansing the skin thoroughly and applying an antiseptic solution.

3. A local anesthetic is infiltrated into the skin.

4. A proper sized needle (often a #14 with 2-inch needle) on a 2-cc. syringe is used to enter the vein, while negative pressure is maintained in the syringe. The nurse who is assisting the doctor should always be alert to signs of pneumothorax.

5. When the doctor determines that the needle is in position, an 8-inch, #16 catheter is inserted into the needle and threaded into the vein.

6. When the catheter is positioned, the proximal end is attached to the intravenous tubing.

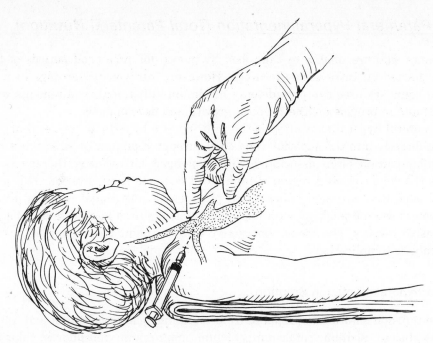

FIGURE 18–26. **Insertion of Catheter**   Note that the child is positioned with the head 15 degrees lower than the feet to allow optimal dilatation of the subclavian vein. Towel roll under the patient's back serves to hyperextend the shoulders. The head is rotated to the side opposite the venipuncture. Sterile gloves and instruments are used.

7. The needle is withdrawn and the I.V. solution is set to flow at the prescribed rate.

8. The doctor secures the catheter to the skin with a silk suture, and a sterile gauze dressing is applied over the site.

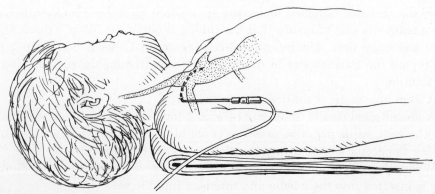

FIGURE 18–27.   The catheter has been inserted into the superior vena cava, the needle is withdrawn its full length, and the I.V. tubing is attached.

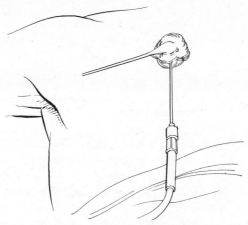

FIGURE 18–28.   The doctor may order an antibiotic ointment to be applied to the site two or three times a week.

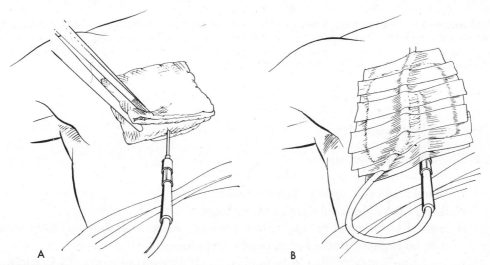

A   B

FIGURE 18–29.   A gauze dressing is secured by adhesive tape to the hub of the needle, allowing the I.V. tubing to be replaced regularly.

9. For an infant, a peristaltic pump is attached to the tubing to keep the I.V. solution flowing freely. This is necessary to prevent backflow of blood into the tubing when the central venous pressure increases as a result of vigorous crying.

10. A millipore filter is inserted between the pump and the catheter to minimize risk of air embolism and bacterial contamination.

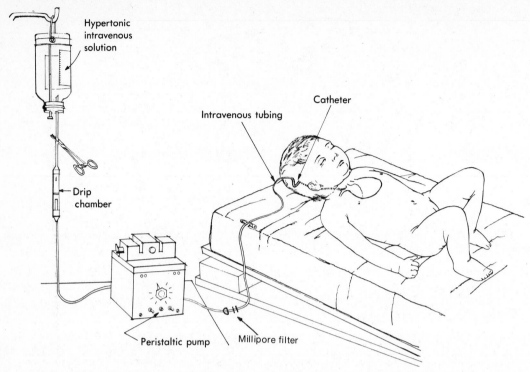

FIGURE 18–30.   Parenteral Hyperalimentation   A peristaltic pump is attached to the I.V. tubing to maintain an even and continuous flow of I.V. solution and to counteract strong back-pressure created when the infant
cries. A sterile dressing should be placed over the catheter insertion site. The tubing should be kept out of the
infant's reach and free from contamination by nasal oral flora.

Nursing Responsibilities

1. The administration set:
   a. Should never be used to administer drugs
   b. Should never be used to sample blood
   c. Should never be used to administer blood
   d. Should be changed *at least* three times per week. Dressing and filter should
   also be changed under strict aseptic technique.
   e. Betadine ointment should be applied to all connecting joints of I.V. tubing.
   f. Any alimentation solution accidentally spilled on the external tubing should be
   washed away promptly to prevent bacterial growth.
2. The dressing over the catheter insertion site should be changed three times a
week and the skin cleansed with Betadine.
3. The catheter should be changed once a month and reinserted by the doctor.
4. The nurse should institute measures to prevent vigorous or prolonged crying by
the child.
5. Carefully observe and record the following:
   a. Inflammation at operative site
   b. Vital signs
   c. Rate of flow of I.V. solution
   d. Signs of dehydration or overhydration

    e. Intake and output
    f. Fractional urine sugar
    g. Body weight
    h. Daily blood chemistry and tests as prescribed

Avoiding Complications of Hyperalimentation

Complication	*Nursing responsibility*
Sepsis	Give meticulous catheter care. Preparation of infusate under sterile conditions.
Excess amino acid can: 1. Produce high urea and cause osmotic diuresis. 2. Produce high ammonia and cause brain toxicity. 3. Produce high free amino acids and cause metabolic acidosis.	Continuous chemical and physiological monitoring is essential in evaluating the response of the child to therapy. The nurse must be aware of normal laboratory values and report deviations promptly.
Hypoglycemia caused by sudden cessation of infusate	Check rate of flow frequently (q1h).
Hyperglycemia from high glucose content which may cause osmotic diuresis and result in dehydration.	Watch for signs of increased diuresis and impending dehydration. Intake and output should be monitored.
Thrombosis, extravasation of fluid, accidental dislodgment of catheter	Check the catheter area carefully. Position and restrain child adequately.
Development of psychological problems due to lack of fulfilling sucking need	Give pacifier to infant while he is not being fed orally.

Changing Hyperalimentation Catheter Dressings

Note: Dressings are usually changed every 48 hours, using *strict sterile* technique.
1. Remove dressings.
2. Don sterile gloves.
3. Cleanse area with sterile sponge moistened in Betadine or other prescribed antiseptic. Hold sponge with sterile clamp. Use circular, outward motion. Repeat as necessary with new sponge each time.
4. Allow area to dry.
5. Apply prescribed ointment with sterile tongueblade to insertion site and all suture sites that are securing the tubing.
6. Cover with sterile gauze.
7. Remove gloves; secure dressing with tape.
8. Be sure loop of catheter is present to avoid tension at insertion site. Record procedure and observations.

BIBLIOGRAPHY

Armstrong, I. L., and Browder, J. J.: *The Nursing Care of Children.* 3rd Edition, F. A. Davis Co., Philadelphia, 1970.

Beaver, W. T.: The Pharmacological Basis For Choice of Analgesic. *Pharmacology for Physicians, 4*:7, 1970.

Bode, H. H., and Warshaw, J. B. (Eds.): *Parenteral Nutrition in Infants and Children.* Plenum Press, New York, 1974.

Catz, C. S., and Giacola, G. P.: Drugs and Breast Milk. *Pediatric Clinics of North America, 19*:151–166, 1972.

Chudzik, G. M., and Yaffe, S. J.: Introduction to Special Problems of Pediatric Drug Therapy. *Drug Therapy, 3*:17, 1973.

Conn, H. F. (Ed.): *Current Therapy 1972.* W. B. Saunders Co., Philadelphia, 1972.

Done, A. K.: Antipyretics. *Pediatrics Clinics of North America, 19*:167–177, 1972.

Driscoll, J. M., Jr., and Heird, W. C., Schullinger, J. N., Gongaware, R. D., and Winters, R. W.: Total Intravenous Alimentation in Low Birth Weight Infants—A Preliminary Report. *Journal of Pediatrics, 81*:145, 1972.

Dudrick, S. J.: Rational Intravenous Therapy. *American Journal of Hospital Pharmacists, 28*:82–91, 1971.

Dudrick, S. J., Copeland, E. M., and MacFadyen, B., Jr.: Long Term Parenteral Nutrition: Its Current Status. *Hospital Practice, 10*:47, 1975.

Gellis, S.: Fibrosis of Quadriceps Following Intramuscular Injection in Premature and Young Infants. *Yearbook of Pediatrics,* p. 361, 1969.

Gellis, S. S., and Kagan, B. M. (Eds.): *Current Pediatric Therapy.* 7th Edition, W. B. Saunders Co., Philadelphia, 1976.

Grossman, M.: Irrigation of the Child's Nose. *Clinical Pediatrics, 13*:229, 1974.

Habersang, R., and Kauffman, R. E.: Drug Doses for Children. *Journal of the Kansas Medical Society, 75*:98–103, 1974.

Heird, W. D., MacMillan, R., and Winters, R.: Total Parenteral Nutrition. Symposium, Wyeth Labs, December, 1973.

Herbert, V., and Jacob, E.: Destruction of Vitamin B_{12} by Ascorbic Acid. *Journal of the American Medical Association, 230*:241, 1974.

Lipman, A.: How Digitalis Glycosides May Interact with Other Agents. *Modern Medicine, 43*:111, 1975.

Lockhart, J. D.: The Information Gap in Pediatric Drug Therapy. *Modern Medicine, 38*:23:56, 1970.

Marlow, D.: *Textbook of Pediatric Nursing.* 4th Edition, W. B. Saunders Co., Philadelphia, 1973.

Meng, H. C., and Law, D. H. (Eds.): Parenteral Nutrition. *Proceedings of an International Symposium.* Charles C Thomas Co., Springfield, Illinois, 1970.

O'Brien, T. E.: Excretion of Drugs in Human Milk. *American Journal of Hospital Pharmacology, 31*:844, 1974.

Winters, R. W., and Hasselmeyer, E. G. (Eds.): *Intravenous Nutrition in the High Risk Infant.* John Wiley & Sons, New York, 1975.

Yaffe, S. J. (Ed.): Symposium on Pediatric Pharmacology. *Pediatric Clinics of North America, 19*:1–256, 1972.

Admixture Study for Fluids in Glass Containers. Travenol Labs, Inc., 1967.

A Shot in the Arm May Beat a Shot . . . Elsewhere. *Infectious Diseases, 5*:5:3, 1975.

Blood Flow Affecting Absorption of I.M. Medications. *Infectious Diseases, 5*:5, 1975.

Injections Show Sex Discrimination. *Medical World News, 16*:23, 1975.

Parenteral Feeding with Fat Emulsion. *Medical World News, 16*:16:1975.

Superjuice Gives New Chance for Life. *Kaiser Permanente Coverage, 1*:2:1975.

Who Should Administer Intravenously Given Drugs? *Journal of the American Medical Association, 230*:1063, 1974.

PRODUCT REFERENCES

Abbott Laboratories, North Chicago, Illinois: Administration set, Scalp-vein set, Pliapak pressure unit, Hemoset.

IVAC Corp., San Diego, California: IVAC unit.

McGaw Laboratories (Division of American Hospital Supply), Irvine, California: Metriset.

Wyeth Laboratories, Philadelphia, Pennsylvania: "The Tubex Closed Injection System."

Chapter Nineteen

POISONING IN INFANTS AND CHILDREN

PRINCIPLES

Ingested poisons (even small amounts) have a chemical action capable of damaging tissues and disturbing body functions.

Identification of the ingested substance aids in determining the specific antidote and therapy.

If poisons can be removed from the stomach, systemic absorption will be minimized.

Lavage does not assure that poisons have not been absorbed into the general system.

Follow-up care is essential to prevent a recurrence of accidental poisoning.

NURSING RESPONSIBILITIES

An accurate habit record of the child may reveal long-term ingestion of poisonous substances (pica).

A poison antidote chart should be posted in the pediatric unit. The Department of Health Poison Control Center may be contacted for specific information regarding the contents of or antidotes to the substance ingested.

The nurse should anticipate and prepare for lavage therapy.

Continuous observation is necessary in regard to:
1. Vital signs
2. Behavior
3. Convulsions
4. Motor ability
5. Intake and output record
6. Urine and blood specimens
Oxygen and suction should be available.

Teaching the parents about prevention of poisoning and referring them to a community agency for follow-up care are advisable.

TECHNIQUES

Poisoning—A Problem at Every Developmental Level in Pediatrics

Poisoning is a leading cause of death in infants and young children. The curious toddler explores the mysterious cabinets in the house only to find an attractive bottle that he decides to "taste"; the wandering young child, who is thought to be safe in the confines of a securely fenced yard, discovers a bright red berry on a bush and decides to eat it. Parents may contribute to the poisoning problem when they pour leftover household cleaners into empty soda bottles, for storage. Even a school age child may accidentally drink what he thinks is leftover soda, only to be poisoned by the cleaner instead. The lead content of the colored sections of newspapers is such that it takes only a few "spitballs" made from them to cause lead poisoning in children. Peashooters or whistles made from the hollow stems of water hemlock can also be poisonous. Neither is the teenager immune to poisoning. In addition to the drug problems often occurring in the adolescent age group, and the problems inherent in making spitballs (as noted above), the innocent teenager on a camping trip may unknowingly pick a branch from an oleander tree to skewer his meat over the fire and will be fatally poisoned when the poison from the branch is transferred to the meat. Any plant on the edges of highly traveled highways can also be highly contaminated with toxic lead. Poisoning is preventable, and the clinic nurse can play a major role in counseling parents and young patients in methods of prevention.

Recent reports indicate that although the management of poisonings has been updated, labels on many household chemicals have not changed, and so many labels provide incorrect data on what to do in case of accidental ingestion. The nurse should urge parents to seek medical aid when a foreign substance is ingested and use poison control centers or "poisindex" information centers when available for guidance in the management of specific poisonings. The telephone numbers of these agencies should be conspicuously posted in the clinic area. This information is available from the Poison Control Center, Department of Health, Education, and Welfare, Washington, D.C. 20201.

Parent education concerning storage of soaps, detergents, bleaches, mothballs, polishes, and medications in order to limit access to children should be initiated by the nurse as part of the well-child visits.

I. Selected Symptoms of Common Poisons

Symptom	Possible Cause
Skin coloring and eruptions	Often caused by long-term ingestion of compounds such as mercury, phenol derivatives, tetracyclines, sulfa drugs, penicillin, ergot preparations, or saccharin

Convulsions	Occur with CNS stimulants, camphor, or substances causing methemoglobinemia such as nitrites, pyridium, methyl alcohol
Muscle spasms	Often caused by atropine, copper salts, bites of black widow spider or scorpion
Coma	CNS depressants, alcohol
Dilated pupils	Atropine, cocaine, ephedrine
Pinpoint pupils	Opiates, physostigmine
Vomiting	Occurs most commonly with metallic, acidic, alkaline, and bacterial poisons
Specific odors of vomitus;	
Sweet	Chloroform, acetone
Bitter almond	Cyanides
Pear	Chloral hydrate
Garlic	Phosphorus, arsenic
Shoepolish	Nitrobenzene
Violet	Turpentine

II.   Goals in the Treatment of Poisoning

1. Remove poison
2. Prevent further absorption
3. Administer antidote
4. Supportive care

III.   The Volume of a Swallow

The volume of a swallow has been estimated to be 0.21 ml. per kg. Thus a child 2 to 3 years of age who takes one swallow may have ingested 4.5 ml. of poison.

IV.   Some Approaches to Emergency Care of Poisoning

Nursing measures include supportive therapy in observing vital signs, maintaining a patent airway, and observing the responses of the child to the ingested poison. The nurse must be prepared to assist with the specific management prescribed. Many hospitals are located near a poison control center and its telephone number should be posted conspicuously. These centers assist in determining specific contents of compounds ingested, and they suggest antidotes.

Induce vomiting.   This may be a lifesaving measure, but it is contraindicated with corrosive or highly irritant poisons, or in the comatose patient.

A. 15 drops ipecac syrup in warm water.

B. Stimulation of posterior pharynx.

C. Lavage stomach by passing gastric tube (See p. 221).

Ipecac syrup.   Can be kept in the home, as it needs no prescription. Doses up to 15 ml. may be given to children more than one year of age with 200 ml. water. It produces vomiting within 15 minutes (should not be used as an antidote for strychnine, alkali corrosives, kerosene, gasoline, paint thinner, or cleaning fluid ingestion).

Activated charcoal with water. Absorbs certain drugs such as strychnine, morphine, atropine and arsenic compounds, pentobarbital, and malathion.

Ipecac and activated charcoal, if given together, will neutralize each other, rendering both ineffective.

Tannic acid. Precipitates alkaloid and metallic poisons.

Magnesium oxide. Used for mineral acid poisonings.

Potassium permanganate (1:5000). Used to oxidize organic poisons.

Milk and eggwhite. Used for metallic poisons.

Calcium lactate. Used to chemically alter oxalic acid.

Gastric lavage or saline cathartics. Used to hasten the removal of poisons from the G.I. tract. Catharsis is contraindicated in phosphorus poisoning.

B.A.L., EDTA, exchange transfusions, dialysis, or peritoneal lavage. Each has value in treatment of serious poisonings. Charts showing indications for use and side effects should be posted in the emergency area of the clinic.

V. Poisoning Due to Plants

Many poisonous plants cause G.I. symptoms, and general supportive care with the prevention of shock is indicated. Some alkaloid-containing plants may cause central nervous system and cardiorespiratory depression or overstimulation. Ensuring an adequate airway, providing oxygen, and observing and reporting vital signs are essential in all cases of plant poisoning. The initial nursing responsibility involves inducing emesis, preparing for lavage, and maintaining and monitoring vital signs.

Many plant poisons cause symptoms similar to specific chemical poisons. Selected examples follow.

Plant	Drugs to Use as Antidotes
Aconitine	
Azalea	Atropine
Baneberry	Physostigmine
Buttercup	Pilocarpine
Christmas rose	Caffeine sodium benzoate
Larkspur	Digoxin
Marigold	Short-acting barbiturates
Monkshood	
Wolfsbane	
Atropine	
Lantana	Sedatives
Jimsonweed	Antipyretics
Pyrocantha	Physostigmine
Stinkweed	Parenteral fluids
	Ephedrine
	Pilocarpine

Colchicine
Autumn crocus
Meadow saffron
Tulip bulbs

Paraldehyde
Barbiturates
10 per cent calcium gluconate I.V.

Curare
Sweetpea
Staggerbush
Black mountain laurel

Mechanical aids to respiration
Atropine
Hypotensive drugs

Cyanide
Apricot pits
Peach pits
Cassava root
Chokecherry
Elderberry
Cherry (except fruit)
Jetberry bush

Amyl nitrite
Sodium nitrite
Sodium thiosulfate
Blood replacement
Methylene blue 1 per cent

Digitalis
Camellia seeds
Dogbane
Foxglove
Lily of the Valley
Oleander
Star of Bethlehem bulb

Quinidine
Na_2EDTA
Magnesium sulfate
Atropine
Potassium

Oxalates
Caladium
Dumbcane
Elephants' ears
Rhubarb leaves
Pokeweeds

Antihistamines
Epinephrine
Intravenous fluids
Calcium gluconate

Phytotoxin
Black locust
Castor beans
Poinsettia
Tung tree

Saline cathartics
Blood transfusions
Urine alkalizers
Sodium bicarbonate

Nitrates
Annual sage
California chicory
Goldenrod
Jimsonweed
Nightshades
Poinsettia
Sweetclover
Wild sunflower

Methylene blue
Antibiotics
Barbiturates
Pilocarpine

Resins
Laurel
Marijuana
Milkweed
Rhododendron
Water hemlock

Barbiturates
Atropine
Hypotensive drugs
Activated charcoal
Meperidine

Salicylates

Acacia	Parenteral fluids
Birch	Sodium lactate
Camellia	
Hyacinth	
Marigold	
Tulips	
Violets	
Willows	

Saponin

Coffeeweed	Paraldehyde
Ivy	Atropine
Holly	Treatment for hemolytic anemia
Pokeweed	
Tung tree	

Miscellaneous

Jessamine	Atropine
Nutmeg	Castor oil, demulcents
Mistletoe	Quinidine, Na_2EDTA
Potato sprouts	Paraldehyde
Wild mushrooms	Atropine, I.V. protein hydrolysate
Yew	Heart stimulants
	Steroids
	Activated charcoal

VI. Poisonous Ingredients of Selected Household Products

Product	Poisonous Ingredient(s)
Absorbine Jr.	Thymol, iodine, menthol
Action bleach	Sodium hypochlorite
AFTA cleaning fluid	Carbon tetrachloride
Airwick	Petroleum distillates
Ajax all-purpose cleaner	Inorganic pyrophosphate
Ajax floor and wall cleaner	Sodium carbonate, tripolyphosphate
Alka-Seltzer	Salicylates
Ant paste	Arsenic
Ant powder	Pyrethrum
Antifreeze	Ethyl alcohol, ethanol, diethylene glycol
Batteries Box	Lead
Flashlight	Zinc
Cigarette lighter fluid	Benzine derivatives
Cold wave hair permanents	Potassium bromate, thioglycolates
Cologne	Denatured ethyl alcohol
Deodorants (home)	Paradichlorobenzine, napthaline, formalin, isopropyl alcohol
Drano	Lye
Flea powder	Rotenone

Crayons	Red and orange are the significantly toxic colors if they are not identified with letters A.P., C.P., or c.s. 130–46 on the label
Fireworks	Antimony, arsenic, barium chlorates, lead, mercury, phosphorus
Flypaper	Arsenic
Furniture polish	Lemon oil, kerosenelike volatile hydrocarbons, castor oil, antimony
Glass cleaners	Propyl alcohol
Ink	Anilene, iron gallate
Indelible ink	Silver nitrate
Listerine	Boric acid, methyl alcohol
Lysol	Cresol, soap solution
Matches	Manganese dioxide, potassium chlorate, sulfur
Mothballs	Napthaline, camphor
Nailpolish	Butyl alcohol
Nailpolish remover	Ethyl alcohol, isopropyl alcohol, acetone
Pipe and drain cleaners	Alkali
Photographers' solutions	Sodium hyposulfite, silver salts
Saniflush	Sodium bisulfate
Snarol snail killer	Arsenic, methaldehyde
Saccharin	A sulfonamide; can affect cardiac rhythm, G.I. tract, photosensitivity and renal toxicity
Toilet cleaners	Acid, sodium bisulfate
Washing powders	Borax, lye, sodium carbonate, sodium hypochlorite, trisodium phosphate
Talcum powder	Contains magnesium silicate that can cause inhalation pneumonia

VII. Gastric Lavage (Gastric Washing)

Equipment Needed for Gastric Lavage

The equipment needed for gastric lavage includes:
1. Restraining sheet
2. Stomach pump or Levin tube
3. 50 cc. syringe
4. 2000 cc. lavage fluid (prescribed by the doctor)
5. Large basin to collect the returns of lavage
6. Water to lubricate the tube
7. Wipes

Technique of Gastric Lavage

1. Assemble the equipment at the bedside.
2. Place the child in a mummy restraint and stabilize his head with your hands.
3. Turn the child's head to one side to prevent aspiration if vomiting occurs.
4. The Levin tube is passed into the stomach by the doctor.

5. The position of the Levin tube may be checked by (a) inverting the tip of the tube in a glass of water (if bubbles appear, the tube is *not* in the stomach) or (b) aspirating the stomach contents.

6. The stomach contents are siphoned by gravity or with a syringe.

7. The lavage fluid is injected slowly into the tube with a 50 cc. syringe. The amount of fluid injected at one time depends upon the age and size of the child.

8. The fluid is then aspirated and discarded into the basin.

9. The procedure is repeated until the return is clear.

10. Save washings for laboratory analysis. Do not routinely discard gastric washings.

The nurse should observe and record the nature of the return and the response of the child. Upon completion of the procedure, the tube should be pinched and removed quickly to prevent the fluid from dripping into the pharynx.

Gastric lavage is contraindicated in corrosive, kerosene, or strychnine poisoning.

BIBLIOGRAPHY

Arena, J. M.: *Poisoning: Toxicology, Symptoms, Treatment.* 3rd Edition, Charles C Thomas, Springfield, Ill., 1973.

Arena, J. M.: Pretty Poisonous Plants. *Consultant, 15*:5:65, 1975.

Coleman, A., and Alpert, J. (Eds.): Poisoning in Children. *Pediatric Clinics of North America, 17*:Aug., 1970.

Gordon, H.: Untoward Reactions to Saccharin. *Cutis,* July, 1972.

Gordon, H.: Hives and Itching: A Diagnostic Challenge. *Consultant, 15*:11:92–94, 1975.

Hardin, J. W., and Arena, J. M.: *Human Poisoning From Native and Cultivated Plants.* 2nd Edition, Duke University Press, Durham, N. C., 1974.

Kingsbury, J. M.: *Poisonous Plants of the U. S. and Canada.* Prentice-Hall, Englewood Cliffs, N. J., 1964.

Marlow, D.: *Textbook of Pediatric Nursing.* 4th Edition, W. B. Saunders Co., Philadelphia, 1973.

Mofenson, H., and Greensher, J.: Keeping Up with Changing Trends in Childhood Poisonings. *Clinical Pediatrics; 14*:621, 1975.

Painter, J. C., Shanor, S. P., and Winek, C. L.: Nutmeg Poisoning: A Case Report. *Clinical Toxicology, 4*:1, 1971.

Vaughn, V. C., III, and McKay, R. J.: *Nelson Textbook of Pediatrics.* 10th Edition, W. B. Saunders Co., Philadelphia, 1975.

Antidotes Listed on Toxic Products Termed Outdated. *Medical Tribune, 16*:2, 1975.

Antifreeze Poisoning is Potentially Lethal. *Modern Medicine, 42*:25:62, 1974.

In Consultation: Dealing with Food Poisoning. *Medical World News, 16*:74, 1975.

Self Poisoning in Adolescents. *Pediatric Digest, 17*:9:9, 1975.

The Sinister Garden: A Guide to the Most Common Poisonous Plants. Wyeth Labs, 1966.

Chapter Twenty

PERITONEAL DIALYSIS

A therapeutic measure used in the treatment of infants and children with acute renal failure, peritoneal dialysis refers to the passing of a solute through a membrane for the purpose of removing toxic substances from the blood. The therapy depends upon the principles of osmosis and diffusion through the semipermeable peritoneal membrane.

The use of an "artificial kidney" refers to *hemo*dialysis, which is another method of accomplishing extrarenal excretion.

PRINCIPLES

In cases of acute renal failure, the peritoneum can be used as a dialyzing membrane to remove diffusible toxins from the body without permitting protein and other large molecules to be lost.

Any therapy involving a surgical incision requires the written consent of the parents.

Maintenance of strict surgical asepsis is essential to prevent peritonitis.

Accurate recording of the urine output is essential. A Foley catheter may be prescribed, or the infant may be "tubed" to facilitate the collection of urine.

NURSING RESPONSIBILITIES

The nurse should assemble the necessary equipment at the bedside, including:
1. Dialysis tubing
2. Dialysis solution
3. Equipment for paracentesis
4. Sterile sutures and dressings
A 50 cc. syringe may also be needed.

Although the consent is obtained by the doctor, the nurse should explain and interpret the therapy to the parents and to the child when possible.

Preparation of the skin is the same as in general preoperative care. A dry sterile dressing is placed over the abdominal wound after the trochar has been inserted into the peritoneal cavity.

The nurse must check the drainage tubes for kinking and prevent obstruction of the tubes by the body weight of the child. An intake and output record must be kept at the bedside.

Diffusion can occur in both directions across the peritoneal membrane. The fluids used must be hypertonic to the plasma of the patient to prevent excessive absorption and overhydration.

The nurse must check the labels of the solutions to be used prior to the initiation of the procedure. The solutions should be labeled "For Peritoneal Dialysis." Since intravenous therapy may be used concurrently with dialysis therapy, intravenous solutions must be kept separate from the dialysis solutions.

The amount of solution drained from the peritoneal cavity should equal or exceed the amount of solution introduced.

The accurate weight of the child should be recorded before and after each treatment. The nurse should measure and record the amount of solution introduced and the amount obtained by drainage.

After the first few exchanges, intermittent peritoneal dialysis can be performed by the nurse. The therapy usually lasts from 12 to 36 hours.

The nurse must be aware of the amount of solution prescribed for each dialysis and the time interval to be allowed between introduction and drainage of the solution.

TECHNIQUES

The abdomen of the child is prepared and draped with sterile sheets. The solution bottles are connected to the tubing, and air is expelled from the tubing, using principles similar to those of intravenous therapy. The doctor inserts the trochar into the peritoneal cavity and initiates the procedure. The doctor may request that certain drugs such as heparin or antibiotics be added to the dialysis solution. The prescribed amount of solution is permitted to flow into the peritoneal cavity as rapidly as possible. The nurse should clamp off the tubing before the bottles are completely empty so that air is prevented from entering the peritoneal cavity and the bottle may serve as a siphon at the time of drainage. When a small amount of solution is introduced, as with newborn infants, a 50 cc. syringe may be used.

The solution is allowed to remain in the abdominal cavity for a prescribed period of time (usually 30 to 90 minutes). During this time, the nurse may prepare the next solution for use. New tubing should be used for each dialysis administration to reduce the infection potential. The head of the bed may be slightly elevated to prevent respiratory distress due to the increased intra-abdominal pressure. Measures should be taken to prevent the child from pulling at the dialysis tubing. The vital signs and the general response of the child should be observed and recorded at frequent intervals. The child's state of consciousness should be accurately described.

After the dialysis solution has remained in the abdominal cavity for the prescribed period of time, the bottles are placed on the floor beside the child's bed and the clamp is released. Aided by gravity, the fluid will drain from the abdominal cavity into the original bottles. Some doctors prefer to use an electric suction pump to facilitate rapid emptying of the peritoneal cavity. All drainage must be measured and an accurate hourly intake and output record must be kept.

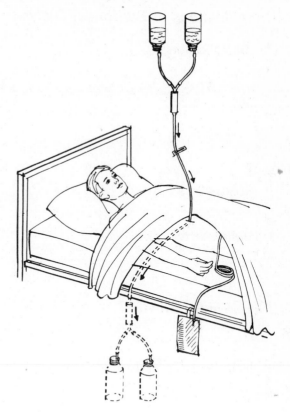

FIGURE 20–1. Peritoneal Dialysis The dotted lines show the placement of the bottles during drainage of the fluid from the peritoneal cavity. Note that the Foley catheter tubing is coiled on the mattress to prevent looping of the distal end and to promote the drainage of urine. The plastic urine collection bag is calibrated in cubic centimeters to facilitate the observation and evaluation of the urine output.

The procedure is then repeated in the same manner for 12 to 36 hours or as specified by the doctor.

Points to observe:

1. The solutions to be administered must be at body temperature.

2. The exact time of administration and drainage of the dialysis solution should be recorded.

3. The abdominal dressing should remain clean and dry throughout the procedure. If leakage occurs, the doctor should be notified promptly.

4. The child must be observed for bleeding.

5. Vital signs should be recorded at frequent intervals, and any deviations promptly reported.

6. An hourly urine output record should be kept, and any *change* in urine output reported.

7. The child should be observed for signs of dehydration or water intoxication.

8. The drainage of dialysis fluid should occur rapidly. If the return flow slows to a drip, the doctor should be notified.

9. The amount of fluid withdrawn from the peritoneal cavity should equal or exceed the amount administered.

10. During the drainage of the dialysis fluid, the child can be turned and coughing may be encouraged.

11. Monitored blood values should be recorded and reported.

Complications of Peritoneal Dialysis

Complication	Signs and symptoms to observe and report
Volume depletion	Tachycardia, hypotension
Perforation of viscus	Cloudy, stained returning fluid with a foul odor, failure of solution to drain from abdomen.
Peritonitis	Leakage around catheter, signs of infection
Digitalis toxicity	If child is on digitalis, the removal of potassium can predispose to toxic symptoms. Special care and recording is essential for *prevention* of this complication.
Diaphragmatic irritation	(Occurs with use of hypertonic solutions) Referred pain to the left shoulder is the common symptom
Sudden changes in body fluid volume	Watch for signs of water intoxication
Pulmonary problems	Watch for signs of pulmonary edema; prevent aspiration pneumonia and atelectasis
Protein loss	Pitting edema of legs, serum protein low (usually a problem of long term therapy)
Difficulty in return drainage	If drainage slows or stops, turn the patient from side to side, elevate the head of the bed, flex the knees, or apply gentle pressure to the abdomen with both hands. If these measures fail to improve drainage, doctor should be notified.

BIBLIOGRAPHY

Chan, J. C. and Campbell, R. A.: Peritoneal Dialysis in Children. A Survey of its Indications and Applications. *Clinical Pediatrics, 12*:131, 1973.

Harmer, B., and Henderson, V.: *The Textbook of the Principles and Practice of Nursing.* 5th Edition, The Macmillan Co., New York, 1970.

Rae, A., and Pendray, M.: Advantages of Peritoneal Dialysis in Chronic Renal Failure. *Journal of the American Medical Association, 235*:937, 1973.

Sabiston, D. C.: *Davis-Christopher Textbook of Surgery.* 10th Edition, W. B. Saunders Co., Philadelphia, 1972. (11th Edition in preparation.)

Varga, C.: *Handbook of Pediatric Medical Emergencies.* 4th Edition. The C. V. Mosby Co., St. Louis, 1968.

Vaughn, V. C., III, and McKay, R. J.: *Nelson Textbook of Pediatrics.* 10th Edition, W. B. Saunders Co., Philadelphia, 1975.

PRODUCT REFERENCES

Abbott Laboratories, North Chicago, Illinois: Imperinol.
McGaw Laboratories, Glendale, California: Peritoneal dialysis solution.
Travenol Laboratories, Deerfield, Illinois: Dialysis solution.

Chapter Twenty One

PRE- AND POSTOPERATIVE CARE FOR INFANTS AND CHILDREN

PRINCIPLES

The goal of preoperative care is to prepare the child for surgery in a manner that will insure optimum tolerance of the procedure and prevent postoperative complications.

NURSING RESPONSIBILITIES

The nurse should observe the child closely, carry out prescribed orders, and maintain communication with the doctor and the anesthetist.

I. Preparation of the Child

The degree of trust and autonomy experienced by the child, his previous experiences, the type of surgery planned, and the number of persons coming in contact with him are factors that affect the child's responses and determine individual preoperative needs.

Children tend to become insecure and apprehensive when separated from their parents and placed in an unfamiliar environment. A child may not have the ability to understand verbal explanations but he can sense tensions present in the atmosphere and overrespond to them.

The nurse can establish a positive nurse-parent-child relationship prior to surgery by providing an opportunity for verbalization and the assessment of individual needs. The nurse should understand and accept aggressive responses from the child.

The nurse may familiarize the child with equipment he will see and let him "play out" his feelings. Older children should be told what to expect after surgery. The nurse should be cheerful, calm, and unhurried. Explanations given whenever possible will aid in gaining the child's confidence. A child may feel more secure if he is allowed to take a favorite toy to the operating reception room.

II. Consents

Prior to surgery, a written consent must be obtained from the parent or guardian. If the operative procedure involves several stages performed at various intervals, a separate consent is necessary for each stage. Consents are legally valid for a period of one month. (See Consents, p. 36.)

A child must not be sent to the operating room without the written consent of the parent or guardian. Since the parents are entitled to a careful explanation of the operation and its implications for the growing child, the doctor is responsible for obtaining consents. The nurse can provide support to the parents by promoting confidence in the doctor and by interpreting his explanations as necessary.

III. Spiritual Needs

The spiritual beliefs of parents must be respected and their faith encouraged and strengthened.

Meeting the spiritual needs of the child and his parents is an essential aspect of the preoperative nursing care plan. The nurse should consult with the parents concerning their preferences. Chaplains of all faiths are available in most hospitals.

IV. Dietary Restrictions

Postoperative complications due to nausea and vomiting may be avoided by allowing the stomach to empty prior to surgery.

Clear fluids pass through the stomach at a much quicker rate than solid foods. Well-hydrated infants are better able to tolerate surgical procedures.

Any oral fluid restriction can cause mild dehydration and fluid and electrolyte disturbance, which can be a serious complication of surgery in infants and children.

Solid foods should be withheld for at least eight hours prior to surgery. Auxiliary personnel must be informed of the food restriction.

Clear liquids with sugar added may be given to infants up to four hours prior to surgery. Juices should not be offered as they cause fermentation within the gastrointestinal tract, precipitating distention.

The nurse should be prepared to carry out the responsibilities of intravenous fluid administration to correct water and electrolyte deficits, especially in emergency surgery.

V. Specific Precautions

Accurate monitoring of ventilation and metabolic status must be initiated prior to surgery to avoid complications, especially in surgery of the newborn.

The nurse should be prepared to assist in taking and reporting of arterial blood values such as pH, $PaCO_2$, electrolytes, and hematocrit.

The deciduous teeth normally loosen and fall out in the preschool and schoolage child. Since the muscles of the throat relax during anesthesia, loose teeth can fall back and be aspirated.

The nurse must be alert to the presence of loose teeth in children scheduled for surgery and report them promptly to the doctor and anesthetist.

An upper respiratory infection may predispose the child to laryngeal complications and impair his ability to withstand anesthesia and surgery.

It is essential that the nurse observe and report the presence of nasal discharges, cough, or any elevation of temperature. The child should be protected from drafts and warmly wrapped for transportation to the operating room.

The dosage of sedatives and anesthetic agents is based upon the weight of the individual child. "Standard doses" do not exist in pediatrics.

The nurse must obtain and record the accurate weight of the child prior to surgery. (See p. 46 for the techniques of weighing infants and children.)

Certain drugs may alter the response of the patient to sedatives and anesthetic agents.

The nurse should report to the doctor and anesthetist if the child is receiving steroids, anticonvulsants, tranquilizers, cardiac drugs, or antihypertensives prior to surgery.

Preanesthetic drugs are administered to allay fear and tension, to reduce secretions that otherwise might be aspirated, and to decrease the amount of anesthesia required during surgery.

The prescribed preoperative medication should be administered on time. (See Chapter 18 for the administration of medications.) The nurse should observe and record the responses of the child. The environment and activity of the child should be planned to foster the goals of the preoperative medications.

VI. Postoperative Care

Following tracheal intubation, children between 6 months and 6 years can develop subglottic edema. Intermittent positive pressure breathing may be prescribed with humidity tents to control this common occurrence.

Constant observation of airway patency, adequacy of ventilation, and circulatory stability is required. Constant monitoring of vital signs is essential and resuscitative equipment must be ready for use.

Umbilical artery catheterization in the newborn provides a means for continuous pressure monitoring and frequent blood sampling. In older children, cannulation of a peripheral artery is often used. An acute rise in $PaCO_2$ over 65 mm. Hg or PaO_2 under 100 mm. Hg at inspired oxygen over 95 per cent usually indicates impending respiratory failure.

The nurse must be aware of her responsibility in the care of infants with umbilical catheters and must report abnormal lab findings immediately. She must also be aware of her responsibilities in the use of oxygen concentration monitors, respiratory monitors, incubators, and humidity tents, often used in the preoperative course with infants and young children (see Chapter 14.)

TECHNIQUES

I. Preoperative Care

The skin surface where the incision is to be made should be washed thoroughly with a bactericidal solution and shaved free of hair that may be present. Oral hygiene is essential to prevent infection and possible pneumonia. The results of routine laboratory tests, such as C.B.C., urinalysis, and bleeding and clotting times should be affixed to the chart. The nurse should observe and chart voiding prior to surgery. An identification band must be secured to the wrist or ankle and checked prior to and following preoperative care. The small infant is wrapped warmly and the older child dressed in laparotomy clothes, which are warmer than ordinary gowns and absorb perspiration. When possible, the nurse should accompany the child to the operating room suite. The principles of safety should be observed during care and transportation of the patient. (See Chapter 8, Transportation of Infants and Children.)

The child between 1 and 4 years of age has special difficulties in understanding the hospital and preoperative experience. Terrifying experiences during the induction of anesthesia can cause disabling psychological problems such as enuresis or night terrors. To minimize psychological trauma the mother should:

1. Explain what is going to happen to the child at a level he can understand.
2. Prepare him for discomforts he can expect.
3. Display confidence and cheerfulness, avoid radiating anxiety.
4. The doctor and anesthetist should visit the child in the presence of the parents so they will not be strangers.

Preanesthetic medication should allow the child to be lightly asleep when transported from his room.

Preoperative Medications Commonly Used in Pediatrics

Age	*Drug*	*Dosage*	*Purpose*
0–6 months	Atropine	*Atropine:* 0.02 mg./kg. to maximum 0.6 mg.	Atropine abolishes the vagal reflex that is so active in infants under one year.
6 months to 1 year	Atropine and pentobarbital	*Pentobarbital:* 3 to 4 mg./kg. to maximum 120 mg.	Pentobarbital is added for sedative effect.
1 year and over	Scopolomine (or atropine) and pentobarbital and Demerol (meperidine) Morphine	*Scopolomine:* 0.02 mg./kg. to maximum 0.6 mg. *Meperidine:* 1 to 2 mg./kg. to maximum 100 mg. *Morphine:* .05 to 1 mg./kg. to maximum 10 mg.	Scopolomine provides better drying of airway secretions and has amnesic effect. Meperidine has a sedative effect and provides easier induction of anesthesia.

II. Postoperative Care

The principles of the postoperative nursing care plan are based upon the diagnosis, the type of anesthesia used, the degree of consciousness, and the age of the child. Constant attention, supervision, and provision of psychological support are essential aspects of postoperative care for the pediatric patient. When the child is recovering from anesthesia, he will need assistance in coping with many new sensations and experiences.

The child may return from the operating room with an airway in place. The airway extends from the outer margin of the lips to a point just above the larynx. It maintains the normal position of the tongue and pharyngeal wall and facilitates a patent airway. Suctioning may be necessary to keep the airway patent.

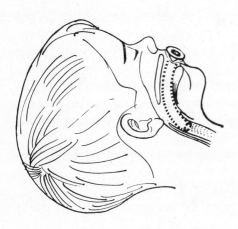

FIGURE 21–1.   An Anesthetized Child with an Airway in Place.

The positioning of the patient is usually ordered by the doctor and depends upon the type of surgery performed and the type of anesthesia used. (See p. 69 for the diaper sling used to relieve abdominal strain for infants with abdominal surgery.) Warmth should be maintained, diapers changed as often as necessary, and measures taken to prevent the child from pulling at his dressing.

The nurse should observe and record the following:
1. Type of operation performed and anesthesia used
2. Position of patient
3. Condition of dressing, drainage
4. Degree of consciousness
5. Presence of cough and gag reflexes
6. Frequent observation of vital signs
7. Voiding, distention
8. Intravenous fluids, rate of flow
9. Responses of the child.

Intravenous therapy may be anticipated postoperatively to maintain protein balance, provide the vitamins necessary for wound healing, and replace electrolytes. An intake and output record should be made routinely, with or without a doctor's order, for at least 24 hours following surgery.

Summary of General Postoperative Care

To this general list of nursing responsibilities, the nurse should add specific responsibilities relating to the particular disease process and the developmental stage of the individual child.

1. Maintain a patent airway
2. Maintain warmth, prevent hyperthermia
3. Monitor vital signs, report deviations
4. Monitor intake and output
5. Change position, prevent aspiration
6. Monitor lab reports, report deviations
7. Maintain general hygiene

III. Chest Surgery

Closed drainage of the pleural cavity is used following chest surgery for the purpose of evacuating fluids and air and aiding in the re-expansion of the lungs. Although the degree and type of suction to be used are determined by the doctor, it is necessary for the nurse to understand the working principles of the drainage apparatus that is used. Negative pressure suction can be regulated by the wall suction (difficult to control), by an electric thoracic pump, a water manometer, or a mercury manometer. The mercury manometer provides a greater degree of suction than the water manometer.

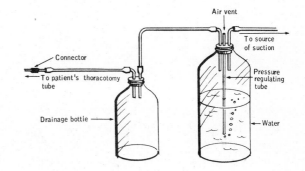

FIGURE 21-2. Underwater Chest and Suction Apparatus The closed drainage system is designed to prevent air from entering the pleural cavity. The long glass tube in the bottle of water is sealed by being immersed in the water. The depth of this tube below the water level determines the amount of negative pressure obtained. If suction is regulated by water for any length of time, the nurse must anticipate some evaporation of the water, and refill the bottle when necessary.

Points to Observe and Record

1. The drainage bottle must be always be below the level of the chest to prevent fluid from entering the pleural cavity.

2. Fluctuation of the water level within the glass tube and intermittent bubbling of the water during the respiratory cycle indicate proper functioning of the apparatus. If there is no fluctuation or bubbling, the nurse should check for kinking of the tube or leakage. Constant bubbling may indicate a small leak from the surface of the lung, or a fistula or leak in the drainage system.

3. The nurse may safely seal all bottle caps with adhesive to prevent leakage or accidental opening. The bottles should be protected against breakage.

4. A Kelly clamp must be kept available at the bedside to clamp the chest tube when the tubing is disconnected or as an emergency measure in case of leakage or breakage of the apparatus.

5. The drainage bottle should be emptied before it is filled to capacity to insure proper functioning of the drainage system. To empty the drainage bottle, seal the chest tube with a Kelly clamp before disconnecting the bottle cap. Before releasing the clamp, be sure the cap is resealed on the drainage bottle. Excess tubing must not loop above site of chest tube insertion nor loop below top of drainage bottle.

6. The chest dressing should be checked frequently. It should be clean, dry, and firmly in place. Loose dressings should be reinforced, and the doctor should be notified.

7. Vital signs should be checked frequently and deviations promptly reported.

8. The type and amount of drainage in the bottle should be recorded every 8 hours. The drainage tube should be "milked" every 2 to 3 hours.

BIBLIOGRAPHY

Shafer, K., Sawyer, J., McCluskey, A., Beck, E., and Phipps, W.: *Medical and Surgical Nursing.* 6th Edition. The C. V. Mosby Co., St. Louis, 1975.

Vaughn, V. C., III, and McKay, R. J.: *Nelson Textbook of Pediatrics.* 10th Edition, W. B. Saunders Co., Philadelphia, 1975.

Chapter Twenty Two

CARE OF A CHILD WITH A FRACTURE

CARE OF A CHILD IN A CAST

PRINCIPLES

Upon admission, minimal handling of the extremity will prevent further trauma at the site of the fracture.

Trauma can cause an increase in circulation that will result in *increased growth* in the length of the bone. Interference with the nerve supply may *retard* bone growth. Damage to the epiphyses may *stop* bone growth.

The rough edges of a plaster cast may traumatize the skin of a child. The pressure of the rim of the cast against the skin will cause bruises.

The extra weight of a plaster cast may cause the mattress to sag.

A plaster cast is porous and will absorb water and urine.

NURSING RESPONSIBILITIES

Upon admission, remove the clothing from the uninjured limb first and then from the injured limb to avoid undue pressure at the site of the trauma.

The nurse must understand the effect of trauma on growing bone, assess problems early, and provide follow-up care and rehabilitation.

Place moleskin or adhesive "petals" along the edges of the cast to prevent skin irritation. Do not lift infants by their legs to change the diaper when a leg or body cast is in place.

A bedboard may be placed under the mattress to prevent sagging.

Since infants and young children cannot control urination, waterproofing the cast is essential.

Waterproofing a cast before it is completely dry will cause mildew to form.

Waterproof a cast in the areas prone to be saturated after the cast is completely dry. Elevate the head of the bed slightly to prevent stool and urine from seeping under the cast.

Providing support to the contours of the cast will prevent flattening or cracking of the cast.

Place small pillows under the curvatures of the cast to provide support.

Pillows under the head or shoulders of a child in a body (spica) cast will thrust the chest forward against the cast, causing discomfort and possible respiratory difficulty.

When elevation of the head is desired, the entire mattress and spring should be elevated at the head of the bed.

Foreign particles under the cast will precipitate skin irritations and infections.

Toys small enough to be pushed under a cast should not be given to the child. Padding the edges of the cast with candy cotton (fluffy cotton padding) will prevent food particles and foreign bodies from being inserted by the child. A small, hand vacuum cleaner may be used to remove crumbs from under the cast.

A plaster cast is not flexible and can inhibit circulation, especially if edema occurs. Characteristically, the infant and child cannot localize pain or discomfort.

The toes or fingers should always be exposed and checked frequently for color and warmth. Cold toes, loss of sensation in the toes, pain, and inability to move the toes should be reported to the doctor. All observations should be charted in detail.

TECHNIQUES

Since infants and children cannot verbalize complaints, the nurse must observe closely and evaluate the child's responses to therapy. When a cast is in place, the toes or fingers should be observed for:
1. Numbness or tingling
2. Color (pale or cyanotic)
3. Warmth to the touch
4. Obvious edema

I. Checking Circulation to the Toes or Fingers

To check circulation, squeeze or press a toe or finger to blanch the skin. When the pressure is released the color should return if the circulation is adequate.

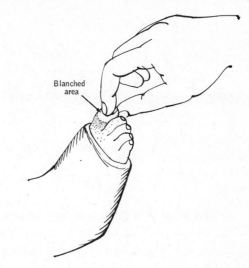

FIGURE 22-1. Checking Circulation to the Toes or Fingers.

1. If the toes do not blanch, congestion may be present and should be reported to the doctor.

2. If the blanching persists after pressure is released, the circulation is impaired. The doctor must be notified.

3. If extreme pain results from touching or moving the toes, report it to the doctor.

Itching

Itching is a common problem with children in casts. When possible, prior to the application of the cast, a strip of gauze may be placed under the cast and used as a mechanical "scratcher." When the strip of gauze becomes soiled, tie a clean length of gauze to one end of the soiled gauze; then pull out the soiled portion from the opposite end.

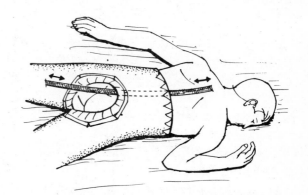

FIGURE 22-2. A Gauze "Scratcher" A strip of gauze, when moved in and out of the cast, serves as a "scratcher" to relieve itching of the skin under the cast.

II. Positioning a Child in a Cast

If a child with a cast is allowed out of bed, he should be placed in a wheelchair. Because the posture and body mechanics of a child differ from those of an adult, the child is more likely to lose his balance or develop muscle strain unless the cast is supported.

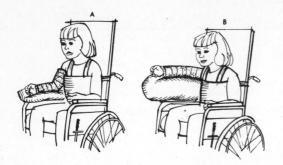

FIGURE 22-3. Correct and Incorrect Positions for a Child in a Wheelchair In the incorrect position (A) the support is too low to relieve local edema. Correctly positioned (B), the arm is elevated, the wrist is higher than the elbow, and the elbow is higher than the shoulder.

The child in a spica cast may be placed on his abdomen on a stretcher for a period of time to enable him to join in supervised play activities with other children. When a child is in a wheelchair or on a stretcher, adequate restraints are necessary to maintain safety.

III.   Turning a Child in a Body Cast

Two people are needed to turn a child in a body cast, one on each side of the bed.

1. Move the child to the edge of the bed as far as possible so that the nurse who will receive the child is farthest away from him.

2. The nurse nearest to the child places one hand under his head and back and one hand under the leg part of the cast and turns the child to the midway point on his side.

3. The nurse farthest away then accepts the support of the child and cast as he is turned completely onto his abdomen.

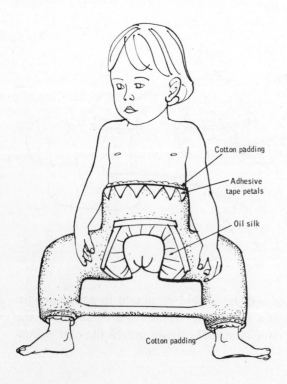

Cotton padding

Adhesive tape petals

Oil silk

Cotton padding

FIGURE 22-4. A Body (Spica) Cast This body cast maintains the legs in a froglike position and is used to treat congenital dislocation of the hip. Note that the child is able to move toes freely. Yellow oil-silk protects the cast from moisture in the diaper area. All edges are padded with candy cotton and protected by adhesive "petals."

The supporting bar between the legs should not be used as a lever when turning the child. All body curvatures should be supported with pillows or sheet rolls. When possible, the older child should be on his abdomen during mealtime to facilitate swallowing and self-feeding.

When placing a child in a body cast on a bedpan, support the upper back and legs with pillows so that body alignment is maintained.

IV. Skin Care After Removal of a Cast

When a cast has been worn for four to six weeks, an accumulation of sebaceous material and dead skin causes the skin to appear brownish and flaky. The skin may be gently washed with pHisoHex and annointed with oil. Vigorous scrubbing of the skin is not advised, as skin trauma may result.

The limb should remain elevated for a few hours each day to minimize the development of edema. Gradual and gentle exercises will relieve joint stiffness.

CARE OF A CHILD IN TRACTION

PRINCIPLES

Traction is designed to maintain the approximation of the fractured segments of bone until union occurs.

The doctor prescribes the type of traction, the amount of weight to be used, and the countertraction needed.

Traction must be kept constant in order to achieve the desired results. The weight of the patient's body provides countertraction to the weights and pulleys. Any change in the countertraction affects the entire traction system.

Traction applied to the skin indirectly affects the bone fragments. The skin must be protected from injury.

Moleskin must fit snugly in order to maintain traction. If edema occurs local circulation may be impaired.

NURSING RESPONSIBILITIES

The extremity must be supported in alignment until union occurs. However, some *body* movement is necessary to prevent hypostatic pneumonia.

The nurse must prepare the prescribed traction and assist the doctor in its application and maintenance.

Weights should not be added or removed without specific doctor's orders. Weights should hang free, not touch the floor or bed. All knotted areas of rope should be wrapped in adhesive tape to prevent slipping. The gatch of the bed should not be elevated at the head or knee without the consent of the physician.

Shave the legs if hair is present, and paint with tincture of benzoin to protect the skin prior to the application of moleskin. Pressure on bony prominences may be minimized by padding with candy cotton.

The nurse must check the circulation to the fingers or toes at frequent intervals.

Detailed skin care is essential to prevent the development of decubitus ulcers in immobilized patients.

All exposed skin areas should be washed and dried thoroughly. Cornstarch will absorb moisture and prevent maceration of the skin.

Atrophy results from the disuse of muscles. A lack of exercise causes an accumulation of waste products in the muscle, resulting in fatigue and discomfort. The effect of therapeutic exercise lasts about four hours.

The nurse should encourage the movement and exercise of the unaffected extremities and provide diversional therapy to the bedridden child. The toes or fingers of the affected limb should also be exercised. Short, frequent periods of muscle exercise should be incorporated into the daily care of an immobilized child.

Prolonged periods of immobilization predispose the child to the development of hypostatic pneumonia and constipation.

The child should be encouraged to breathe deeply at intervals. Constipation is best prevented or relieved by dietary modifications.

TECHNIQUES

I. Preparing for Traction

A basic traction-bar setup should be affixed to one empty bed in the unit at all times. When skin traction is to be applied, the equipment assembled at the bedside should include:

1. Strips of moleskin (to extend above the knee on each side of the leg)
2. Adhesive tape
3. Leg roll
4. A square wooden block
5. Ropes, weights, pulleys

Traction bars should be affixed to the bed as shown in the illustrations in this chapter.

II. Cutting Rope for Use in Traction

The ropes used to maintain traction must be cut to an appropriate length. The proper cutting technique can prevent fraying of the rope end and weakening of the rope fiber.

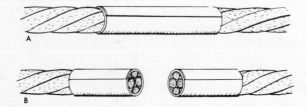

FIGURE 22–5. Cutting Rope for Use in Traction 1. Determine the length of rope needed. Wrap adhesive tape around the rope in the area to be cut (A). 2. Cut *through* the adhesive tape to obtain the desired length (B). This technique is designed to prevent fraying and weakening of the rope fiber.

III.   Maintaining the Position of the Bed

When the doctor orders the bed gatch to be raised to a specific level in order to maintain countertraction, it is wise to apply adhesive tape to the bed gatch so that ambulatory children will not raise or lower the bed level by turning the gatch during play. In the pediatric unit, posted signs warning against raising or lowering the bed often go unheeded.

IV.   Charting

The nurse should record the following observations, in detail, on the patient's chart:
1. Color, temperature, and warmth of toes or fingers
2. Evidence of local edema
3. Condition of the skin
4. Offensive odors
5. Functioning of the traction ropes, pulleys, and weights
6. Steps taken to prevent or relieve pressure at bony prominences
7. Alignment of the body
8. Response of the child to therapy

V.   Types of Traction

Skeletal traction is traction applied directly to the bone. Skin traction refers to traction applied to the skin. The goals of therapy for both methods are the same. The doctor selects the type of traction to be used, based upon the bone pathology and the age of the child. Congenital or acquired bone disease can affect the growth of the bone. Adequate nutrition, nursing care, and rehabilitation are vital to a favorable prognosis.

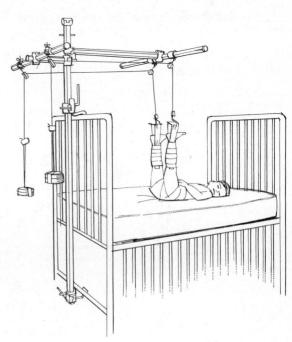

FIGURE 22–6. Bryant's Traction Note that the buttocks are slightly elevated from the mattress and all weights are out of the child's reach. An increased fluid intake and roughage in the diet will aid in preventing constipation in a child immobilized in Bryant's traction.

Bryant's Traction

Bryant's traction (Fig. 22–6) is used for children who weigh less than 40 pounds and involves the application of vertical traction to the fractured limb. This traction is more effective than the Buck's extension commonly seen in adult units, because children cannot provide sufficient countertraction with the weight of their bodies against the *horizontal* pull of the weights. This skin traction is applied to both legs in order to minimize potential trauma to the affected limb and maintain the stability of the position. The child's weight serves as countertraction to the *vertical* pull of the weights.

Points to observe and record:

1. The hips should be flexed at right angles to the body.
2. The buttocks should be slightly raised from the mattress.
3. The ankles should be padded to prevent trauma and the heel left free from pressure.
4. Padding should be in place between the wooden block spreader and the foot to prevent foot drop.
5. Circulation to the toes should be checked and recorded at regular intervals. (See page 236.)
6. A jacket restraint may be applied to prevent the child from turning.
7. Diversional therapy (toys) should be provided.
8. The weights should be out of the child's reach.
9. The weights should not hang directly over the body of the child.
10. The weights should hang free—not rest on the bed frame or the floor.
11. The weights should be secured in place with adhesive tape.
12. The ropes should rest securely within the pulley to minimize friction.
13. Adhesive tape should cover all knots to prevent slipping.

The Thomas Splint

The doctor may select the Thomas splint (Fig. 22–7) for the older child in order to achieve desired hip and knee flexion. This balanced traction also allows the child more liberal movement. Balanced traction eliminates the need for countertraction by body weight, and therefore the position of the bed is usually level. A Pearson attachment is

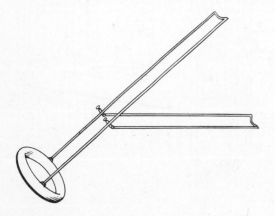

FIGURE 22–7. The Thomas Splint and Pearson Attachment The circumference of the ring of the splint should be large enough to accommodate the circumference of the thigh, without creating pressure on the skin. The leather ring may be covered with waterproof material (such as plastic) to prevent soiling by urine or feces. Strips of muslin or roller gauze are wrapped around the frame of the splint to provide leg support. Padding with candy cotton will provide comfort and lessen skin friction.

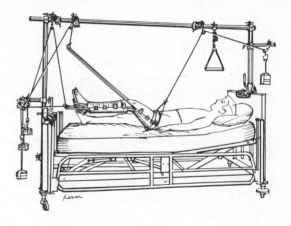

FIGURE 22–8. Balanced Skin Traction with the Thomas Splint and Pearson Attachment. Note that all traction bars in contact with the bed are padded with rubber to protect the bed surface. All weights are hanging free and away from the child. The body is in alignment.

usually used with a Thomas splint for the purpose of supporting the lower leg. The Pearson attachment is affixed to the Thomas splint at the point of the child's knee joint (see Fig. 22–8). The nurse should select a size of splint compatible with the anatomy of the child, so that pressure on soft tissue is avoided. The appropriate size of the leather ring may be determined by measuring the circumference of the unaffected thigh and allowing some room for possible edema.

Points to observe and record:

1. All weights are taped securely and hanging free.

2. The muslin or gauze support does not extend beyond the heel in order to prevent the development of decubiti.

3. The foot is at right angles with the ankle to prevent foot drop.

4. The ring of the Thomas splint does not press on the perineum.

5. The bed linen, mattress, or bed frame does not contact any part of the Thomas splint, since it could alter the degree of flexion of the hip or knee.

6. All knots are taped to prevent slipping.

The Bohler-Braun Splint

The Bohler-Braun splint (Fig. 22–9) may be used for preadolescents and adolescents. The use of this frame eliminates the need for overhead traction bars. Muslin or rolled gauze is wrapped around the frame prior to use. Paddings with candy cotton will increase comfort.

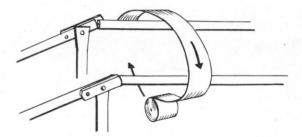

FIGURE 22–9. The Bohler-Braun Splint Wrap gauze securely around the thigh and calf area of the splint to provide rigid support. Roller gauze may be secured in place with adhesive tape. The knee angle of the frame should not be wrapped with gauze or padded.

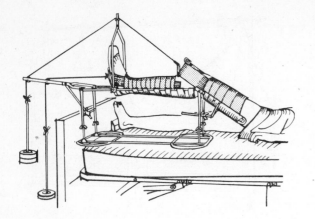

FIGURE 22–10. Traction with the Bohler-Braun Splint Note the space free of padding at the popliteal area. The heel and Achilles tendon are free of pressure from the muslin supports. All metal parts of the underframe should be padded to prevent injury to the unaffected leg as the child moves.

Points to observe:

1. The knee should be directly over the angle of the frame.

2. A space under the popliteal area (knee) is free of padding to prevent pressure at this site.

3. The heel extends beyond the gauze support.

4. The metal frame does not press on the perineum.

5. The foot is at a right angle to the ankle to prevent foot drop.

Traction on the Humerus

Traction on the humerus requires the application of traction bars to the lateral frame of the bed. The use of clamps is the preferred method of safely securing the traction bars to the bed (see Fig. 22–11). Some traction bars depend on the weight of the patient's body on the mattress to stabilize the position of the bars. In pediatrics, however, the weight of the child may not be an effective means of stabilization.

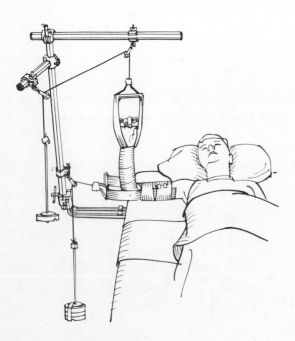

FIGURE 22–11. Traction on the Humerus Note that the arm is extended at a 90 degree angle from the body and is level with the chest. The wrist is not flexed. A pajama top or hospital gown may be placed over the child, with the affected arm left exposed. Circulation to the fingers should be checked frequently.

Points to observe:

1. The forearm should be flexed and extended at a 90 degree angle from the body.

2. The forearm should be in the same plane as, or level with, the chest. (The level is controlled by the head gatch of the bed.)

3. The wrist and hand should be in a neutral position, and prolonged flexion or hyperextension should be avoided.

4. The weights should be hanging free — unobstructed by the bed frame or the floor.

5. The ropes should not touch the mattress or the metal bars.

If traction weights pull the child to the side of the bed, a rolled blanket may be placed between the spring and mattress to aid in tilting the child's body and maintaining countertraction.

Cervical Traction

Cervical traction may be applied directly or indirectly. Direct traction is applied to the skull bone by means of a Crutchfeld tong. Indirect traction is accomplished by using a "head halter." Principles of nursing care are the same with skeletal or skin traction.

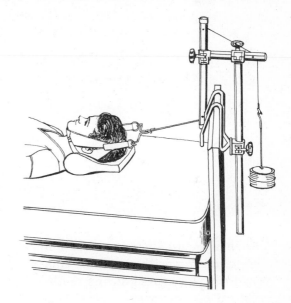

FIGURE 22–12.   Cervical Traction (Skin Traction)   The level of the head of the bed is prescribed by the doctor. Note the adhesive tape securing the weights in place. The rope does not touch the child's skin. Candy cotton padding may be placed under the chin halter to alleviate pressure on the skin.

Points to observe:

1. The position of the bed should be flat unless otherwise prescribed by the doctor. Raising the head of the bed increases countertraction, which may be undesirable.

2. The child must be flat on his back. Occasionally a Stryker frame bed may be used to facilitate turning the patient if cervical traction is planned for a long period of time.

3. The position of a head halter should be checked as follows: (A) The halter should not press on the ears, (B) the rope should not be resting against the skin, and (C) the chin piece should not press on the throat.

Hyperextension may be accomplished by placing a rolled towel under the child's shoulders. Avoid lifting the head or flexing the neck during feedings. The chin halter must be protected when feeding the child, as a soiled or wet halter can irritate the skin. Cornstarch should be substituted for powder for skin care under and around the halter, so that "caking" will be minimized.

VI. The Balkan Frame Bed

The Balkan frame bed is designed to protect the injured limb from the pressure of bedclothes and prevent unnecessary exposure of the child's body. School age children, preadolescents, and adolescents are characteristically modest, and psychological trauma may result from undue exposure of the body.

The foundation of the bed is made in the usual way. A top sheet is folded in half across the width, and a blanket is inserted between the folds. The sheet and blanket are placed over the child, extending from the hips to the shoulder. The open ends of the sheet are at the shoulder line. Another topsheet is folded in the same manner, and placed at the foot of the bed, extending *under* the suspended limb and *over* the unaffected limb. The open ends of the sheet are toward the foot of the bed. The excess is tucked under the mattress at the foot of the bed. The upper and lower portions of the top linen are pinned securely at the hip line, with the open ends of the safety pins away from the skin. The Balkan frame bed may be used for a child with a fracture of the lower extremity that is in traction or in a cast.

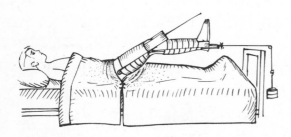

FIGURE 22–13. The Balkan Frame Bed Pinning the edges of the upper and lower portions of the top linen prevents undue exposure of the body. The toes are exposed so that they may be observed for impaired circulation. A stockinet may be used to cover the toes if the child feels cold. Although the Balkan frame bed refers specifically to a bed facilitating traction, this modification of the linen may be adapted to the child in a leg cast.

VII. Changing Linen

During routine nursing care, minimal handling of the fractured limb is desirable. Since traction must be kept constant in order to achieve the desired results, weights should not be removed during routine care. Foundation linen on the bed of any immobilized patient must be kept clean, dry, and free from wrinkles and crumbs. The preadolescent and adolescent child characteristically perspires more than an adult or a small infant because of the developmental status of his skin glands. The school age child's play habits and toilet habits are also reasons why a daily change of foundation linen is essential for any child confined to bed.

When the injured limb is suspended above the mattress, as in the Thomas splint, the technique of changing the foundation linen does not differ from the conventional method. However, when the affected limb or the equipment supporting the limb rests on the mattress, as in Buck's extension, the Bohler frame, a cast, or traction to the humerus, a modification of technique is necessary. Lifting or turning the affected limb or pushing linen under the limb will result in injury to the skin and discomfort to the patient. A supporting frame, such as the Bohler frame, should not be lifted or tilted.

If the nurse uses the proper techniques during routine care, she will contribute to the child's adjustment to his temporary handicap. The correct method is to fold the sheet in half (lengthwise) and place it on the edge of the bed with the fold toward the center of the bed (Fig. 22–14). *Roll* the top half of the sheet close to the affected limb.

Place one hand, palm up, under the affected limb and *support it in position*. With the free hand, *depress the mattress* and unroll the linen under the affected limb, toward the opposite side of the bed (Fig. 22–15).

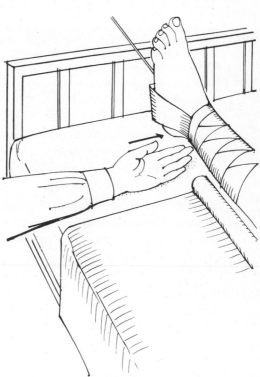

FIGURE 22–14.   Changing Linen Under the Affected Limb.

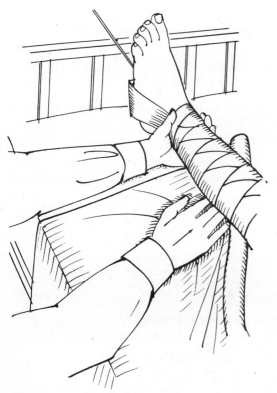

FIGURE 22–15.   Unrolling Clean Linen Under the Affected Limb.

The nurse may repeat this procedure at the ankle and knee, depending on the size of the patient. The linen is then pulled tight and the foundation completed in the usual way. Leg support should be provided at the joints, rather than under a muscle group, to prevent painful muscle spasm.

Diversional therapy for the bedridden child is discussed in Chapter 24.

VIII. Prevention and Treatment of Bedsores

Any bedridden patient is prone to the development of bedsores. Only good nursing care can prevent bedsores.

Prevention:
1. Interrupt sustained skin pressure that comes from lying in one position.
   A. Reposition patient every two hours
   B. Use a rubber foam cushion to relieve pressure
   C. Keep two sheets of polyethylene under bony prominences
   D. Keep skin clean and dry
   E. Use a water mattress
2. Correct protein deficits.
   A. Provide an appetizing, nutritious diet
   B. Prevent and correct anemia
   C. Watch for and prevent protein deficits

Treatment:
1. Soaks. Commonly prescribed soaks include:
   A. 1:40 dilution of Burow's solution 20 min. T.I.D.
   B. Organic iodine compounds and acetic acid compresses (depending on culture findings)
   C. Fresh hydrogen peroxide washes if anaerobic organisms are present
2. Topical enzymes following debridement.
3. Antibiotic or steroid creams are usually prescribed.
4. Honey under a dry dressing packed with sugar may be prescribed for bedsores that do not respond to routine therapy.
5. Whirlpool or infrared therapy may also be prescribed.
6. Skin grafting may be necessary in severe cases.

BIBLIOGRAPHY

Bank, H. (Ed.): Symposium on Musculoskeletal Disorders. *Pediatric Clinics of North America, 14*(3), 1967.

Larson, C., and Gould, M.: *Orthopedic Nursing,* 8th Edition, The C. V. Mosby Co., St. Louis, 1974.

Marlow, D.: *Textbook of Pediatric Nursing.* 4th Edition, W. B. Saunders Co., Philadelphia, 1973.

Vaughn, V. C., III, and McKay, R. J.: *Nelson Textbook of Pediatrics.* 10th Edition, W. B. Saunders Co., Philadelphia, 1975.

Zimmerbook: Traction Handbook. Zimmer Manufacturing Co., Warsaw, Indiana, 1975.

Chapter Twenty Three

BURN THERAPY

PRINCIPLES

In a child, a burn involving 15 per cent of the body area or more usually requires admission to the hospital.

Nursing personnel should consider any burn as an open wound.

NURSING RESPONSIBILITIES

As soon as the nurse knows that a burn patient is to be admitted, she should prepare the equipment needed for the unit.

Maintenance of strict medical aseptic technique is essential in the care of children with burns. A private room is preferable (if available), as isolation technique is essential to prevent secondary infections.

I. Anticipated Therapy

Medication for maintenance of vital signs, blood volume, prevention of infections, etc., is given as soon as possible. Dosage is dependent upon the size of the patient and the extent of the injury.

Fluid and electrolyte imbalance and shock frequently occur in children with extensive burns.

Reduced blood volume is reflected by changes in blood chemistry.

Respiratory complications may be anticipated, especially if fumes or flames have been inhaled.

The child should be weighed and his length measured upon admission, before *and* after dressings are applied.

Intravenous therapy may be anticipated.

The nurse should assemble the equipment necessary for the collection of blood specimens. The specimens should be sent to the laboratory for immediate analysis.

Oxygen and a tracheotomy tray should be available within the unit.

When burns are treated by the "open" method, a black crust (eschar) will form. Close observation and recording by the nurse will facilitate the accurate evaluation of the child's progress by the medical team.

The nurse should observe and record:
1. Eschar formation
2. Edema
3. Symptoms of acidosis
4. Symptoms of infection
5. Symptoms of toxicity
   a. Vomiting
   b. Abnormalities in vital signs
   c. Oliguria
6. Temperature of the unit

Excessive heat in the burn tent may dilate peripheral vessels and aggravate the circulatory disturbance, and also provide a medium for the growth of pathogenic organisms.

The temperature within the burn tent should be checked every 8 hours. The temperature may be controlled by increasing or limiting the number of bulbs used to provide heat.

Severe burns may cause renal failure.

An intake and output record must be kept for any child admitted with extensive burns.

Burns allow plasma loss, which in turn causes a reduction of blood volume, blood flow, and cardiac output.

The nurse must observe and record vital signs every 4 hours. (See p. 41 for the observation of vital signs for infants and children.)

From the second to the fifth day following extensive burns is a period of sodium retention, whereas from the fifth to the fourteenth day is a period of nitrogen loss. An increased fluid intake aids in the elimination of toxins.

Oral administration of *pure water* will cause water intoxication in the early stages of a burn. The doctor will order special electrolyte solutions to be administered by mouth. A high protein diet may be indicated after the fifth day of burn therapy.

Edema frequently occurs in the early stages of a burn. The healing and scarring of a burn may cause contractures.

Burned extremities should be elevated to minimize edema, and anatomical positions should be maintained to prevent contractures.

Necrotic tissue may be soaked off to promote healing.

A tub bath or saline soaks may be prescribed by the doctor. All equipment used must be sterile. Only unburned areas of the skin may be washed with soap and water.

Plastic surgery, physical therapy, and early rehabilitation will reduce the disfigurement and handicaps resulting from extensive burns.

The nurse should explain to the parents and the child the plan of long-term care and rehabilitation. Nursing care should be designed to prevent contractures and minimize deformities.

TECHNIQUES

I. The Rule of Nines

The body surface area of an infant differs from that of an adult. The modification of the "rule of nines" shown in Figure 23–1 aids the doctor in evaluating the percentage of burned surface and determining the therapeutic needs.

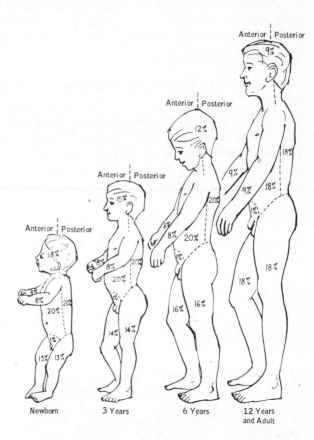

FIGURE 23–1. The "Rule of Nines" to Determine the Percentage of Burned Body Surface in Infants and Children.

Burns may be treated by the "open" or "closed" method. When the "open" method of treatment is selected, the doctor may request that the child be placed in a burn tent. When the "closed" method of treatment is selected, pressure dressings are applied in the operating room, and a burn tent is not used. A cradle affixed to the bed frame will relieve pressure from the bedclothes. Sterile linen should be used when caring for any child with extensive burns.

II. Anticipated Therapy

The doctor may order wet soaks or tub soaks to the burned area. Wet soaks are done at the bedside, using a bulb syringe and sterile gauze dressings.

III. Tub Soaks for Body Burns

1. The clean tub is filled to half capacity with the solution ordered by the doctor.

2. The child may be lifted from the bed onto a stretcher draped with a sterile sheet. A sterile sheet can be used to lift the child, maintaining body alignment.

3. The child is immersed in the tub, using the sterile sheet to support the body at a controlled depth.

4. One nurse should support the child's head, for reasons of safety.

5. The nurse should observe the responses of the child.

6. The treatment should be terminated after 20 minutes.

Accurate charting concerning the type of bath given and the response of the child is essential.

IV. The Burn Tent

A burn tent may be assembled by attaching traction bars to the four corners of the bed or crib, being sure to secure them with crossbars at the ends and midsection of the bed. Only approved lighting facilities should be used to provide warmth for the patient. Blue light bulbs, enclosed in metal frames for safety, should be available. Lights should be checked by the electrician immediately before use. Canopies may be autoclaved as needed or improvised with sterile bed linen.

The burn tent frame is set up over the bed and fastened securely as illustrated in Figure 23–2.

1. Be sure there are crossbars (A and B) at the ends and midsection of the frame.

2. Tie the light bulbs (in their metal frames) to the center bar, or string them from all the crossbars. Be sure that the lights are out of the reach of the child.

3. Extend the cord attached to the lights to the corner of the burn tent frame and bandage it down the side of the frame. Plug it into the appropriate outlet.

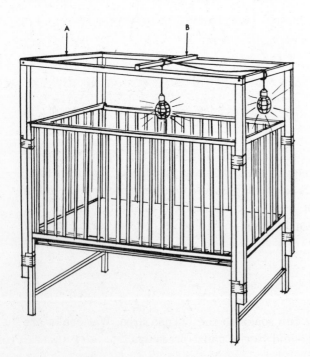

FIGURE 23–2.   The Burn Tent Frame.

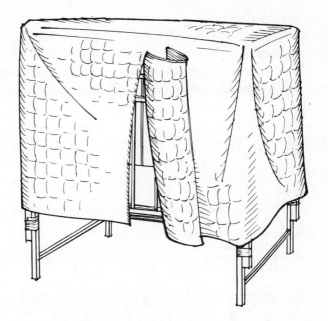

FIGURE 23–3. Burn Tent Frame with Canopy in Place.

4. Place the quilted canopy over the top of the frame and allow the quilt to extend a few inches below the mattress (but not to touch the floor). The openings of the quilt should be at the center of the bed on both sides.

A thermometer may be secured to the burn tent frame at the head of the bed. The temperature should be 85 to 100° F. If increased humidity is desired, a jar of water may be fastened to the inside of the frame of the bed. Side rails must be secured to the bed for reasons of safety.

V. Semiclosed Dressings

Semiclosed methods of treating burns, which eliminate large bulky dressings, have recently proved most successful in decreasing infections and providing early ambulation and uninterrupted activity. Early ambulation has definite psychological implications as

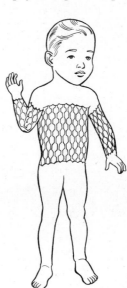

FIGURE 23–4. Tubular Elasticized Netting over a Burn Dressing.

well as increasing joint mobility, which limits contracture formation. Topical agents and biologic (animal skin) dressings are held in place with a thin layer of sterile, fine mesh gauze, which is secured in place with a tubular elasticized netting (see Fig. 23-4). The netting allows maximum aeration with minimum constriction. Dressings are usually changed once a day.

BIBLIOGRAPHY

Armstrong, I. L., and Browder, J. J.: *The Nursing Care of Children.* 3rd Edition, F. A. Davis Co., Philadelphia, 1970.

Gellis, S. S., and Kagan, B. M. (Eds.): *Current Pediatric Therapy.* 7th Edition, W. B. Saunders Co., Philadelphia, 1976.

Marlow, D.: *Textbook of Pediatric Nursing.* 4th Edition, W. B. Saunders Co., Philadelphia, 1973.

PRODUCT REFERENCE

Diffusan Sales, Inc., Woodmere, New York: Elasticized netting.

Chapter Twenty Four

DIVERSIONAL THERAPY FOR HOSPITALIZED INFANTS AND CHILDREN

PRINCIPLES

Play is an essential part of a child's life and is an important aspect in fostering growth and development.

Toys are the "tools" of play and provide a more "natural" environment for a child. The proper selection and use of toys can reduce the traumatic effects of a hospitalization experience and aid in the recovery phase of illness.

A favorable nurse-child rapport can be established if the happy experiences of the child are related to the nurse, who is also often responsible for administering painful therapy.

The child can find acceptable outlets for hostilities through play activities.

The proper selection of toys can provide constructive, educational, stimulating, relaxing, diversional, or therapeutic values.

NURSING RESPONSIBILITIES

Organization of the day's activities for a hospitalized child should provide opportunities for play.

To achieve optimum benefits, toys should be selected by the professional nurse with deep thought and consideration of the child's age, special interests, developmental status, activity limitations, and their therapeutic value.

The nurse should assume a major role in initiating play therapy and should observe the child at play. Toys can serve as a channel of communication between the child and the nurse.

A little time spent in planning and initiating play activities will save much time which would otherwise be spent in coping with behavior problems.

The nurse should use stable criteria for the selection of toys for the hospitalized child.

The physical therapist is specially trained to analyze and evaluate muscle activities involved in the handling of specific toys.

The nurse should work closely with the physical therapist in selecting toys for the handicapped child in order to achieve optimum therapeutic values and provide continuity of care.

The inaccessibility of toys locked in a central area will force the busy nurse to leave the full responsibility for play activities to a volunteer worker.

Toys should be located in an area easily accessible to the nurse.

An excessive number of toys can produce overstimulation, frustration, and confusion and may hamper the goal of play therapy.

It is the responsibility of the nurse to discuss and plan play therapy with the parents, who may wish to bring toys during visiting hours.

Some toys can present a danger to a hospitalized child.

All toys should be screened by a nurse or other designated person for safety.

TECHNIQUES

I. Selection of Toys

The selection of toys should be based upon the special interests of the child, the age of the child, the level of activity allowed, and the level of activity involved in the play material. Toys for handicapped or palsied children should not be classified by chronological age groups, but should be selected in terms of the capacity of the child and the developmental or therapeutic purposes served.

Generally speaking, a toy that encourages imagination and allows the child to become involved in the activity is more desirable than a mechanical toy that plays "for" the child. Safety is of primary importance. Some general criteria for the selection of toys include:

1. Toys should not have sharp edges.
2. Toys should not have removable parts that can be swallowed or pushed into a cast.
3. Toys that may burn, explode, or produce a shock should not be given to a hospitalized child.
4. Friction toys or toys that produce sparks should not be given to a child in an oxygen-enriched environment.
5. Toys with attached ropes or loops present a potential danger to a hospitalized child.
6. Toys should be lead-free.
7. Toys should be easy to clean, easy to store, and preferably nonspillable.

Toys for the handicapped child should be evaluated in terms of:

1. Their interest value
2. Durability

3. Variety of motions required for their manipulation

4. The degree of mental and physical stimulation provided

The nurse must also consider physical facilities and limitations when selecting play activities.

II. The Bedridden Child

Quiet or moderate activity for a bedridden child may include picture books, drawing books, clay, squeeker toys, large beads, weaving, jointed figures, and puppets. A ball on a string can be dropped over the bedside and pulled back. Miniature autos can be pushed back and forth on the mattress.

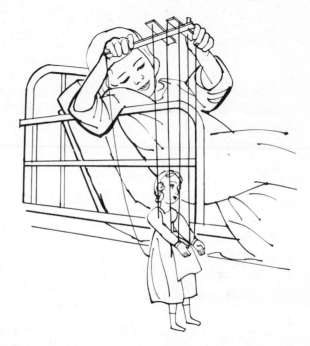

FIGURE 24-1. Puppets provide moderate activity for a bedridden child.

A child who sits up in bed must have adequate body support. A box placed behind the pillow will provide a makeshift back support for a child confined to a crib. A bed tray makes a suitable stable, flat surface for play, and a shopping bag may be hung on the bedpost or a nearby chair as a "catch-all" for toys and cutouts.

Selected Toys of Interest to Specific Age Groups

The toys in the following list are useful to divert children of various ages.

Infants:
    Bright hanging objects
    Rattles
    Toy animals
    Plastic keys

Toddlers:
    Blocks

Toddlers continued:
    Dolls
    Pots and pans
    Cloth books
    Pull-toys
    Toy telephone
    Music boxes

Preschool:

    Crayons

    Clay

    Cuddly toy animals

    Doll furniture

    Plastic tools

    Toy telephone

    Record player

    Toy trucks and cars

    Books

    Housekeeping toys

School age:

    Cutouts

    Doll house

    Puzzles

School age continued:

    Simple hobbies

    Toy housewares

    Dress-up clothes

Preadolescent:

    Clay

    Cutouts

    Books

    Crafts

    Checkers, chess, dominoes

    Magic tricks

    Dolls

    Hobbies

    Sewing, knitting

    Weaving looms

Many studies concerning the use of toys for hospitalized children have been conducted. Table 24–1 reports observational data adapted from one of these studies. The results of this study show the type of toy that is most likely to hold the interest of a hospitalized child.

TABLE 24–1.   Suitable Toys for Hospitalized Children*

Play Material		Age Group	Approximate Range of Play Time (in minutes)
1. Active play toys			
	Baby crib toys	4–15 months	2–10
	Bench with pegs	3½–5 years	20–30
2. Constructive toys			
	Wooden blocks, trains	4–11 years	45–120
3. Imaginary toys			
	Nurse-doctor kits	4–12 years	60–120
	Dolls	4–11 years	15–120
	Telephones	2½–10 years	10–60
4. Manipulative toys			
	Jointed figures	4–11 years	5–15
	Simple puzzles	7–11 years	10–30

*Adapted from Gips, C.: A Study of Toys for Hospitalized Children. Child Development, *21*:149, 1950.

III.   *Therapeutic Values of Selected Toys**

Toys can be of definite therapeutic value if selected by the professional nurse or the physical therapist.

Clarinet.   The clarinet is good for finger flexion and extension in older children. Blowing is an excellent basis for speech therapy.

---

*Adapted from Langdon, M., Ream, C. T., and Doebler, M. H.: Report of a Study on the Use of Toys in Work with Cerebral Palsied Children. National Society for Crippled Children and Adults, February, 1955.

Color xylophone. This toy aids in developing rhythm, requires hand-eye coordination and hand grasp. The sound and random movements provide satisfaction to the child.

Junior floor train. The train teaches reaching grasp, encourages hand-eye coordination and placement values.

Push-pull toys. Encourage walking and crawling as well as imaginative play. Children may try to imitate the sounds, thus aiding in speech and vocalization.

Rocking horse. A rocking horse aids in maintaining sitting balance. It also provides for bilateral arm movements, reach, and grasp.

Take-apart train. This toy encourages the use of both hands, requires hand-eye coordination, and encourages form perception. It teaches reach and placement; it is also a highly imaginative toy.

Tot's tool box. Tools are good for the hand grasp, supination, and pronation. They increase hand-eye coordination and form perception.

Tricycle. The tricycle provides reciprocal motions, hand grasp, leg-muscle exercise and dorsiflexion of the ankle. It also provides a highly imaginative form of group or individual play.

Wagon. A wagon provides hand grasp, trunk control, dorsiflexion and plantar flexion of the ankles, hip and leg flexion and extension.

Selected toys may also be used to teach color discrimination, size discrimination and shape discrimination.

BIBLIOGRAPHY

Brooks, M. M.: Why Play in the Hospital? *Nursing Clinics of North America,* 5:431, 1970.
Frantzen, J. OTR.: Toys—The Tools of Children. National Society for Crippled Children and Adults, Chicago, Illinois.

Chapter Twenty Five

THE USE OF VISITING HOURS: TEACHING THE PARENTS

PRINCIPLES

Studies have shown that parents play a major role in the recovery and rehabilitation phase of pediatric therapy.

If parents are aware of the disease process and its implications for the growing child, efforts to promote a gradual return to a state of positive health will be more easily facilitated.

The nurse must recognize her limitations in the amount and kind of information she may safely impart.

The nurse must be aware of the resources and sources of information available within the hospital and the community.

Teaching is defined as "the imparting of knowledge." Factors affecting learning are:

NURSING RESPONSIBILITIES

Parents must be greeted as guests, not intruders. With the help of the nurse, parents can be encouraged to provide continuity of care and foster the growth and development of the child.

The nurse must plan time for teaching parents. Rapport is best developed by maintaining an unhurried atmosphere and exhibiting sincere interest. The trend in many hospitals toward providing increased facilities for parent-child contacts during hospitalization provides an excellent opportunity for teaching and guidance of parents.

The nurse may interpret explanations given by the pediatrician. The individual needs and responses of the parent should guide the nurse in planning her teaching and referrals.

If the nurse cannot answer a particular question, she should refer the parents to the proper source.

A plan of teaching must be preceded by psychological support and the development of a positive nurse-parent relation-

260

1. The desire to learn
2. The intellectual capacity of the parents
3. The response of the parents to the teaching

An awareness of the parent's interpretations or misinterpretations of facts will enable the nurse to present her teaching on a more individualized basis.

Parents who think they understand the care of the child may become insecure when actually confronted with the problem at home.

ship. Information must be presented at the intellectual level of the parent, and the responses of the parent should be noted. Recording the progress of the parent's learning will facilitate continuity and prevent duplication of information.

"Telling" is not "teaching." *Listening* and involving the parent in the plan of care for the child is an essential part of teaching the parent.

Printed teaching aids, written diets, etc., provided by the nurse, will offer parents a ready reference at home and aid in the transition phase after discharge.

TECHNIQUES

The general excitement occurring on the discharge day can inhibit the effective concentration that is necessary for the assimilation of new teaching. Education of parents should be initiated long before the discharge date to facilitate evaluation of the teaching and assure continuity of care. Teaching should contain general information as well as the factors specific to the disease process and follow-up needs. The interest and motivation of the parents should be the determining factors in the sequence of the teaching plan (see Chapter 27 for teaching the outpatient).

I. General Factors in Teaching Parents

Growth and Development

Since the changing needs of children are attributed to the pattern of growth and development, parents will be better able to meet these needs if they understand the developmental process. Many books and pamphlets concerning growth and development are available to the nurse, free of charge, for distribution to parents. The nurse should maintain a library of these teaching aids and select and distribute them as needed.

Immunizations

The value of routine inoculations to guard children against infections should be discussed with parents. Although cleanliness, fresh air, exercise, rest, and nutrition build up the natural resistance to disease, community health measures, in the form of routine immunizations, can protect the child from serious epidemic diseases. The plan for routine protective immunizations, based upon the recommendations of the American Academy of Pediatrics, is given in Table 25–1.

TABLE 25–1.   Plan for Routine Protective Immunizations*

Approximate Age	Immunizations Given
6–8 weeks of age	First diphtheria, pertussis, and tetanus vaccine, (DPT) and oral polio vaccine
6 weeks later	Second DPT and oral polio vaccine
6 weeks later	Third DPT and oral polio vaccine
12 months of age	Measles vaccine, rubella vaccine, mumps vaccine; tuberculin test
18 months of age	Booster DPT and oral polio vaccine
4 years of age (preschool)	Booster DPT and oral polio vaccine
14–16 years of age	Diphtheria and tetanus toxoid
Every 10 years thereafter	Tetanus toxoid

*Injections are given I.M. into the lateral thigh in infants or deltoid muscles of older children. Deep injection and massage reduce postinjection problems. In breast fed infants, oral polio vaccine may be deferred until weaning to insure effective vaccination.

The parent may be referred to a private physician or a local child health station for immunizations. The school nurse will guide parents concerning the "booster shots" necessary for the school age child. Immunizations are rarely given to a hospitalized child because of the danger of vaccinia reactions.

General Nutrition

General nutrition for infants and children, and techniques of feeding are discussed in Chapter 13.

General Hygiene

General principles of child care concerning weaning, teething, bathing, rest, and dental care should be discussed with parents. The Department of Health offers many publications free of charge for distribution to parents.

Accident Prevention

Teaching the parents about accident prevention is classified as general teaching but it can be considered a specific teaching need when dealing with the parents of children hospitalized because of physical trauma.

The teaching of safety in child care should be correlated with the teaching of growth and development because the behavior patterns occurring at various phases of development predispose the child to specific potential hazards. This relationship is illustrated in Table 25–2. The goal of teaching safety in child care is to protect the child from potential hazards rather than change his behavior patterns during any developmental phase.

II.   Specific Factors in Teaching Parents

The nurse should include factors specific to the illness of and therapy for the individual child in her teaching plan. Consideration of the disease process as it may affect nutritional needs, bodily functions, and activity limitations should be discussed. If any

TABLE 25–2.   A Guide to Accident Prevention at Various Age Levels*

Age	Developmental Behavior	Typical Accident	Precautions to Teach Parents
Birth–1 year	Can roll over	Falls	Do not leave child unattended on bassinet table, etc., and keep crib sides up.
	Places objects in mouth	Aspiration of foreign bodies	Avoid the use of small toys with removable parts.
	Can creep and is curious	Poisoning, burns	Keep harmful substances out of reach.
	Helpless in water	Drowning	Supervise in wading pools and bathtub.
	Can squirm	Choking	Avoid the use of restraints with long straps that can entangle and choke the child.
1–2 years	Able to walk	Falls	Keep windows screened securely.
	Puts objects into mouth	Poisoning	Keep medicines and poisons out of reach.
	Helpless in water	Drowning	Supervise in pools and tub.
	Spatial judgment is poor	Car accidents	Keep gate closed at top of stairway, supervise outdoor play.
	Curiosity motivates exploring	Burns	Keep handles of pots on stove away from edge, cover unused electrical outlets.
3–4 years	Runs and climbs, poor spatial judgment	Falls	Keep windows screened securely.
	Opens doors, investigates closets, etc.	Asphyxiation	Keep doors locked and keep dangerous objects out of sight and reach of child.
	Throws balls	Lacerations	Teach the child the danger of throwing sharp or harmful objects.
	Rides tricycle	Car accidents	Teach child how to cross the street safely.
5–9 years	Is adventurous and has large muscle control	Car accidents, drowning	Teach child rules for bicycle, encourage swimming skills.
	Has interest in group play and partakes in "hero worship"	Burns, fractures	Know the leader of the child's group and encourage leadership qualities rather than allow the child to be easily influenced.
10–14 years	Needs strenuous physical activity	Falls	Teach safety in sports.
	Seeks peer approval, plays in hazardous areas	Car accidents, burns fractures	Teach rules of pedestrian safety, provide safe area for socialization and play.

*Adapted from Shaffer, T. E.: *Pediatric Clinics of North America.* 1:426, 1954.

special equipment is required for home care of the child, the parents should be familiarized with its use and referred for financial assistance as needed. Various community agencies may be called upon to assist and guide parents in caring for their convalescent or chronically ill child at home. (See Chapter 26.)

III. Principles of Reassuring the Hospitalized Child

The responses of a child to hospitalization vary according to the age of the child, but skillful psychological management can avoid damage to the developing personality. Three general rules for reassuring a hospitalized child include:

1. Establish a personal involvement with the child in order to offer reassurance.

2. Never lie to a child.

3. Show that you understand and accept the fears of the child before offering reassurance.

Effective utilization of these principles implies that the nurse has an underlying understanding of growth and development and of the types of fears common to each age group, as well as the ability to accurately analyze the individual situation.

BIBLIOGRAPHY

American Academy of Pediatrics: *Accidents in Children.* Committee on Accident Prevention, Evanston, Illinois, 1968.
American Academy of Pediatrics: *Care of Children in Hospitals.* Committee on Hospital Care, Evanston, Illinois, 1971.
Meeks, J.: Dispelling the Fears of the Hospitalized Child. Hospital Medicine, 6:77, 1970.
Tunnesson, W., Jr.: Questions New Mothers Ask and How I Answer Them. *Consultant,* March, 1971.
Vaughn, V. C., III, and McKay, R. J.: *Nelson Textbook of Pediatrics.* 10th Edition, W. B. Saunders Co., Philadelphia, 1975.

Chapter Twenty Six

DISCHARGE OF INFANTS AND CHILDREN

PRINCIPLES	NURSING RESPONSIBILITIES

I. Carrying out the Doctor's Order

The doctor must write the order for discharge and complete the summary record of the infant's chart.

The nurse notifies the information office of the discharge and notifies social service agencies when indicated.

II. Planning Follow-up Care

Instructions concerning follow-up care and clinic visits must be written for the parents and reinforced by oral explanation.

The nurse should obtain the information concerning follow-up care and the instructions to be given to the parents from the doctor. A doctor-nurse-parent conference would be helpful.

III. Teaching the Parents

The nurse must determine whether the parents understand the care that may be necessary for the child.

The nurse should allow the parent to handle and dress the child but should remain available to talk with the parent. Clinic referral and the importance of follow-up care should be explained.

IV. Identification

A child must be returned to the proper family. Family court decisions regarding custody of the child must be considered.

The nurse must check the identification supplied by the parent and record the type of identification shown. The identification band of the child should be checked prior to his discharge.

V. Records

All records of nursing and therapeutic care must be kept on file in the hospital after discharge of the patient.

The nurse should:
1. Assemble the chart
2. Record the discharge note, including:
   a. Time of discharge
   b. Identification shown by parent
   c. To whom discharged
   d. Instructions given
   e. Condition of patient
   f. Property taken

VI. Other Responsibilities

The nurse is responsible for the child until he leaves the hospital building. All outdated cards should be removed from the files. A permanent record of admissions and discharges must be kept.

The nurse should assign a staff member to accompany the parent and child to the discharge office. She should then dispose of the medicine tickets, formula card, Kardex, and bed card, and record the discharge in the census book.

TECHNIQUES

The nurse should be guided by the individual hospital's policy concerning the type of identification required prior to the discharge of infants and children. The supervisor is available for assistance when the nurse is in doubt concerning the adequacy of identification. The infant's birth certificate or the driver's license of the parent is usually considered acceptable identification.

The proper office is notified concerning the discharge of the child and the parents are requested to bring the required identification and the child's clothing.

Clinic appointment slips and the prescriptions for medication should be given to the parents as well as written instructions for general follow-up care and special diets. A health team–parent conference should be planned whenever possible prior to the discharge of the child.

The chart should be assembled and a discharge note recorded. The completed chart should be forwarded to the record room of the hospital at the time of discharge.

I. Follow-up Care

It is a nursing responsibility to identify high risk infants and provide long-term follow-up care to assess the development, detect persistent chronic problems, plan necessary intervention, and provide appropriate referrals. The nurse should work as part of a team, along with the doctor, social worker, and public health agency, in planning follow-up care.

Analysis of the infant's level of development at various key ages and physical and psychological stages can provide a developmental profile predictive of the child's future. It may be able to assist in later vocational preparation and guidance to enable the child to function within his capacity.

II.   Transfer of a Premature Infant to a Premature Unit

The establishment of specialized units for the care of premature infants has contributed significantly to the survival rate of these infants.

Premature units are usually centrally controlled by the public health agency of the city. When a doctor requests the transfer of a premature infant to a premature unit, the head nurse should phone the appropriate center and provide the necessary information concerning the condition of the infant.

When the public health nurse arrives to take the infant, the nurse should obtain proper identification, dress the baby and assist in placing it in the portable incubator supplied by the public health nurse. She should then chart the transfer as a "discharge" (to the premature center), forward the chart to the record room, and enter the name in the census book as a "discharge" to the premature center.

General Nursing Responsibilities

1. Preparation of a report of the infant's condition, including:
   A. A copy of infant's chart and a summary of the mother's chart.
   B. Reports of cord blood, blood glucose, and hematocrit.
   C. A tube sample of the mother's blood.
   D. X-ray of infant and placenta.
2. Parental consent and emotional preparation for separation.
3. Nursing intervention to help parents accept I.C.U. care for the newborn.
4. Preparation for maintenance of oxygen levels and body warmth during transportation procedure.
5. Being sure identification tags are securely in place on infant.

Note: Parents should be informed as to the purpose and time of the transfer and the location of the premature unit.

III.   Discharge of an Infant to the Bureau of Child Welfare

A hospital or its staff should not participate in matters related to adoption.

When a child is in need of the services of the Bureau of Child Welfare he should be referred to the hospital social service department as soon as possible. The social worker works with the Bureau of Child Welfare in arranging for the care of the child. The nurse notifies the social worker when the child is medically ready for discharge and the doctor writes a discharge order on the order sheet. The social worker fills out the required forms and obtains the written approval of the medical superintendent of the hospital.

The social worker will notify the nurse when the placement arrangements are completed. The social worker aids the nurse with the identification of the Bureau of Child Welfare representative who comes for the child. The nurse should record the discharge notes on the chart and enter the name in the census book as a "discharge" (to the Bureau of Child Welfare).

IV. Community Agency Referrals

Purpose

Referral to a community agency provides continuity of nursing care after discharge from the hospital and is an essential nursing responsibility. The nurse may call upon the physician and the social worker to assist with providing the information necessary for the community agency. The choice of agencies should be made with the problems of the child in mind, and recommendations which will provide continuity of care should be included. Follow-up care is considered part of the matrix of total child care.

Types of Agencies Available Within Most Communities

Visiting nurse service.   A child may be referred to the Visiting Nurse Service for follow-up care following hospitalization. The fee charged by the agency is usually based upon the patient's ability to pay and is adjusted on a sliding scale basis.

Indications for referral.   A referral should be initiated for any child who can be expected to profit by such a plan.

1. Newborns:
   Neonates with a birth weight under 5 1/2 pounds
   A neonate with a congenital anomaly
   A neonate with a birth injury
   A neonate born out of wedlock and taken home by the mother
   A neonate with a health problem
   Parents who need guidance in caring for the neonate

2. Infants and children: This includes infants and children who require nursing care in the home and parents who require instruction in the treatments to be done at home such as:
   Temperature, pulse, respiration
   Dressings
   Medication by injection
   Colostomy care
   Testing of urine
   Rehabilitation exercises

3. Also eligible are those infants and children whose parents need guidance in understanding and following special diets such as:
   P.K.U. diet
   Diabetic diet
   Allergy diet
   Feeding and diet supplements for the infant prior to a scheduled appointment at the health station

4. Infants and children who need help in adjusting to limitations imposed by a handicap may also be referred. They include:
   Cerebral palsy
   Cleft palate
   Paralysis

Procedure for referral to the Visiting Nurse Service

1. The nurse on the pediatric unit initiates the referral. Orders for medication, treatments, or diet must be written by the doctor.

2. The interagency referral forms are filled out by the nurse and doctor, and sent to the local office of the Visiting Nurse Service.

3. The nurse on the pediatric unit may make a telephone request when the patient requires a visit within the next day or two, but a written referral form signed by the physician should be submitted following the telephone request.

4. The V.N.S. will maintain communication with the hospital concerning the progress of the patient after the discharge of the child.

Board of education.   The Board of Education in most cities provides individual tutors for homebound children of elementary and high school ages, free of charge. The nurse may initiate the referral by contacting the hospital school teacher or the social worker.

Public health agency.   The public health nursing agency identifies the health problems of families with individual or multiple health problems. The public health nurse may be called upon to visit and guide persons who have had contact with a communicable disease. The public health nurse may also serve as a school nurse in some communities. The school nurse plans continuity of care for the school aged child who returns to the public school after hospitalization.

Child health stations.   These stations provide medical guidance and immunizations for healthy children under school age.

Hospital clinics.   Clinics provide medical guidance on an outpatient basis to patients requiring medical follow-up care. An appointment at a hospital clinic should be given to the family at the time of the child's discharge.

Home care programs.   The child should be referred for home care services prior to the time of discharge. Home care is a part of the hospital service whereby hospital doctors provide medical guidance in the home of the individual patient who is unable to travel to the clinic and does not require hospitalization. (See also Chapter 27.)

The Department of Public Welfare.   The Department of Public Welfare provides financial aid for children with financial or social problems. Day nursery care may be planned for the accident prone child whose parents both work. A child in need of welfare services should be referred through the social service worker of the hospital.

Convalescent homes.   The nurse should refer the child to the social service department prior to the date of discharge. The social service worker will assist the nurse in completing the required forms and will arrange for placement of the child in a suitable convalescent home.

Dental services.   The nurse may refer a child who is in need of dental services to the social service department. The social service worker will determine the child's eligibility and arrange appointments at an approved dental clinic.

The division of handicapped children.   The Handicapped Children's Home Service provides recreation and diversional services to homebound handicapped children. Referral is initiated for children with such handicaps as polio, cerebral palsy, muscular dystrophy, heart disease, cancer, and nephritis. This agency charges a nominal fee for services rendered.

The division of crippled children.   Provides clinic treatment for children with musculoskeletal conditions, epilepsy, hearing defects, etc.

Other voluntary agencies.   The nurse may, at her discretion, refer a child and his family to a voluntary agency for such diseases as:

1. Epilepsy
2. Cardiac diseases
3. Diabetes

The telephone numbers and the locations of the various agencies are listed in the public telephone directory. The nurse's primary purpose is to make the patient (or his parents) aware of the nature of the services available to him through voluntary agencies.

BIBLIOGRAPHY

Marlow, D.: *Textbook of Pediatric Nursing.* 4th Edition, W. B. Saunders Co., Philadelphia, 1973.

Chapter Twenty Seven

THE PEDIATRIC OUTPATIENT AND THE CLINIC NURSE

PRINCIPLES	NURSING RESPONSIBILITIES
I. Preventative Care and Screening	
A schedule of well-child visits should be planned for each child to detect deviations, provide immunizations, assess growth and development, and provide health teaching and anticipatory guidance.	The clinic nurse should emphasize the need for well-child visits, and follow-up should be provided for delinquent parents.
II. Home Care of Illness	
When illness is diagnosed and treatment prescribed, the principles of home care should be discussed with parent and patient.	The diagnosis, treatment, and home care of the specific illness should be discussed with the parent. Interpretation of medication prescribed and other directions and the need for specific follow-up visits should be reinforced.
III. Health Teaching and Referral	
Motivation and readiness for learning is often present in the patient or parent who is seeking help for a medical problem in a clinic or office setting.	The nurse can utilize office waiting room time to provide health teaching and anticipatory guidance. Family interrelationships can be observed, and progress of chronic problems can be assessed. All information should be recorded on the chart. Proper referrals can then be made.

IV.   Dental Care

The main goal of oral care is achievement of an intact, balanced permanent dentition.

Untreated dental caries and malocclusion in childhood can predispose to periodontal disease in adulthood.

During eruption of the teeth, as the teeth penetrate the gums, inflammation and sensitivity can occur. The child may become irritable, and salivation increases.

Delayed eruption of all teeth may indicate a systemic or nutritional disturbance such as hypopituitarism, hypothyroidism, rickets, or cleidocranial dysostosis. If the entire dentition is early for sex and age, an endocrine disorder such as hyperpituitarism may be responsible.

In early infancy, when the enamel of the outer third of the permanent incisors, cuspids, and first molars is forming, illness or malnutrition can affect dentition.

Dental caries is a bacterial disease that, in combination with fermentable, carbohydrates, especially sucrose, cause destruction of the tooth structure. Children 4 to 8 years and 12 to 18 years are most susceptible.

Parents should be encouraged to take their child to the dentist by the age of 3 years.

Referral to proper agencies for dental care is essential when private dental care is not available to the family. The nurse should review proper methods of daily oral hygiene with parent and child (see p. 52).

The nurse may guide the parent in selecting a safe, firm, blunt object for the infant to bite on. Counseling about methods of relieving teething discomfort can help the infant and save parents many sleepless nights.

The nurse must be aware of the average time of eruption and shedding of primary and permanent teeth. Variations from the expected time of eruption can be normal, but the nurse must also be aware of deviations from normal and must refer and counsel the parent accordingly.

The nurse should counsel the parents concerning proper nutrition of the young infant and prevention of illness as well as early care of dental problems that may occur.

Between-meal snacks containing sucrose, particularly in forms that cling, like taffy, or those requiring prolonged contact, such as lollipops and lozenges, contribute to formation of dental caries. The practice of putting small children to sleep with a bottle also contributes to formation of dental caries. Counseling parents about dietary habits is essential.

TECHNIQUES

I.   Introduction

To avoid repetition and duplication of material, cross references are provided to information covered in sections concerning the hospitalized child that is also applicable to the pediatric outpatient. Emphasis is placed upon the independent nursing responsibilities of the clinic nurse rather than the dependent functions and those, such as weighing infants and preparing and assisting with doctor's examinations, which are covered in other areas of the text.

II. Emergency and Preventative Care

Snakebites

The incidence of snakebites in the United States is about 3 to 4 per 100,000 population, with 48 per cent occurring in children of school age or younger. Although most cases occur in Arizona, Florida, Georgia, Texas, and Alabama, modern means of rapid transportation and frequent travel make it mandatory for medical personnel in all states to be aware of the emergency care of snakebites. A child can be bitten by a snake while on vacation in Texas and can travel to New York via plane before severe symptoms occur and motivate his parents to seek medical care. Each case of snakebite is serious and should be treated rapidly with the primary goal of preventing death.

Grading and treating snakebites. Table 27–1 can serve as a guide in the grading and treatment of snakebites.

TABLE 27–1.   Grading and Treating Snakebites

Grade	Symptoms	Suggested Treatment
0	History of suspected snakebite. Presence of fang wounds. No signs of poisoning.	Clean wound. Provide standard care for puncture wounds. Have child seen by the doctor.
1 (Minimal)	Symptoms as above. Moderate pain or throbbing at site; swelling around the wound.	Immobilize affected part. Place patient on bedrest to prevent rapid distribution of poison into circulation. Seek medical aid immediately.
2 (Moderate)	Same as grade 1. Swelling more severe, progressing toward trunk. Nausea; vomiting; discoloration of wound; low-grade temperature.	Immobilize part, place patient on bedrest. Seek medical aid immediately.
3 (Severe)	Same as grade 2. Shock; general discoloration; temperature subnormal; Collapse.	The nurse should administer antivenin serum without delay. The smaller the child, the larger the dose required, as children have less resistance and less body fluid to dilute the venom. The patient may then be taken to a doctor.

Emergency Care of Dental Injuries

Problem

Dental injuries are a common occurrence caused by accidents or vigorous sports activities.

Nursing responsibility

Dental therapy should precede soft tissue treatment when possible. Completely avulsed teeth should be placed in saline and taken immediately to the dentist. Temporary reimplantation allows dental structures to mature before prosthesis is prescribed.

Tongue injuries or burns are common in children.

Ice can be used to reduce swelling. Food should be cool and in liquid form while the patient is in the painful stage of tongue lesions. Saline mouthwashes are soothing.

Salivary flow rates can be decreased by medication, disease, or irradiation, and can increase formation of dental caries.

Good oral hygiene is essential for the ill child as well as for the healthy child (see Chapter 7).

Preparing the Child for Foreign Travel

General requirements of international health regulations include vaccinations against smallpox, yellow fever, and cholera. Smallpox and cholera vaccinations may be given by a physician and authenticated by the local health department on an approved form, but yellow fever vaccinations are given only by special health centers in the United States. Children under 12 months of age may be accepted into a country without immunization, except in cases of epidemic or endemic when the age is lowered to 6 months. Many countries will vary their requirements for immunization from time to time, depending on the health problems existing within that country. The state health department can help the international traveler interpret the immunizations necessary for international family travel. If there is a contraindication to a required immunization, a doctor's written statement may be accepted but does not insure that a child will be allowed into a country without a period of quarantine. Even if vaccination is given at the border of a country, entrance may be denied for a period of time. A child should, as part of general health care, be up to date on diphtheria, tetanus, pertussis, measles and polio immunizations prior to foreign travel.

Properly documented vaccination certificates are usually valid for three years beginning eight days after date of vaccination. A general rule of thumb is to obtain immunization for diseases the child is likely to contact in the countries in which he will travel or reside. The risk of exposure should be evaluated in all cases, and immunization should be planned to protect the individual, not only to meet international requirements.

Passports.   All children are required to have a passport for foreign travel. A child may have his own passport or share the passport of the parent with whom he travels. The nurse should offer a word of advice for the traveling family—they should carefully plan their trip before obtaining a passport. If a child shares the mother's passport, then he cannot travel alone with the father and vice versa. Problems at borders will be avoided with adequate planning.

Screening

The following is an example of a routine schedule of well-child visits:
Births to 6 months—Monthly visits
6 Months to 1 year—Visit every 2 months
Second year—4 visits per year
2 to 6 years—1 or 2 visits per year
After 6 years—Annual visit

Vision and hearing defects should be diagnosed well before school age, or school problems will ensue with serious effects upon the growth and development of the child.

Vision testing.   Before 2 years of age, test the response of child to a toy or small keys dangled. Observe the ability to watch a light with each eye. If behavior changes occur when one eye is covered, vision may be reduced in that eye. Between 2 and 6 years, the Snellen E chart can be used. If there is difficulty in completing the visual screening test in preschool children it may indicate behavioral or perceptual problems, and the child should be referred for a more detailed examination.

Hearing tests.   Hearing can be tested informally as early as 4 to 6 months of age by having the child sit on the mother's lap facing away from the nurse. The nurse can crackle a paper or spin a rattle and the child will turn his head toward the noise. After this age, a history of hearing problems should be taken, including a history of turning up the volume on radio or television, repeated ear infections, or defects in speech patterns. Formal hearing tests should be given in a quiet atmosphere, probably a specially designated area. The noisy clinic is not the the best area for an audiometer test.

Screening for lead poisoning or sickle cell trait.   Screening is recommended for children 18 months to 5 years in high risk populations.

Growth screening.   A height-weight chart should be made for each child. The *recumbent* length is more accurate than a standing height for children under 5 years of age. A head circumference is usually taken until 3 years of age. The presence of specific growth problems will dictate need for other measurements.

System 80.   System 80 consists of an audiovisual unit which utilizes programmed instruction materials. These instructional materials present tasks in a simple, step by step progression. It is designed to measure ability or teach basic concepts. The material is presented in such a way that the child is immediately appraised of the correctness or error of his response. Once a specific learning weakness has been identified in the child, the system can also be used to define that weakness in behavioral terms so that specific learning tasks can be designed to help correct it. Gifted children can also be readily identified, enabling an early, educationally stimulating program to be planned to meet his developmental needs. The advantage of this system is that a trained administrator is not an essential part of these tests, decreasing the cost of testing children in the preschool or primary school age group. This type of individualized program can be utilized in the clinic, doctor's office, preschool center, or public school system.

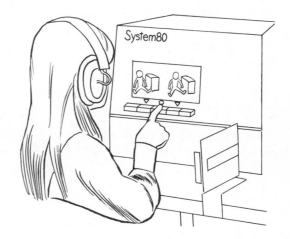

FIGURE 27–1.   System 80 is a diagnostic and therapeutic tool that can be used with preschool or school age children to identify strengths and weaknesses or to enhance learning. The child listens to a record that asks her to select and press a button that best answers the question illustrated on the screen. A hole is punched in the paper tab inserted into the machine for each incorrect response, providing a score for each program. This machine may be used with or without earphones.

Use of Over-the-Counter Medications

Advantages   *Disadvantages*

Aspirin
Antipyretic   Frequent administration over a period of
Anti-inflammatory   time can cause a cumulative effect and
Analgesic   can result in overdosage since elimina-
                                              tion of aspirin from the body is slow
                                              when high doses are used. It is not avail-
                                              able in liquid form because of its insolu-
                                              bility.

Acetaminophen
Antipyretic   Keep out of reach of children, as acute
Analgesic   toxicity can cause hepatic necrosis. It is
Available in liquid form, thus making   not a "harmless drug."
dosage more accurate in infants.

Tylenol (Tempra)
It may be used in children who are allergic to salicylates.

Salicylamide (Liquiprin)
Pharmacologically not related to salicy-   Not very effective as an antipyretic
lates   agent.

The nurse can discuss the advantages and disadvantages of using over-the-counter medications. The above list outlines a few analgesic antipyretics. Similar discussions should include individually related cultural and health practices of the family, especially relating to interaction with prescribed medication (see Chapter 18). The nurse should instruct the parent that fever is an important factor in diagnosis, and therefore should not be vigorously medicated without consulting a doctor. Self-medication is often the cause for overdosage.

III. Home Care of Illness

Home Care of Communicable Diseases

Principles   *Parent teaching*
Patients with contagious diseases should   Provide a separate room and bed for the
be isolated to limit distribution of the   child away from other members of the
disease and to protect them from second-   family. Limit visitors. Provide toys that
ary infections.   are washable for his exclusive use.

See specific principles (Chapter 12).   Adequate handwashing technique before
                                              and after contact with the child should
                                              be discussed. The hot cycle of most home
                                              laundry machines is usually adequate for
                                              care of contaminated linens and clothing.
                                              Paper bags should be provided for dis-
                                              posal of used tissues.

Contagious Periods of Selected Infections Usually Cared for in the Home*

Infectious Period	*Isolation*
Measles (Rubeola)	
Five days of incubation through several days of rash.	Onset of catarrhal stage to third day of rash.
German measles (Rubella)	
Seven days before rash through five days after (up to 12 months for congenital type).	None. Women in first trimester of pregnancy should not be exposed.
Chickenpox (Varicella)	
One day before rash to 5 to 6 days after, when all lesions are crusted.	Until all lesions are crusted (5 to 6 days). Elderly persons with herpes problems should not be exposed.
Pertussis	
Catarrhal stage through fourth week.	Four weeks. Until cough ceases.
Mumps	
Seven days before and nine days after parotitis symptoms.	Until swelling subsides.

Principles involving prevention of contamination, cleaning of articles used, care of the room, and family togetherness should be discussed, based upon the above information and geared to meet the individual family needs.

Administration of Eye Drops by an Unassisted Parent

Eyedrops prescribed by a clinic doctor are often not instilled as frequently or as effectively as desired because it is a difficult and often frustrating task for the parent, who is usually confronted by an uncooperative child. A simple technique to adequately restrain the child and permit quick and effective instillation of eyedrops is illustrated in Figure 27-2.

---

*Adapted from Report of Committee on Infectious Diseases, Red Book, 17th Edition, American Academy of Pediatrics, Evanston, Illinois, 1974.

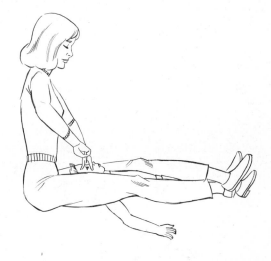

FIGURE 27-2. Note that the arms of the child are restrained by the parent's thigh and the lower body is restrained by the parent's legs. The parent's hands are free to open the eyelid and instill the eyedrops.

Maintaining an Allergy-Free Room

Specific instruction should be geared to meet the individual needs of the family in relation to their culture and life style. General instructions for maintaining an allergy-free room include:

1. Encourage parents to set up at least one room (bedroom) for the allergic child.
2. Avoid: wool rugs; feather pillows; upholstered furniture; drapes; venetian blinds.
3. Close all holes and cracks in walls, ceilings, and floor.
4. Clean thoroughly with vacuum and *damp* cloth.
5. Cover mattress and pillow with plastic.
6. Use cotton blankets between two sheets.
7. Keep windows and doors closed except at night.
8. Keep a screen door on door of room.
9. Use the room only for sleeping, no other activity.
10. Do not use stuffed toys.

Toilet Training a Child with Constipation or Hirschsprung's Disease

A mother who is advised to "give fluids and fruit" to avoid constipation may give *milk* as the fluid and *applesauce* as the fruit — both are constipating! Directions must be specific. For toilet training:

1. The child *must* squat. The upper rectum will be squeezed first as the child "pushes" and helps expel the feces. If a child is not squatting, the increased intra-abdominal pressure will result in the moving of the feces in *both* directions.
2. Provide a suitable toilet chair. An adequate squat cannot be achieved if the child is placed on a toilet with feet dangling. A small "potty" chair will enable the child to squat with his feet on the floor, which is essential in toilet training a constipation-prone child.
3. The doctor may prescribe mineral oil as a lubricant — not a laxative — to enable the child to pass soft stool and overcome the fear of toileting.
4. Sit the child on the potty once or twice a day regularly to achieve conditioning.
5. Use praise for success. Develop a positive attitude and avoid stress.

IV. Health Education

The President's Committee on Health Education in 1973 defined health education as "a process that bridges the gap between health information and health practices." Thus health education involves more than just supplementing information. Careful listening to the patient can serve as a guide to planning health teaching. Patient teaching may be general in nature, for example, the warning signs of cancer or heart disease. Some teaching must be specifically related to individual diagnosis and therapy as they affect daily functions of living within a certain culture and lifestyle. As modern care becomes more complex, the treatment of chronic illness and the prevention of illness depend largely upon the cooperation and understanding of the patient, the family, and the community. Noncompliance becomes increasingly significant and increases the probability of remission. Cultural practices and the widespread use of nonprescription medication can be assessed in terms of its negative or positive effect with prescribed therapy and dealt with in the health education setting.

The best person to initiate and maintain an organized health education program is the clinic or office nurse. She often is the first person to see the well or sick child and his parents in a nonacute setting. The waiting room of the clinic or doctor's office provides a natural time and place for health education. Motivation and readiness for learning are likely to be present since the parents have already sought help for a medical problem.

Suggested educational methods include:

1. Assessment of the patient's knowledge before and after the program.

2. Audiovisual instruction followed by a question and answer session. There are many free films available.

3. Reference materials for home use.

4. Patient library in the waiting area.

5. Box of mini-toys each labeled with therapeutic or developmental purpose (see p. 258).

These approaches can be followed by parent instruction and discussion. Once a "self-teaching" area has been established in the waiting room, a health teaching program will take surprisingly little nursing time in relation to the results achieved.

Counseling

Anticipatory guidance is the basic principle of parent counseling. Preventative counseling through application of knowledge of growth and development can assist mothers to cope with developmental problems such as feeding, toilet training, and accident prevention. At each visit, a history of behavior, illness, accidents, eating, sleeping, elimination, current family situation, school, and dental care should be recorded and discussed with the parent. Much of this information can be taken while the parent is waiting for the doctor or during a nurse practitioner's scheduled visit.

For adolescent patients, the nurse should include discussions of smoking, drugs, and peer relationships, and should assess the status of sex education and personal hygiene. Privacy during counseling is essential for the adolescents. Parents should be interviewed separately from the adolescent child.

Food Cultists and Dietary Patterns

Malnutrition does not necessarily result from the lack of an available food source, or money to purchase it, but in families who are vegetarians or members of various food "cults," the deliberate elimination of specific foods from the diet can also be the cause. It is not difficult to treat the illness, but gaining the cooperation of the family is often quite difficult. Some examples of food cults are described here.

General vegetarian.   The general vegetarian diet is usually adequate when supplemented with dairy or poultry products. This can be a bulky diet. The quality of amino acids may be inferior. Body protein can become a calorie source unless care is taken to prevent this.

Vegan cult.   Excludes animal products including dairy and eggs. There is risk of vitamin B_{12} deficiency that is masked by a high folic acid intake. Thus, degeneration of the spinal cord, anemia, and menstrual irregularities may be advanced before they are recognized. Vitamin B_{12} supplements can prevent this problem.

Krishna cult.   Excludes meat and eggs but not dairy products. Iron deficiency anemia is usually a problem with those rigidly following this type of diet.

Zen macrobiotic.   Limits fluid intake severely while eating foods rich in sodium. Intake of calories, calcium, iron, vitamins C and D is low, with a diet consisting mainly of cereal grains and vegetables. This diet, rigidly followed, can create a major health problem including hypoproteinemia, scurvey, hypocalcemia and even starvation.

If the nurse wishes to help the food cultists and their families, she must understand the cult philosophy and understand their principles of food selection. Maintenance of effective communication between the parent, the patient, and the health team is the key to success in dealing with food cultists and their children. The goal in treating these children should be to provide adequate nutrition to maintain health until they are old enough to determine their own goals in life.

The Use of Water-Softened Water

Sodium chloride is often used to regenerate the synthetic ion exchange resin in home water softeners. One liter of water-softened water supplies as much as 500 mg. sodium chloride. This may be significant to any patient with severely restricted sodium intake.

Caffeine Content of Beverages

Caffeine has a systemic stimulant effect that may be contraindicated in specific medical conditions.

Percolated coffee yields the greatest amount of caffeine, (120 mg. per 5 oz. serving), although the longer it is boiled, the more caffeine is extracted. Tea has about half the caffeine content of coffee. Cola drinks contain about 30 mg. per serving. Chocolate, although low in caffeine, is high in theobromine, another type of stimulant. Ovaltine is caffeine free and contains only a small amount of theobromine.

Assessing Adolescent Maturity

Rates of maturation differ during the adolescent years but the adolescent is especially sensitive to being "different" from his peers. Therefore, the psychological effect on those at the early or late end of the normal range must be taken into consideration when dealing with the adolescent. Factors such as disease, nutrition, and physical and emotional stress will alter normal patterns of growth and development and should be considered in the assessment of the individual child.

Factors to consider in assessing adolescent physiological maturity

1. *Family history.* Heredity plays an important role in determining the age of onset of puberty.

2. *Skeletal age.* Assessment of bone age is used when clinical problems present. Bone age is more closely correlated with maturity than chronologic age. The more retarded the bone age, the more potential for growth can be expected.

3. *Growth spurt.* A growth spurt including an increase in height between 4 and 12 inches usually precedes pubertal changes by a year or two. During this growth spurt,

the growth of the trunk is more rapid than the legs. Therefore, the later puberty occurs, the longer the period of leg growth and the taller the person will be. It is important to know that maximum muscle strength is achieved a year or two after muscle mass has reached maturity. Muscle skill requires muscle mass. In girls the growth spurt occurs between $9\frac{1}{2}$ and $14\frac{1}{2}$ years of age. In boys the growth spurt occurs between $10\frac{1}{2}$ and $17\frac{1}{2}$ years of age.

4. *Secondary sexual characteristics.* In boys, enlargement of the testes and penis, and the appearance of pubic hair is a satisfactory criteria of sexual maturity. It usually starts between 11 and 18 years. In girls assessment of the stage of breast development is a satisfactory criteria. Breast development and pubic hair usually start developing between 10 and 14 years of age. The menarch usually occurs between 10 and 16 years of age.

Understanding the maturing adolescent. During the process of psychological maturing, the adolescent passes through normal stages that may be characterized by behavior changes. Discussing these behavior changes with the parents can help them to understand their adolescent and better cope with the problems within the family caused by them.

Maturing process	*Associated behavior change*
Relinquish the infantile nature of relationship with parents.	Sever close emotional ties with the parents by becoming negativistic, noncommunicative, etc.
Have emotional needs met by peers rather than parents.	Boys turn to boys and try to prove manhood. Girls develop attachments for unattainable men such as movie stars.
Accept gender and develop stable identity.	Establishment of heterosexual relationships and successful experiences with peers, job, or school provides positive behavioral changes to the adult level.

Often, the adolescent view of the world and its problems as those of a sinking ship is a cause of despair and "dropouts." Principles of approach to the adolescent:

1. Do not chase him unless you are sure you can catch him, or your energy is wasted.

2. Don't make threats you cannot or will not carry out.

3. Do: standby, tell the facts, express your stand, listen to his stand, and hope he will listen to you.

V.   Play Activities and Their Role in Promoting Growth and Development

To an adult, play is recreation, *taking time out* from daily routines of life for enjoyment before returning to the routines of daily living. To a child, play is not time out from daily living, but rather an *essential part* of it that enables him to grow and mature through various stages of the develovmental process.

Analysis of A Play Activity

One common play activity will be analyzed here to demonstrate the mastery of skills essential to the developmental process involved in it. Other play activities should be analyzed in the same fashion and used as a guide in selecting toys and play activities to meet the specific needs of individual children.

Riding a Tricycle

Vision, touch, curiosity, language.   Used in investigating parts of the cycle—rubber wheels, shiny handle bars, soft seat, etc.

Balance.   Must climb on seat and arrange himself properly.

Mobility.   Learns to synchronize foot activity to achieve mobility.

Foot pressure, hand steering.   Necessary to achieve his destination.

Coordination.   Develops when riding on smooth or rough surfaces, grass, curves, and small hills.

Comprehension of space, size, or form.   The child must avoid fixed obstacles to achieve his destination.

Communication via fantasy.   Often, the tricycle becomes a train, bus, or spaceship, and the child assumes a role in cooperative play adventures.

Emotional growth.   Socially accepted forms of emotional growth occur as a child comforts another who has fallen off a bike, or helps another to ride a bike.

Problem solving, self confidence.   The child learns to take turns, set limits and accept them, and channels aggressions into constructive play.

Safety.   Roles assumed transform traffic safety into a learning experience.

APPROACH TO THE HANDICAPPED CHILD

There is a great need for everyone—nurse, therapist, teacher, and parent—to know and be aware of the medical, neurological, and physiological deficiencies that can affect the intellectual performance and abilities of children.

To the observer, some handicaps are very apparent such as Down's syndrome (mongolism), celebral palsy, and the profoundly retarded. Others are not as obvious and hence many children who have not been identified sometimes present problems at school and home. These are generally the neurologically handicapped who have normal, near normal, or even above normal intelligence with learning or behavior disabilities. Among this group there is a great diversity in the degree and way they are affected.

If a professional nurse has a patient who seems to lag in development of the motor, language, or perceptual areas, she should note the signs indicative of the deficiency and inform the doctor and social worker, who can then see that proper tests are made and a specific diagnosis reached.

When this has been accomplished, the child and parent can be referred to special clinics, centers, or classes, and the skilled professionals there, after a period of observation and evaluation, will set up a special prescriptive program, which can be used at school and home.

I. General Objectives in the Approach to a Handicapped Child

1. Evaluate the teacher's report carefully. In many states the salary of the teacher is directly related to student scores on state achievement exams. Therefore, some teachers may wish to remove disruptive children and are quick to "label" MBD (minimal brain damage).

2. Change the pattern of a child's failure to a pattern of success.

3. Work at developing a better mother-child relationship and medical–social agency team care.

4. Use community resources to meet individual family needs.

II. Observing the Handicapped Child

Area of Development	Observe
Coordination Gross Motor	Walk poor (13–15 months); inability to skip correctly (4–5 years) Clumsiness in gait (after 2 years) Inability to ride with ease correctly (after 3 years) tricycle or bike (parent may relate this) Loses balance easily, not able to stand on one foot (after 3 years)
Fine Motor and Eye-Hand Coordination	Has trouble buttoning (3 years) Has trouble with zippers (3 years) Has trouble turning pages in book Handwriting or drawings poorly spaced and messy (5 years) Cannot use scissors (after 4 years)
Abnormal Motor Activity	Overactive Slow moving in everything Talk is excessive and disorganized
Language-Speech	Delayed speech or no speech Hard to understand Does not comprehend what is said to him
Perceptual	Has trouble with simple shape puzzles (3 years) Reverses letter or words when writing or reading (5–6 years) Misinterprets what is said to him; does not seem to hear correctly, though hearing is normal (3 years) Has no concept of size; can not differentiate large-small or tall-short (after 3 years)
Attention span	Very short attention span on things he needs to do Easily distracted by noise or others

Behavior   Quick temper
                                            Tantrums
                                            Overly sensitive
                                            Must touch everything and everyone
                                            Moody
                                            Cannot tolerate frustration or failure
                                            Irritable
                                            Unmanageable

Basically, everyone with a handicap is more *like* a so-called normal person than different. They have the same physical, emotional and social needs. Far too much stress is put on the disability and too little on the child as a person. Too much notice has been taken of where he fails. The need for success is important to everyone, but these children need it more.

In order for the child to have a taste of success, it is necessary to build up a prescriptive program where he can succeed. Start with tasks that he can perform with ease and skill, gradually adding more difficult ones.

A general sensorimotor program can be set up for all with more attention given in the area or areas needed by each child so he will not regress. A handicapped child must have a planned program of games and toys, especially if he is confined to bed at home or in the hospital for any period of time.

Almost all children with handicaps or learning disabilities have a very poor concept of themselves. They know (unless the handicap is a very severe one) that they do not and cannot perform. Each child senses the feelings of failure, displeasure, unhappiness, and confusion of parents, family, and others involved with them. They know they do not come up to the expectation set for them. The child needs to be aware of himself as a person of worth.

III.   Goals of Play Therapy for a Handicapped Child

Recreation should have as its goal the promotion of positive aspects of growth and development and de-emphasis of the chronicity or terminal nature of the disease. Table 27–2 describes a program of recreation and encouragement that can be initiated by the nurse or by parents.

1. Maintain a positive self-image by developing an activity in which he can excel and experience success, such as playing musical instruments, or arts and crafts.

2. Provide activities that foster social growth and development, such as scouting, social clubs, church groups, or drama groups.

3. Develop hobbies, such as gardening, model building, chess or checkers, cooking, or collecting things to avoid television addiction.

4. The level of activity allowed should be communicated between doctor, teacher, patient, and parents, and should serve as a guide to the selection of recreational activities.

Toys

It is very important that safe toys are selected which will have the characteristics listed on p. 288.

TABLE 27–2.   A Multi Sensory Program

To Develop	Nursing Activity	
	Say or Do To Child	Examples of Toys—Tasks—Books
I. AWARENESS OF SELF		
A. As a person of value	"You're a pretty girl." "You're a handsome boy." "You have nice blue eyes" (or long hair, etc.). Honest, true feelings only; smile of acceptance, with stroke on cheek.	How Do I Feel (book) Free To Be—You and Me (book) Fun For Chris (book) (simple story explains skin color differences) Feelings (book)
B. Able to give pleasure to others by helpfulness, love, or just their company	"My, it's so good to see such a happy face!" "You were helpful because *you* waited your turn," etc. Repeat *often*: Have some special thing each child does that is really helpful. Stroke of the arm of child.	Do You Want to be My Friend? (book) Making Friends (book) Amigo (book)
C. Able to learn many things	"Good! *You* worked that puzzle." "You have learned lots of new words." "My! That's a pretty picture you drew!" *Sincere* praise over and over and over again. Touch or pat hand.	Puzzle of vehicles (crepe foam) 3–6 years. Golden Book Dictionary (pictures and words) The Very Hungry Caterpillar (book)
D. Able to be successful in some ways and some things	"*You* did a good job washing your hands." "*You* always say 'thank you' so nicely." "*You* put your puzzle away neatly." Smile with approval. Give a hug.	What Do I Do? (book) What Do I Say? (book)
E. Know that he cannot be successful in everything	Show acceptance even when he fails. Say, "Well once in a while you just can't do it." "Do you know *I* have trouble sweeping the floor?" (Anything you might not succeed at). Blow a kiss to let him know you love him even when he fails.	Is It Hard—Is It Easy? (book)
II. AWARENESS OF OTHERS		
A. Other people are of great value	"Dr. Hartston is so nice. He wants to help all the people. "Nurse Gloria has such a nice smile." Pick out people he knows, say it with appreciation and approval.	Going to the Doctor (book) Doctors Kit (toy) Mother–Dad (book) Some One Always Needs a Policeman (book)
B. Other people have needs	"Fred looks tired and needs to go to sleep. Let's turn down the light and be quiet so he can sleep." "Amos is hungry. Let's get him some crackers and milk." "He needs a friend." Say with love and concern.	Rest-Land Time (record) Everybody has a House and Everybody Eats (book)

TABLE 27–2.   A Multi Sensory Program

To Develop	Nursing Activity	
	Say or Do To Child	Examples of Toys—Tasks—Books
C. Other people succeed and fail, too.	"John worked *that* puzzle, but *this* one was too hard for him." "John tried to comb his hair but he's too little to do a good job." "We should tell him it was a good try though."	He is My Brother (book about learning disabilities) My Father can Fix Anything (book)
III. AWARENESS OF BODY PARTS	At bath time when washing and also when drying, *name* the body parts. Have child *repeat* the names when you touch the part again.	My Five Senses (book)
	Make up a game having children put both hands on the parts you name: "Put your hands on your ears." "Put your hands on your knee," etc.	Look in the Mirror
IV. MOTOR SKILLS A. Gross motor, large muscles, body balance	"Here's a game that's fun— put your foot on each footprint."	Mosier Foot Rug; Crossing the Midline; Space Rug I
	"Can you balance yourself on this?"	Balance Board.
	"Walk on this board and look at the picture here on the wall."	Walking Board.
	"Watch Barry jump on this and then you try it."	Trampo mat (34 in. × 34 in.) (mat—25 in. × 25 in.), height 6 in.
	"Take the red trike and go the way the blue arrows (marked on pavement) go."	Tricycle
B. Fine motor skills	"What can you build with these?"	Very small building blocks (various shapes)
	"Try to unscrew these nuts."	Nuts and bolts (large plastic)
	"Squeeze these sticks and see the man move."	Trapeze artist (figure that moves when two sticks are squeezed)
C. Eye-hand coordination	"This is the way to weave." (demonstrate)	Weaving looms
	"This doll has a zipper to zip, try it."	Dolls with buttons, buckles, zippers and laces
	"Use the screw driver here and turn to take out a screw." (demonstrate)	Wooden tools and box
	"You can sew a button like this." (demonstrate)	Large buttons with thick thread or cord; use blunt needles
	"This opens like a scissor and it moves this part here so I can pick up this small piece of yarn." (demonstrate) "You try it now—open . . . close it."	Reach Extender (toy; found in grocery store, toy display or toy stores)

TABLE 27–2.   A Multi Sensory Program

To Develop	Nursing Activity	
	Say or Do To Child	Examples of Toys — Tasks — Books
V. PERCEPTUAL SKILLS (Visual, tactile, auditory)	"Can you work this puzzle?"	Wood board with geometric shapes
	"Put the blue ones in the blue box and the red ones in the red box like this."	Sorting boxes with different colored discs
	"Touch this and find another that feels like it."	Feel and match textures
	"Shake this tube and shake the others to find one that sounds the same."	Box of sound tubes
	"Can you put your thumb on the thumb on this rug?" "Find your hand on this rug— find one that is larger," etc.	Mosier Hand Rugs (left-right training) (size)
VI. LANGUAGE SKILLS	"See if you can say what this says."	Talking toys (example: phone with record disc)
	"Listen to the songs on this record and sing with it."	American Negro Folk and Work Songs, Rhythms (record)
	"Here is a flute to play."	Plastic song flute
	"Find the letters in your name" (Print name on paper and say "letters" as you do it).	Box of letters (capital and lower case)
VII. CREATIVE SKILLS	"Here's a rolling pin and clay—what can you make?"	Reusable clay (colored) with cookie cutters and rolling pin
	"Paste some of these things on this paper and make a pretty picture."	Collage (scraps of paper, tissue paper, cloth, lace, etc.) Library paste, (school) scissor.
	"Draw a picture and tell me about it."	Crayons (nontoxic) and paper.
	"Try some finger painting on this blue paper."	Finger paint (soap flakes with small amount of water), colored construction paper
	"Draw a horse." "Draw a picture of your family."	Felt tip pens (nontoxic, odorless)

Educational input
Moral building qualities
Encouraging increased rapport with others
Stimulating and able to hold interest over a period of time
Appropriate to the needs of each child taking into account age and abilities (gross motor, perceptual, etc.)

Storage and Care of Toys

1. Toys should be kept together and marked as according to the skills they develop—Gross motor, Fine motor, etc. Small toys should be put in a large (18 in. × 12 in. × 4 in.), soft, vinyl covered box.

2. Toys may be washed since they are rubber, vinyl, plastic, wood, or metal, or cleaned with an antiseptic solution.

IV. Community Agency Referrals

The care and management of a child's acute or chronic illness in the home has an impact on every aspect of family life, and in order to preserve the normalcy of that family life some assistance with the care and understanding of the illness and support in facing the emotional and financial stresses is essential. The need for assistance crosses socioeconomic lines, and therefore, the poor are not the only group requiring referral. Often the clinic nurse serving a higher socioeconomic group overlooks the need for referral and does her patient a grave injustice. The diagnosis of a child's illness is a time of crisis, and community resource personnel can help a family adjust to the initial impact and to the long-term stresses involved.

The child is often an uncooperative patient and the parents need assistance in devising ways to give medications or daily treatments, to prepare special diets within the family budget and cultural habits, and to maintain school progress. Parents must also be helped by understanding the implications of the illness upon the family.

A directory of community services is often published by the local county medical association or a community group. Listings will include location and functions of area groups such as those listed here. A current copy of community services should be available to all clinic nurses for use as a referral source. The lists and description of services should be updated periodically.

American Heart Association
American Cancer Society
American Institute of Family Relations
American Red Cross
Association for Retarded Children
Association for the Visually Handi-
    capped
Braille Institute of America
Bureau of Child Care and Foster Homes
Cerebral Palsey Center
Child Care Placement
Children's Home Society

City Recreation Department
Crippled Children's Society
Community Welfare Funds
County Bureau of Adoptions
County Bureau of Public Assistance
Cystic Fibrosis Foundation
Epilepsy Society
Family Aide Programs
Hearing and Speech centers
Homes for Children
Muscular Dystrophy Association
Mental health groups
Parent-teacher groups
Planned Parenthood
Project Headstart
Public Library
Social Security Agency
Social welfare departments
State rehabilitation centers
Suicide prevention centers
Visiting Nurse Association

BIBLIOGRAPHY

Barsch, R.: *Enriching Perception and Cognition: Techniques for Teachers.* Special Child Publications Inc., Seattle, Washington, 1968.
Beaver, W. T.: The Pharmacologic Basis for Choice of Analgesic. Pharmacology for Physicians, 4:1–7, 1970.
Carlson, B., and Ginglend, D. R.: Play Activities for the Retarded Child. Abigdon Press, Nashville, Tennessee, 1961.
Chang, T.: Immunization: Weighing the Ounce of Prevention. *Modern Medicine, 41*:16:22, 1973.
Done, A. K.: Antipyretics. *Pediatric Clinics of North America, 19*:167–177, 1972.
Frank, D. J., and Drobish, N. L.: Toy Safety in the Hospital or Beware of Parents Bearing Gifts. *Clinical Pediatrics; 14*:400, 1975.
Gellis, S. S., and Kagan, B. M. (Eds.): *Current Pediatric Therapy.* 7th Edition, W. B. Saunders Co., Philadelphia, 1976.
Glass, T. G., Jr.: Early Debridement in Pit Viper Bite. *Surgery, Gynecology and Obstetrics, 136*:744, 1973.
Hatcher, E. D., and Mullin, H.: *More Than Words—Movement Activities for Children.* Parents for Movement Publications, Pasadena, California, 1967.
Jamplis, R. W.: The Practicing Physician and Patient Education. *Hospital Practice, 10*:10:3, 1975.
Marlow, D.: *Textbook of Pediatric Nursing.* 4th Edition, W. B. Saunders Co., Philadelphia, 1973.
Schiff, J. L., and Day, B.: *All My Children.* M. Evans & Co., Philadelphia, 1970.
Schropp, M. L.: Patient Education: Brink of a Boom. *Group Practice,* September/October, 1974.
Simonds, S. K.: President's Committee on Health Education. *Hospitals, 47*:55, 1973.
Sunderlin, S. (Ed.): Bits and Pieces: Imaginary uses for Children's Learning. Association for Childhood Education, International, Washington, D.C., 1967.
Banned Products. U. S. Department of Health, Education, and Welfare, Food and Drug Administration, Bureau of Product Safety, Vol. 2, Part I. January, 1973.
Immunization. Report to the Committee on Infectious Diseases. *Medical Opinion; 5*:1:63, 1976.
Playing Safe in Toyland. Department of Health, Education and Welfare, Public Health Service, Food and Drug Administration, Pub. #72-7009, 1971.
Proceedings, Annual Medical Symposium on Current Pediatric Therapy, Variety Children's Hospital, Miami, Florida, 1976.
Proceedings, Fourth National Symposium on Creative Communication, Orff-Schviwerk, Symposium Planning Group, Bellflower, California, 1970.
Snakefarm. Science Division, The Thai Red Cross Society, Queen Saovabha Memorial Institute. Swicharn Press, Bankok, Thailand, 1969.

PRODUCT REFERENCES

Borg-Warner Educational System, Arlington Heights, Illinois: System 80.
Childcraft Education Corp., Edison, New Jersey: Childcraft—The Growing Years.
The Judy Co., Morristown, New Jersey: Early Childhood Catalogue.
Lakeshore Curriculum Materials Co., Los Angeles, California: Preschool through elementary toys.
Mosier Materials, San Bernardino, California: Sensorimotor games, rug games.

Chapter Twenty Eight

MINI-REVIEW: SELECTED PEDIATRIC DISORDERS, AND THEIR NURSING RESPONSIBILITIES

Achalasia: A spasm of the cardiac sphincter of the esophagus resulting in a decreased ability to pass food and fluids into the stomach.

Nursing responsibilities include feeding the child slowly in an upright position. Frequent small feedings are recommended. The child should be cuddled during the feeding process.

Adjuvant feedings: The inclusion of foods in an infant's diet that supplement formula or breast feedings.

Nursing responsibilities include the proper selection of foods, proper size portions, and the addition to the diet of one new food at a time. Adjuvant feedings should be offered *before* the bottle or breast, when the appetite is at its peak.

Amebiasis: An infection of the colon caused by a protozoan parasite.

Nursing responsibilities include proper disposal of stool and linen to prevent the spread of this disease, the maintenance of nutrition with a bland diet, observation for untoward responses to the drug therapy prescribed, and general hygienic care. Stool specimens for laboratory examination must be freshly obtained and should not be left standing at room temperature. Parent teaching con-

cerning the need for follow-up care and the examination of all members of the family are essential. Community agencies should be utilized.

Anoxia: A state of oxygen deprivation within the body.

Nursing responsibilities include: The maintenance of a patent airway, the administration of a safe concentration of oxygen, and the maintenance of body warmth.

Anterior fontanel: A characteristic "soft spot" or space between the bones of the infant's skull. Bounded by the frontal and parietal bones, this fontanel is diamond-shaped and closes by the time the child is 18 months of age.

Nursing responsibilities include observation for sunken or bulging fontanels, which are associated with dehydration and increased intracranial pressure.

Arnold-Chiari syndrome: A congenital defect in which a portion of the brain is forced through a bony canal (foramen magnum), blocking the flow of cerebrospinal fluid.

Nursing responsibilities include accurate observation and reporting of vital signs and neurologic signs. Prevention of upper respiratory tract infection is essential, since surgery is the only known treatment.

Ascariasis: A roundworm infestation.

Nursing responsibilities include observation for characteristic symptoms such as cough, vomiting, abdominal pain, lethargy, and anorexia. The linen should be treated as in isolation cases. The need for stool specimens for laboratory tests should be anticipated. Pinning the diaper snugly at the thigh will prevent the child from contaminating his fingers with fecal matter. Teaching the patient and his parents concerning hygienic habits and referral of the *family* for follow-up care are essential.

Atelectasis: Incomplete expansion of the alveoli of the lungs.

Nursing responsibilities include the observation of vital signs, skin color, and symptoms of respiratory distress. It is essential to maintain a patent airway and body warmth and to prevent upper respiratory infections. The position of the child should be changed frequently, and the head of the bed kept slightly elevated. The child should be fed slowly and burped frequently to prevent abdominal distention. Short periods of crying will aid in the expansion of the lungs, but crying should not be induced immediately after feedings.

Athrepsia: Extreme malnutrition, also known as marasmus.

Nursing responsibilities include the maintenance of body warmth, detailed skin care, frequent changes of position, and the taking of accurate daily weights. The nurse may anticipate parenteral fluid therapy. Parent teaching concerning the dietary needs of the child and referral for follow-up care are essential.

Atresia: A congenital anomaly in which a normal anatomical opening is absent. For example, atresia of the esophagus prevents food from being transported to the stomach, and choanal atresia prevents nasal breathing.

Nursing responsibilities include appraisal of the newborn and general supportive care. Surgical correction should be anticipated.

Bezoars: The accumulation of an undigestible mass that forms an intestinal obstruction. It is caused by repeated ingestion of substances such as fur, hair, or paper.

Nursing responsibilities include the observation and reporting of stools and abdominal distress. Surgery may be anticipated. Furry and hairy objects should be removed from the child's environment and long hair should be braided and affixed to the top of the head. Teaching the parents concerning the need for follow-up care is essential to prevent recurrence of this condition.

Bradford frame: An apparatus that consists of narrow strips of canvas attached to a metal frame which is supported by blocks to elevate it from the mattress. It is most often used for corrective positioning of the spine.

Nursing responsibilities include providing support for the arms (pillows) and using a restraint jacket to maintain the position and for safety. A bedpan should be placed *under* the frame to facilitate defecation and urination without moving the patient. Pillows under the head should be avoided. Elevation of the head may be accomplished by placing the mattress of the crib in Fowler's position or by elevating the *base* of the Bradford frame.

Caput succedaneum: Edema of the scalp usually associated with the birth process. Discoloration due to subcutaneous hemorrhage may be present. This condition differs clinically from cephalohematoma in that the swelling is *not* limited to the surface of one cranial bone.

Nursing responsibilities include assuring the parents that this condition will disappear without treatment.

Cardiac catheterization: A diagnostic procedure which involves passing a catheter through a cut-down site, directly into the heart and large vessels, in order to obtain a blood specimen and measure pressure within the heart chamber.

Nursing responsibilities include checking for preoperative consent, providing psychological support, and observing the responses of the child during the procedure. Postoperative nursing responsibilities include frequent checking of vital signs and observation of the cut-down site for evidence of bleeding. The pulse distal to the cut-down site should be taken to observe for arteriospasm. It is essential to instruct the parents in care of the cut-down site and the need for follow-up care.

Celiac syndrome: An impaired ability to absorb fats, resulting in malnutrition, vitamin deficiency, and symptoms such as foul, bulky stools and a distended abdomen. *Celiac disease* involves an intolerance to gluten; *mucoviscidosis* involves pancreatic lesions, and the development of abnormally viscous mucous secretions. Both diseases (classified under the general term "celiac syndrome") are thought to be of genetic origin.

Nursing responsibilities include accurate recording of stools in relation to food intake, adherence to dietary restrictions, prevention of upper respiratory infection, and referral for follow-up care. The use of parenteral and aerosol therapy and postural drainage may be anticipated. When collecting a stool specimen, avoid contamination by urine.

Cephalohematoma: A subperiosteal hemorrhage usually associated with the birth process. The swelling is limited to the surface of one cranial bone.

Nursing responsibilities include observation for symptoms of skull fracture and resulting neurological signs. Parents need reassurance that the condition will clear up without treatment.

Cerebral palsy: A disorder of the motor centers and pathways of the brain. It may be congenital or acquired before the central nervous system matures.

Nursing responsibilities include fostering developmental capacities, providing continuity of rehabilitation programs, nutritional maintenance, and prevention of contractures and injury due to lack of neuromuscular coordination. Parents should be provided with psychological support, and plans for long-term goals should be discussed. The intelligence potential of the child is not necessarily diminished by this condition. Available community resources should be used, and the nurse must function as a member of the interdisciplinary health team.

Chordee: A fibrous strand of tissue extending from the scrotum to the penis,

preventing urination with the penis in the normal elevated position. Chordee is commonly associated with a congenital anomaly known as hypospadias. Surgical repair is usually initiated before the child is of school age.

Nursing responsibilities include preparation for surgery and providing psychological support to the parents and the child.

Clapping: Clapping the cupped hands on the chest wall over a segment of lung to be drained is thought to set up vibrations that are transmitted to the bronchi, where they help dislodge and move secretions. The cupped hand traps a cushion of air, softening the impact of the clap and making an effective impulse or vibration. It should be done over soft comfortable clothing. It is done for 1 to 2 minutes over each lung segment for a total of 30 minutes. Patients should be encouraged to cough after each clapping.

Cleft lip and palate: A congenital anomaly due to a partial or complete nonunion of the maxillary bone, palatal bone, and upper lip. The cleft lip is usually repaired surgically before the age of 1 month, and the cleft palate before the age of two years.

Nursing responsibilities include prevention of aspiration during feeding, maintenance of oral hygiene, prevention of upper respiratory infection, and provision of psychological support to the parents. Nursing measures should be instituted to prevent straining or contamination of the suture line postoperatively. Referral for follow-up care and speech therapy may be indicated.

Club foot: A congenital orthopedic anomaly in which the shape or contour of the foot is distorted.

Nursing responsibilities include teaching the parents the purpose and techniques of the prescribed therapy and providing psychological support. The patient should be referred for follow-up care.

Craniotabes: A condition which involves a softening and resultant deformity of the skull bones. Although the condition may be considered normal in premature and newborn infants, it is usually associated with rickets or other bone diseases.

Nursing responsibilities include observation for bulging fontanels, frequent changes of position, and safety measures.

Croup: An inflammation of the larynx. Laryngotracheobronchitis is the most serious form of croup.

Nursing responsibilities include the maintenance of a patent airway, provision of increased environmental humidity, and frequent observations of vital signs. Prevention of fatigue, maintenance of body warmth, and attention to an adequate fluid intake are vital aspects of the nursing care. An emergency tracheotomy set should be available.

Cryptorchidism: A condition in which the testicles fail to descend into the scrotum. Also known as "undescended testicles." Hormonal or surgical therapy is usually instituted prior to puberty in order to preserve the fertility of the child.

Nursing responsibilities include the psychological preparation of the child for surgery, since the operation may be performed at a time when the child's awareness of his body is keen. Contamination by urine and feces at the operative site must be prevented.

Denis Browne splint: An orthopedic appliance, used for children with club foot, consisting of two separate foot plates attached by a cross bar. The foot plates are fitted to the child's shoes to maintain a corrective position.

Nursing responsibilities include teaching the parents the purpose and proper use of the appliance.

Down's syndrome: Also known as mongolism; a chromosomal anomaly that causes a form of mental retardation.

Nursing responsibilities include the prevention of upper respiratory infection, general supportive care and referral for vocational guidance.

Ductus arteriosus (patent): A congenital anomaly in which the opening between the aorta and the pulmonary artery fails to close after birth.

Nursing responsibilities include the prevention of fatigue, observation for dyspnea and cardiac failure, and frequent observation of vital signs. Surgical correction may be anticipated. The nurse must provide psychological support to the parents.

Eczema: An inflammatory skin condition most often associated with allergic responses to food proteins.

Nursing responsibilities include the use of elbow restraints to prevent scratching and subsequent secondary infection of lesions; adherence to the dietary restrictions prescribed; and selection of diversional therapy, using nonallergenic toys. The use of heavy plastic sheets will prevent absorption of skin ointment by the bed linen. The use of soap should be avoided and articles containing wool should not be used. It is important to instruct the parents concerning diet, skin care, and the prevention of infection.

Enuresis: The inability to control urination in a child over 3 years of age, due to an organic or psychological problem. (Bladder control is usually established by the third year of life, unless a disease condition exists.)

Nursing responsibilities include fostering a positive attitude in parent and child and guiding them in the identification of the underlying cause.

Enterobiasis: A pinworm infestation; also known as oxyuriasis.

Nursing responsibilities include teaching hygienic habits, pinning the diaper snugly at the thigh to prevent contamination of the infant's fingers, and isolation of all linen. The nurse must be alert for symptoms of abdominal distress, local infection, and nocturnal perianal itching.

Epistaxis: "Nose-bleeding." This condition may be caused by local or systemic factors.

Nursing responsibilities include the placement of the child in a semi-Fowler's position in a quiet environment. The clothing around the neck should be loosened and blowing the nose should be avoided. The nurse should also watch for and teach the prevention of trauma which may be caused by placing foreign bodies in the nares or "picking" the nose. Each episode of epistaxis must be reported to the physician.

Erb-Duchenne paralysis: A condition which is the result of injury to the brachial plexus incurred during the birth process, and involving damage to the fifth and sixth cervical nerves. Signs and symptoms include a unilateral Moro reflex and a characteristic position of the affected arm.

Nursing responsibilities include maintaining the position of the hand and arm as prescribed and explaining the therapy to the parents.

Eructation: Synonymous with "belching." Eructation differs from "bubbling" in that it takes place at a time other than when the infant is held upright and patted on the back.

Erythroblastosis: A physiological hemolytic anemia that results from a blood incompatibility. This condition is usually associated with the offspring of Rh positive fathers and Rh negative mothers.

Nursing responsibilities include the maintenance of nutrition and body warmth, prevention of upper respiratory infection, and observation and reporting of jaundice or edema. Deviations in vital signs or signs of central nervous system involvement should be promptly reported. Exchange transfusion therapy may be anticipated.

Exanthem subitum: See *Roseola infantum.*

Exstrophy of the bladder: A congenital defect in which the lower urinary tract is everted and exposed on the abdominal wall.

Nursing responsibilities include the prevention and relief of skin excoriation, prevention of infection of the exposed tissues, and referral for rehabilitation and follow-up care.

Fibroplasia, retrolental: A spasm of the retinal vessels resulting from high concentrations of oxygen administered to a newborn, causing permanent blindness.

The true nursing responsibility lies in the prevention of this condition by the judicious use of oxygen in the newborn nursery. Oxygen concentrations exceeding 40 per cent may cause this condition in the newborn.

Fontanels: Openings at the point of union of skull bones, often referred to as "soft spots" on the infant's head. The posterior fontanel is often difficult to palpate in the newborn because of the molding that takes place during the birth process. The anterior fontanel usually closes by the age of 18 months.

Nursing responsibilities include the prevention of trauma and observation and prompt reporting of bulging or depressed fontanels.

Foramen ovale (patent): An opening in the septum between the right and left atria of the heart that remains patent after birth. Cardiac catheterization may be performed for diagnostic purposes. Surgery may or may not be indicated.

Nursing responsibilities include the observation and reporting of cyanosis, prevention of fatigue, and referral for follow-up care after discharge.

Fredjka splint: An apparatus used to maintain flexion and abduction of the hips and knees in the treatment of a congenital dislocation of the hip.

Nursing responsibilities include detailed skin care, maintenance of the prescribed position, and selection of appropriate articles for diversional therapy.

Gastroenteritis: An inflammation of the gastrointestinal tract characterized by vomiting and diarrhea.

Nursing responsibilities include the maintenance of medical aseptic technique, maintenance of body warmth, observation and reporting of signs of dehydration and acidosis, recording of intake and output, skin care, and adherence to dietary restrictions. Parenteral therapy should be anticipated.

Gaucher's disease: A congenital defect in the metabolism of specific fatty acids resulting in an increase of the acid phosphatase in the blood. Symptoms include development of strabismus (crossed eyes), retroflexion of the head, respiratory problems, abdominal enlargement, and pathological bone fractures.

Nursing responsibilities include observation for bleeding tendencies, prevention of injury, prevention of standing and weight-bearing, prevention of upper respiratory infection, and maintenance of nutrition. Psychological support is essential in the care of any child with a neurological handicap or long-term illness.

Ghon complex: The initial lung lesion (or lesions) involving the regional lymph nodes associated with the development of miliary tuberculosis.

Nursing responsibilities include providing adequate rest and adequate diet, the prevention of upper respiratory infection, and maintenance of isolation precautions.

Hemangioma: A benign tumor of the skin involving blood vessels.

Nursing responsibilities include preventing trauma to the lesion and providing psychological support to the parents.

Hemophilia: An inherited disease which is characterized by an abnormal tendency to bleed.

Nursing responsibilities include maintenance of a safe environment, careful selection of toys, padding of the crib, and vocational guidance. Parents must be instructed concerning the prevention of trauma.

Hiccups: Spasms of the diaphragm which cause short, noisy inspiratory coughs.

Nursing responsibilities include the avoidance of overfeeding and minimal handling of the infant after feedings as a preventative measure.

Hirschsprung's disease: Also known as "megacolon"; a condition in which the colon is enlarged without evidence of mechanical obstruction. Congenital absence of ganglionic cells in the distal segment of the colon is a frequent cause of this condition.

Nursing responsibilities include maintaining adequate nutrition with a low residue diet, accurate observation and recording of stools, and maintaining a semi-Fowler's position to avoid respiratory distress. Solutions other than normal saline should be avoided for enema therapy.

Hyaline membrane disease: The development of a membranous substance lining the alveoli of the lung and preventing adequate gaseous exchange. It occurs most often in premature babies, newborns of diabetic mothers, or newborns delivered by cesarean section.

Nursing responsibilities include maintenance of body warmth, maintenance of a patent airway, and maintenance of the prescribed body position for postural drainage. Progressive symptoms of respiratory distress must be reported promptly. Tube feedings, oxygen therapy, or hyperbaric oxygen therapy may be anticipated.

Hydrocephalus: A congenital cerebral anomaly resulting in an excess of cerebrospinal fluid within the ventricles of the brain.

Nursing responsibilities include the observation of vital signs, prevention of decubitus ulcers, and maintenance of adequate nutrition. The head must be supported when moving or lifting the child to avoid muscle strain. Psychological support to the parents is essential. Surgical correction is possible in some cases.

Hydrops fetalis: A generalized edema of the newborn due to cardiac failure and/or hypoproteinemia. The condition is often associated with erythroblastosis fetalis.

Nursing responsibilities include the maintenance of body warmth, frequent observation of vital signs, and observation for jaundice and neurological symptoms. The general principles of caring for the cardiac patient and the patient with a hemolytic disease should be followed.

Hyperalimentation: The infusion of a nutrient solution directly into the vena cava to maintain a positive nitrogen balance and to maintain growth and development during prolonged illness.

Nursing responsibilities include recording daily weight, fractional urines, and blood tests as ordered, maintaining aseptic technique to prevent infection at the infusion site, observing and recording signs of overhydration or dehydration, and keeping strict intake and output records.

Hyperbaric oxygen therapy: The administration of oxygen under increased atmospheric pressure to increase the oxygen pressure within the blood. The patient and the nurse must be enclosed in a sealed chamber to achieve the goals of this therapy. The effects of gas under pressure require modification of nursing techniques which includes the use of flameproof linens and uniforms. Standard closed-system supplies must be protected against "implosions." After leaving the pressurized unit, the nurse should not reenter it within a 12 hour period to prevent the development of nitrogen toxicity.

Hypospadias: A congenital anomaly in which the urethra opens on the lower surface of the penis in males or into the vagina in females. Circumcision of male infants with hypospadias should be postponed.

Nursing responsibilities include providing psychological support to the patient and his parents. Surgical correction may be anticipated.

Immunization: The process of rendering a child resistant to a disease by the injection of antitoxins or toxoids.

Nursing responsibilities include teaching the parents concerning the need for various immunizations during childhood and referral to community agencies as necessary.

Impetigo neonatorum: A highly communicable skin disease caused by streptococcic or staphylococcic organisms.

Nursing responsibilities include maintenance of strict isolation techniques and detailed skin care.

Intertrigo: Chafing of the skin where two skin surfaces come in close contact.

Nursing responsibilities include providing detailed skin care, particularly in the folds of the skin.

Intussusception: A condition in which one portion of the intestine "telescopes" into an adjacent portion of the intestine, causing a mechanical obstruction.

Nursing responsibilities include the observation and description of stools and observation of vital signs. Nursing care should be designed to conserve the energy of the child. Parenteral therapy and gastric suction may be anticipated.

Jaundice: A symptom characterized by a yellowish tinge of the skin and sclera. If associated with lethargy, dehydration, and increased serum bilirubin levels, jaundice may have serious implications.

Nursing responsibilities include observation for jaundice in daylight. Physiological jaundice may be a normal occurrence in the newborn (icterus neonatorum), but since the nurse cannot make a medical diagnosis she must consider all jaundice pathological and report it immediately to the doctor.

Kernicterus: Staining of the basal ganglia of the brain, which occurs as a result of increased serum bilirubin. It is associated with hemolytic disease of the newborn and infant.

Nursing responsibilities include observing and reporting jaundice and neurological symptoms. Exchange transfusion or phototherapy may be anticipated for newborns with high blood bilirubin levels.

Klumpke's paralysis: An injury to the seventh and eighth cervical nerves incurred during the birth process. Signs and symptoms include a unilateral Moro reflex and a characteristic position of the affected hand.

Nursing responsibilities include maintaining the arm in the prescribed position and providing continuity of physical therapy.

Laryngotracheobronchitis: A serious form of croup involving an inflammation of the larynx, trachea, and bronchi.

Nursing responsibilities include a knowledge of the principles of caring for a child in a Croupette humidity tent, the observation of vital signs, conservation of energy, maintenance of a patent airway, and frequent change of position.

Lead poisoning: Also known as plumbism; a toxic response of the body to lead which may have been ingested or inhaled. A marked degree of toxicity may cause severe and permanent brain damage.

Nursing responsibilities include observation for respiratory distress, convulsions, and signs of central nervous system involvement. It is essential that parents be instructed concerning the elimination of sources of lead in the child's environment.

Leukemia: A blood disease characterized by a massive increase in white blood cells.

Nursing responsibilities include observation for bleeding, prevention of infection, and general supportive care. The nurse must be familiar with the effects of the drug prescribed. Referral for follow-up care is necessary.

Lipidosis: A group of symptoms resulting from a congenital defect that causes increased fat content of tissues or serum. This condition produces an enlargement of the viscera and is often accompanied by impaired neurological functions.

Nursing responsibilities include observation of vital signs and maintenance of the safety measures necessary for the neurologically handicapped.

Lues (congenital): Syphilis acquired by the fetus through the placenta of an infected mother. Clinically, this condition in the newborn is similar to the secondary stage of syphilis in the adult and is characterized by various anatomical defects.

Nursing responsibilities include isolation of the newborn from other newborn infants, suctioning of the nose prior to feedings, and provision for follow-up care.

Marasmus: See *Athrepsia.*

Megacolon: See *Hirschsprung's disease.*

Meningocele: A congenital anomaly characterized by a protrusion of the meninges through an opening in the spinal column.

For nursing responsibilities see *Meningomyelocele.*

Meningomyelocele: A congenital anomaly characterized by a protrusion of the meninges *and the spinal cord* through an opening in the spinal column.

Nursing responsibilities include prevention of trauma and infection at the site of the defect, detailed skin care, maintenance of nutrition, and observation of developmental motor abilities. Postoperative rehabilitation, referral for follow-up care, and psychological support to the parents are essential.

Miliaria: Also known as prickly heat, this inflammatory skin condition is caused by an obstruction of the sweat ducts.

Nursing responsibilities include maintenance of an optimum environmental temperature and instruction to the parents concerning proper clothing for the infant, especially during warm weather.

Mongolism: See *Down's syndrome.*

Mucoviscidosis: See *Celiac syndrome.*

Myoclonic seizures (infantile): A convulsive seizure characterized by a sudden drooping of the head and flexion of the arms that may be repeated several hundred times a day.

Nursing responsibilities include maintenance of environmental safety, accurate observation and reporting of seizures, and referral for follow-up care.

Nevi: A congenital lesion of the skin causing functional or cosmetic problems. Hemangiomas and strawberry marks are types of nevi.

Nursing responsibilities include providing psychological support to the parents, referral for the follow-up care indicated by the specific defects, and interpretation of the planned therapy to the parents.

Omphalocele: A herniation of abdominal contents into the umbilical cord.

Nursing responsibilities include prevention of infection and drying of the umbilical cord and tissues. The nurse may anticipate and prepare for surgical correction.

Ophthalmia neonatorum: A highly communicable disease also known as gonorrheal conjunctivitis.

Nursing responsibilities include observing and reporting eye discharges and the use of strict isolation techniques. The nurse may contribute to the prevention of this disease by using proper techniques when instilling prophylactic eye drops at birth.

Oxyuriasis: See *Enterobiasis.*

Paraphimosis: Impaired, circulation to the uncircumcised penis, due to retraction of the foreskin beyond the corona.

Nursing responsibilities include observation for voiding and preparation for surgery. This condition may be prevented by gentle retraction and replacement of the foreskin during daily care.

Parotitis, infectious: Mumps, a highly communicable viral disease affecting the salivary glands.

Nursing responsibilities include maintaining isolation techniques, providing for adequate rest, and maintaining adequate nutrition with a soft or liquid bland diet. Abdominal pain, fever, vomiting, or the development of cerebral symptoms should be promptly reported.

Perthes' disease: Legg-Calve-Perthes disease is an aseptic necrosis of the epiphysis of the femur.

Nursing responsibilities include the

prevention of weight bearing on the affected leg and the initiation of a long-term plan for therapy.

Pertussis: A highly communicable disease of the respiratory tract, also known as whooping cough.

Nursing responsibilities include observation and reporting of dyspnea and fever, support of the abdominal muscles during coughing paroxysms, maintenance of body warmth, maintenance of a patent airway, and conservation of energy. Teaching parents the importance of early immunization is an aspect of preventative nursing care.

Phenylketonuria (P.K.U.): A congenital metabolic defect in which the ability to metabolize a specific amino acid is impaired. The resulting rise in phenylalanine in the blood affects skin pigmentation and causes irreversible mental retardation.

Nursing responsibilities include teaching the parents concerning dietary restrictions and referral for follow-up care.

Phimosis: A narrowing of the prepuce of the uncircumcised penis.

Nursing responsibilities include observation for voiding and preparation for surgical correction by circumcision. Following surgery, the nurse must observe for voiding and report bleeding.

Postural drainage: A physical method to aid pulmonary hygiene and relieve bronchial obstructions caused by accumulated secretions. Indications for this treatment include conditions of increased production, increased viscosity and inadequate removal of bronchial secretions. The technique employs gravity to assist in drainage from the tracheobronchial tree. The patient should be instructed to cough following the procedure; he can be suctioned or can expectorate into disposable tissues. In the head-down position, infants and children should be supported by a pillow to prevent slipping.

Purpura: See *Schoenlein-Henoch syndrome.*

Pyloric stenosis: A congenital narrowing of the pylorus of the stomach caused by a hypertrophied muscle.

Nursing responsibilities include observation and recording of tolerance to food ingested, recording of daily weights, and reporting symptoms of dehydration. Gentle handling, slow and careful feeding of a thickened formula, and maintenance of Fowler's position following feedings are essential (see the diaper sling, p. 69). Surgical correction may be anticipated.

Regurgitation: The act of returning food to the mouth from the stomach immediately after ingestion. It is neither forceful nor associated with nausea.

Nursing responsibilities include evaluation of feeding techniques, frequent burping during feedings, and avoidance of large nipple holes. The infant should be placed in Fowler's position after feedings.

Retrolental fibroplasia: See *Fibroplasia, retrolental.*

Rheumatic fever: A collagen disease associated with group A streptococci and characterized by migratory polyarthritis, Sydenham's chorea, and carditis. This disease can cause severe cardiac damage.

Nursing responsibilities include maintenance of adequate nutrition, limitation of physical activity, and observation of responses to drug therapy. Teaching the parents concerning the need for follow-up care is essential.

Roseola infantum: Also known as *Exanthem subitum;* this viral disease is characterized by a period of high fever abruptly terminated with the eruption of a generalized maculopapular rash.

Nursing responsibilities include frequent observation and reporting of pyrexia, provision of the prescribed therapy to reduce fever and prevent febrile convulsions, observation and accurate description of rash, and general supportive care.

Rubella: Also known as German measles; this viral communicable disease is common to children and is characterized by a tender enlargement of the cervical nodes, a maculopapular rash and general flushing of the skin.

Nursing responsibilities include accurate observation and recording of the rash and general supportive care.

Rubeola: Also known as measles;

this highly communicable viral disease is manifested by catarrhal symptoms, a maculopapular rash, and fever.

Nursing responsibilities include prevention of secondary infection, meticulous oral hygiene, protection of the eyes from strain and strong light, and provision for adequate food intake. Symptoms of ear, cardiac, or cerebral involvement should be promptly reported.

Scarlet fever: An acute allergic reaction to a hemolytic streptococcal infection.

Nursing responsibilities include maintenance of bed rest with minimal activity, provision of adequate fluids, a soft, bland diet, and symptomatic care. Observations for cardiac and renal complications are essential.

Schistosomiasis: A parasitic infestation caused by the blood fluke. The eggs are passed in the stool and urine.

Nursing responsibilities include proper disposal of contaminated urine and stool, prevention of skin irritation, maintenance of adequate nutrition, and observation for jaundice and hematuria. Teaching the parents concerning general hygiene, the sanitary disposal of urine and feces, and the choice of swimming areas free from contaminated water is essential in the prevention of this disease.

Schoenlein-Henoch syndrome: An inflammation of the blood vessels resulting in arthralgia and typical purpuric skin rash.

Nursing responsibilities include observation for hematuria, frequent observation of vital signs, and provision for adequate rest.

Spina bifida: A congenital defect in which the bony portion of the spinal column fails to close.

For nursing responsibilities see *Meningocele* and *Meningomyelocele.*

Strabismus: An imbalance of the extraocular muscles causing "crossed eyes."

Nursing responsibilities include teaching the parents concerning the prescribed therapy. Prevention of sight defects and psychological trauma by early treatment should be stressed. Safety is of utmost importance for a young child who must wear glasses or a patch over one eye.

Strawberry mark: See *Nevi.*

Tay-Sachs disease: A congenital lipid metabolic defect, also known as infantile amaurotic familial idiocy. Signs and symptoms include apathy, retardation of growth and development, visual disturbances, spasticity, and cerebral seizures. The developmental retardation is usually noticed by the sixth month in life.

Nursing responsibilities include general supportive care with special consideration to skin care, maintenance of nutrition, and prevention of hypostatic pneumonia. Environmental stimulation should be kept to a minimum. Observation of cerebral seizures and accurate recording of developmental abilities are essential to the evaluation of the child's progress.

Tetany: An increased neuromuscular irritability associated with a deficiency of vitamin D or calcium.

Nursing responsibilities include general precautions against convulsions, observation for neurological symptoms, and maintenance of a patent airway. Intramuscular calcium should not be given, as necrosis may occur at the site of injection.

Tetralogy of Fallot: A congenital heart defect, involving pulmonary stenosis, dextroposition of the aorta, right ventricular hypertrophy, and intraventricular septal defect.

Nursing responsibilities include limitation of activities to avoid fatigue, prevention of upper respiratory infection, and frequent observation of vital signs. Chest surgery may be anticipated.

Thalassemia: A hemolytic type of anemia of genetic origin.

Nursing responsibilities include adherence to the principles of long-term care and provision for follow-up care by the health team. Transfusion therapy may be anticipated.

Thrush: A mild fungus infection of the skin and mucous membranes of the mouth characterized by pearly white, curdlike lesions.

Nursing responsibilities include the maintenance of medical aseptic techniques. Detailed oral hygiene is essential.

Tinea: A highly contagious fungus

infection, also known as ringworm. Tinea capitis involves the head, while tinea corporis involves the skin, and tinea pedis is "athlete's foot."

Nursing responsibilities include cleansing the affected area as prescribed and teaching the patient and parents concerning general hygienic habits.

Tonguetie: A congenital short fold underneath the tongue, resulting in limitation of its motion.

Nursing responsibilities include the observation of sucking abilities. If this condition interferes with sucking or speech, surgery may be anticipated.

Toxoplasmosis: A congenital or acquired protozoan parasitic infection, characterized by pathological changes in the eyes, cerebral involvement, psychomotor retardation, and convulsions.

Nursing responsibilities include observation and recording of the vital signs, rash, convulsions, and developmental abilities. Environmental safety must be maintained. Psychological support to the parents is essential, as it is in any long-term handicap-producing disease.

Varicella: Also known as chickenpox, this communicable viral disease is characterized by a vesiculopustular rash.

Nursing responsibilities include maintenance of medical aseptic techniques, prevention of scratching, and prevention of secondary infections.

Variola: Also known as smallpox, this highly communicable viral infection causes general sepsis and is characterized by a vesicular rash.

Nursing responsibilities include maintenance of strict medical aseptic techniques, prevention of secondary skin infection, prevention of scratching, and stress on oral hygiene. Frequent observation of vital signs and reporting of cerebral symptoms are essential. Teaching the parents concerning early vaccination is an important aspect of preventative care.

Vibration: Helps stimulate flow of secretions during expiration. Press firmly with flat or cupped hands on the chest wall. Vibration is performed during exhalation with patient exhaling as completely as possible and making a *sss* sound. Usually used with clapping and postural drainage therapy.

Volvulus: A twisting of the mobile loops of the small intestine, causing intestinal obstruction.

Nursing responsibilities include the observation and recording of stools and reporting of abdominal distention. Preoperative preparation may be anticipated.

Wilm's tumor: A malignant tumor of the kidney.

Nursing responsibilities include observation and reporting of hematuria and elevated blood pressure. Frequent palpation of the tumor should be avoided. Surgery and radiation therapy may be anticipated.

Xanthoma: A skin eruption associated with a lipid disturbance or increased serum cholesterol level. The lesion is a circumscribed elevated papule which may appear in clusters and has yellow, orange, brown, or red tinges of color. The lesion may appear on any part of the body.

Nursing responsibilities include the observation and accurate reporting of any new lesions and symptomatic care.

BIBLIOGRAPHY

Gellis, S. S., and Kagan, B. M.: *Current Pediatric Therapy.* 7th Edition, W. B. Saunders Co., Philadelphia, 1976.

Marlow, D.: *Textbook of Pediatric Nursing.* 4th Edition, W. B. Saunders Co., Philadelphia, 1973.

Vaughn, V. C., III, and McKay, R. J.: *Nelson Textbook of Pediatrics.* 10th Edition, W. B. Saunders Co., Philadelphia, 1975.

APPENDIX

_____

Urine Output of Infants and Children

An understanding of the normal urine output in infants and children will aid the nurse in identifying deviations from normal.

The amount of urine excreted by infants and children is influenced by diet, environmental temperature, and the status of the central nervous and digestive systems. Before bladder control is established, the frequency of urination may be as high as 40 times within 24 hours. After bladder control has been established, frequency varies from six to eight times within 24 hours.

TABLE A–1. Average Daily Excretion of Urine*

Age	Amount (cc.)
Birth–2 months	30–400
2 months–1 year	400–500
1 year–3 years	500–600
3 years–5 years	600–700
5 years–8 years	650–1000
8 years–14 years	800–1400

*Adapted from Nelson, W.: *Textbook of Pediatrics*. 10th Edition, W. B. Saunders Co., Philadelphia, 1975.

Some Laboratory Values the Intensive Care Nurse Must Know

	Age	Normal range
Bilirubin (total)	Cord	under 2 mg./dl.
	0–1 day	under 6 mg./dl.
	3–5 days	under 12 mg./dl.
	after 5 days	under 1 mg./dl.

	Age	*Normal range*
PO_2	Neonate	60–90 mm. Hg
pCO_2	(Venous)	40–50 mm. Hg
Fibrinogen	Newborn	150–300 mg./dl.
	after 1 month	200–400 mg./dl.
Fasting blood sugar	Premature	30–60 mg./dl.
	Newborn	30–80 mg./dl.
	Child	60–100 mg./dl.
	after	70–110 mg./dl.

Note: In newborn, under 30 mg. per cent means hypoglycemia. After 72 hours, under 40 mg. per cent means hypoglycemia.

Potassium	Premature cord	5.0–10.2 mEq./l.
	Premature 48 hours	3.0–6.0 mEq./l.
	Term newborn	5.0–7.7 mEq./l.
	Infant	4.1–5.3 mEq./l.
	Child	3.5–4.7 mEq./l.
	after	3.4–5.6 mEq./l.
Sodium	Premature 48 hours	128–148 mEq./l.
	Newborn	139–162 mEq./l.
	Infant	139–146 mEq./l.
	Child	138–145 mEq./l.
	Older	135–151 mEq./l.
BUN	0–infant	5–15 mg./dl.
	older	10–20 mg./dl.
pH	0–1 week	7.30–7.40
Chloride		95–110 mEq./l.
Calcium	Newborn	8.0–10.5 mg./100 ml.
Magnesium	Newborn	1–2 mg./100 ml.
Phosphorus	Newborn	3.5–8 mg./ml.

TABLE A–2.   Tests Used for Phenylketonuria (P.K.U.)

Test	*Method*	*Advantage or Disadvantage*
Diaper test	10% ferric chloride dropped on freshly saturated diaper. A green spot indicates a positive reaction.	Inexpensive. Not of value until infant is over 6 weeks of age.
Phenistix	Phenistix is pressed against wet diaper or dipped in urine. A green reaction is positive.	More accurate than diaper test but more expensive. Used after 6 weeks of age.
Blood tests	Require blood drawn from patient or finger puncture. Is done by a laboratory technician.	Used to confirm diagnosis. Results above 8 ml./100. cc. considered a positive P.K.U. diagnosis.

TABLE A–3.   Normal Cerebrospinal Fluid Values for Infants and Children*

	Age	*Normal Value*
Cell count	Under 1 year	Up to 10 cells per cu. mm.
	1–4 years	Up to 8 cells per cu. mm.
	5–12 years	0–5 cells per cu. mm.
Chloride	7 days–3 months	636–716 mg./100 ml.
		(108.8–122.5 mEq./liter)
	4–12 months	659–742 mg./100 ml.
		(112.7–128.5 mEq./liter)
	13 months–12 years	638–763 mg./100 ml.
		(116.8–130.5 mEq./liter)
Glucose	6 months–10 years	71–90 mg./100 ml.
	over 10 years	50–80 mg./100 ml.

*Adapted from Nelson, W.: *Textbook of Pediatrics*. 9th Edition, W. B. Saunders Co., Philadelphia, 1969.

TABLE A–4.   Average Normal Blood Values at Different Age Levels*

	Birth	*2 Days*	*14 Days*	*3 Months*	*1 Year*	*2 Years*	*4 Years*	*8–12 Years*
RBC per cu. mm. (in millions)	5.1	5.3	5.0	4.3	4.7	4.8	4.8	5.1
Hgb. (gm. per 100 ml.)	17–20	18	17	10–12	12.2	12.9	13.1	14.1
WBC per cu. mm. (in thousands)	15	21	11	9.5	9	8.5	8	8
Platelets per cu. mm. (in thousands)	350	400	300	260	250	250	250	250
Polymorphonuclear neutrophils	45	55	36	35	40	40	50	60
Eosinophils	3	5	3	3	2	2	2	2
Lymphocytes	30	20	53	55	53	50	40	30
Monocytes	12	15	8	7	5	8	8	8
Immature white blood cells	10	5	–	–	–	–	–	–
% nucleated red blood cells	1–5	2	–	–	–	–	–	–
% reticulocytes in RBC	2	3	1	.5	1	1	1	1
Hematocrit	43–63	–	–	28–40	32–40	–	36–44	39–47
CO₂ content (arterial)	–	–	–	–	15–20 mEq./l.	18–20	mEq./l.	19–21 mEq./l.
Total protein	6.1 gm./100 ml.	–	–	–	6.9 gm./100 ml.			7.1 gm./ 100 ml.

Cholesterol	50–100 mg./100 ml. newborns
	70–125 mg./100 ml. infants
	150–250 mg./100 ml. over 6 years

Alkaline phosphatase	5–10 B.U. infants
	3–13 B.U. children

*Adapted from Nelson, W.: *Textbook of Pediatrics*, W. B. Saunders Co., Philadelphia, 1964, page 1007.

Selecting the Proper Size Catheter

The selection of an appropriate size catheter for purposes of catheterization, suction, or gavage is a nursing responsibility. If the catheter is too large or too small, the therapeutic goals will not be achieved. The size of the orifice to be entered, the type of fluid that must pass through the catheter, and the purpose of the therapy should be the bases for determining the optimum size of the catheter.

Since many catheters are labeled in French sizes, the Table A–5 is presented to aid the nurse in selecting the most appropriate size catheter for use.

TABLE A–5.   Table for Converting French Size into Millimeters or Inches*

French Size	Diameter (mm.)	Diameter (in.)
1	$\frac{1}{3}$	0.013
2	$\frac{2}{3}$	0.026
3	1	0.039
4	$1\frac{1}{3}$	0.052
5	$1\frac{2}{3}$	0.065
6	2	0.078
7	$2\frac{1}{3}$	0.091
8	$2\frac{2}{3}$	0.104
9	3	0.118
10	$3\frac{1}{3}$	0.131
11	$3\frac{2}{3}$	0.144
12	4	0.157
13	$4\frac{1}{3}$	0.170
14	$4\frac{2}{3}$	0.183
15	5	0.196
16	$5\frac{1}{3}$	0.209
17	$5\frac{2}{3}$	0.223
18	6	0.236
19	$6\frac{1}{3}$	0.249
20	$6\frac{2}{3}$	0.262
21	7	0.275
22	$7\frac{1}{3}$	0.288
23	$7\frac{2}{3}$	0.301
24	8	0.314
25	$8\frac{1}{3}$	0.328
26	$8\frac{2}{3}$	0.341
27	9	0.354
28	$9\frac{1}{3}$	0.367
29	$9\frac{2}{3}$	0.380
30	10	0.393

*Courtesy of Sterilon Corporation, Buffalo, New York.

Conversion of Apothecary Measures to Metric Equivalents

Apothecary	Metric
3/4 grain	45 mg.
1/2 grain	30 mg.
3/8 grain	23 mg.
1/4 grain	15 mg.

Conversion of Apothecary Measures to Metric Equivalents (Continued)

Apothecary	Metric
1/6 grain	10 mg.
1/8 grain	8 mg.
1/10 grain	6 mg.
1/15 grain	4 mg.
1/30 grain	2 mg.
1/60 grain	1 mg.
1/100 grain	0.6 mg.
1/250 grain	0.25 mg.
1/300 grain	0.2 mg.
1/1000 grain	0.06 mg.
1 grain	60 mg. (.06 gm.)
2 grains	120 mg. (.12 gm.)
3 grains	180 mg. (.2 gm.)
5 grains	300 mg. (.3 gm.)
15 grains	1000 mg. (1 gm.)
240 grains	15,000 mg. (15 gm.)

INDEX

Note: *Italicized* numbers refer to illustrations;
numbers followed by (t) indicate tables.

DATE LOANED

MAR 3 0 1979			
JUN 9 1980			
APR 1 7 1981			